www.bma.org.uk/library

D1345438

WITHDRAWN FROM
BRITISH MEDICAL ASSOCIATION

0919901

Migration and Mental Health

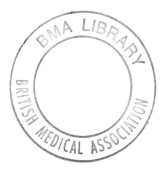
BMA LIBRARY
BRITISH MEDICAL ASSOCIATION

Migration and Mental Health

Edited by

Dinesh Bhugra
Professor of Mental Health and Cultural Diversity, Health Service and Population Research Department, Institute of Psychiatry, King's College London, UK

and

Susham Gupta
Consultant Psychiatrist, East London NHS Foundation Trust, London, UK

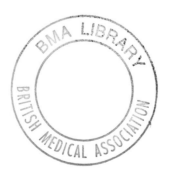

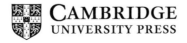
CAMBRIDGE
UNIVERSITY PRESS

CAMBRIDGE UNIVERSITY PRESS
Cambridge, New York, Melbourne, Madrid, Cape Town, Singapore,
São Paulo, Delhi, Dubai, Tokyo, Mexico City

Cambridge University Press
The Edinburgh Building, Cambridge CB2 8RU, UK

Published in the United States of America by Cambridge University Press, New York

www.cambridge.org
Information on this title: www.cambridge.org/9780521190770

© Cambridge University Press 2011

This publication is in copyright. Subject to statutory exception
and to the provisions of relevant collective licensing agreements,
no reproduction of any part may take place without the written
permission of Cambridge University Press.

First published 2011

Printed in the United Kingdom at the University Press, Cambridge

A catalogue record for this publication is available from the British Library

Library of Congress Cataloguing in Publication data
Migration in mental health / edited by Dinesh Bhugra and Susham Gupta.
    p. ; cm.
Includes bibliographical references and index.
ISBN 978-0-521-19077-0 (hardback)
1. Emigration and immigration – Mental health.   2. Psychotherapy.   I. Bhugra, Dinesh.
II. Gupta, Susham.
[DNLM: 1. Transients and Migrants – psychology.   2. Acculturation.   3. Emigrants and Immigrants –
psychology.   4. Mental Disorders – therapy.   5. Mental Health Services – organization &
administration.   6. Refugees – psychology. WA 305.1]
RC451.4.E45M53   2011
362.2086′91–dc22

                                                                                            2010030608

ISBN 978-0-521-19077-0 Hardback

Cambridge University Press has no responsibility for the persistence or
accuracy of URLs for external or third-party internet websites referred to
in this publication, and does not guarantee that any content on such
websites is, or will remain, accurate or appropriate.

Every effort has been made in preparing this book to provide accurate and up-to-date information which is in
accord with accepted standards and practice at the time of publication. Although case histories are drawn
from actual cases, every effort has been made to disguise the identities of the individuals involved.
Nevertheless, the authors, editors and publishers can make no warranties that the information contained
herein is totally free from error, not least because clinical standards are constantly changing through research
and regulation. The authors, editors and publishers therefore disclaim all liability for direct or consequential
damages resulting from the use of material contained in this book. Readers are strongly advised to pay careful
attention to information provided by the manufacturer of any drugs or equipment that they plan to use.

Dedicated to
the memory of Mrs Deepti Gupta
and to
Dr Samir K. Gupta

Contents

Foreword

The World Psychiatric Association (WPA) identified mental health and mental healthcare in migrants as one of the priority issues to be addressed in its guidances (Thornicroft *et al.*, 2010; Sartorius *et al.*, in press; Bhugra *et al.*, in press; Brockington *et al.*, in press), which are being published in its official journal *World Psychiatry*. Dinesh Bhugra was asked to chair the relevant task force, and the document was finalized in May 2010 (Bhugra *et al.*, in press). This book is in part the product of the work of that task force.

There are several reasons why the WPA decided to focus on this issue. The first is that in our present multicultural world it is the rule that psychiatrists come into contact with first or second generation migrants in their professional activity, and this poses significant problems that have to be addressed in a rational and effective way.

Diagnosis and differential diagnosis of mental disorders in migrants is one of the most sensitive areas of these problems. Psychiatric diagnosis is based on the experiences that the service user shares with the psychiatrist, and the behaviour the psychiatrist observes. The role of laboratory and instrumental tests is, in our specialty, very limited. But the sharing and the interpretation of the user's experiences may be problematic if there are language barriers and significant cultural differences in the idiom of distress between the user and the psychiatrist, and several behavioural manifestations may have very different meanings across cultures. There is an urgent need for good quality information and continuing education in this area, and the WPA guidance and this book should be very useful in this respect.

Access to mental health services is another sensitive issue. There is evidence that several groups of migrants in various countries have difficulties with contacting health services in general, and mental health services in particular, owing to a variety of barriers and limitations. Furthermore, there are data suggesting that some particularly restrictive modalities of psychiatric care, such as compulsory admission, may be used with a high frequency in some groups of migrants, probably in part because of the above-mentioned problems in communication. A greater awareness of these problems and some guidance about how to address them is urgently needed.

Furthermore, a variety of difficulties is emerging in the implementation of all the most common psychiatric treatments in migrant populations. Pharmacological treatment is complicated by ethnic differences in the pharmacokinetics and pharmacodynamics of some psychotropic drugs, but also by users' problems in understanding and adhering to the prescriptions, and by the interference of dietary habits, religious practices (such as complete fasting in certain periods) and the concomitant use of traditional remedies. On the other hand, the delivery of all psychotherapies is complicated by users' difficulties in establishing an effective therapeutic relationship with professionals, in accepting some basic assumptions of the various techniques, and in agreeing with the proposed outcome indicators. Finally, all psychosocial interventions are made more difficult in migrants by the frequent lack of an efficient social network, by stigma and discrimination, and by objective obstacles to social inclusion.

A second reason that the WPA identified mental health in migrants as a priority is that research in this area has an enormous potential, which up to now has been only partially explored. The study of the epidemiology of mental disorders in migrants may provide precious information on the role of gene–environment interactions in the development of the various disorders, on the impact of coping strategies and resilience factors, on the genesis of the comorbidity between mental and physical diseases, on the determinants of attempted and completed suicide, and on the factors affecting the course and outcome of the various disorders. Currently available research already provides some interesting hints, but findings are often inconsistent and difficult to interpret, owing to a variety of methodological problems that it will be important and instructive to address and solve. A review of the available research evidence and of its limitations, such as that provided in this book, may be of great use.

Finally, another reason that the WPA gave priority to this issue is that we need to incorporate the mental health of migrants into the curricula of medical students and residents in psychiatry. This topic does not deserve just a formal and marginal attention. Addressing mental health in migrants in the curricula provides the means to emphasise the more general issue of the role of culture in the genesis, manifestation and management of mental disorders, an element which has been lacking in the education of almost all psychiatrists practising today.

We hope that this book, and the WPA guidance produced by the task force led by Dinesh Bhugra, will call the attention of psychiatrists, other mental health professionals, policymakers and the general public to this challenging and fascinating area, and will generate improved practices and innovative research.

Professor Mario Maj
President, World Psychiatric Association

References

Bhugra D, Gupta S, Bhui K *et al.* (2011). WPA guidance on mental health and mental health care in migrants. *World Psychiatry* (in press).

Brockington I, Chandra P, Dubowitz H *et al.* (2011). WPA guidance on the protection and promotion of mental health in children of persons with severe mental disorders. *World Psychiatry* (in press).

Sartorius N, Gaebel W, Cleveland H-R *et al.* (2011). WPA guidance on how to combat stigmatization of psychiatry and psychiatrists. *World Psychiatry* (in press).

Thornicroft G, Alem A, Antunes Dos Santos R *et al.* (2010). WPA guidance on steps, obstacles and mistakes to avoid in the implementation of community mental health care. *World Psychiatry*, **9**, 67–77.

Preface

Human beings have migrated from one place to another for millennia. As we are discovering, the human race originated in Africa and gradually spread all over the globe. The reasons for such a movement are both personal and social. Individuals move for betterment – be it educational, financial or social – and may take their families with them or they may follow a primary migrant. Social reasons may include disasters, political turmoil and other factors. The adjustment to the new culture and society will depend upon both personal and social factors. Acculturation will allow the individual to settle down and contribute to the economy both of the new country and of their own. A vast majority of migrants will not suffer from any mental distress but some will, and their responses will depend upon a number of personal, social and cultural factors. Women, children, the elderly, lesbian, gay and transgender individuals will have additional hurdles to overcome, both in the process of migration and in postmigration stages. There is considerable evidence in the literature to suggest that some migrant groups are more prone to certain types of mental illness than others, though aetiological factors still remain unexplained. Managing people with mental illness from other cultures needs a level of awareness and sensitivity which is the hallmark of good clinical practice. Clinicians must be aware of subtle cultural nuances, cultural norms and explanations so that patients and their families can engage in the therapeutic process. Countries around the globe have experienced increasing levels of migration as a result of globalisation and resulting global interconnectedness. Globalisation has also contributed to migration from rural areas to urban areas, with a resulting increase in urbanisation: this has highlighted problems of changing family structures and social support systems and also overcrowding and strains on infrastructure.

The idea of this book emerged as a result of an invitation from the President of the World Psychiatric Association, Professor Mario Maj, made to the senior editor to chair a task force on Migration and Mental Health. The guidance emerging from this task force is being published separately. Some of the authors contributed both to the guidance and to this book; in addition, several chapters were commissioned separately for the book. Putting together and editing this book has been a great pleasure and indeed an honour. We are immensely grateful to all our contributors, who contributed on time in spite of their busy schedules and made our task seriously enjoyable. Inevitably, there is overlap between some chapters and we have deliberately left this in place, first to ensure that the themes of the chapters are not disturbed and, secondly, so that these can be read independently of each other.

Our thanks go to Richard Marley and his team at CUP for their enthusiastic support for the project. We are also thankful to Professor Mario Maj for his direction and support, and for writing the Foreword. Andrea Livingstone did a sterling job of coordinating and pulling the book together, and for this we are immensely grateful.

Dinesh Bhugra
Susham Gupta

Contributors

Mohamed Agoub
Professor of Psychiatry
Department of Psychiatry
Ibn Rushd University Psychiatric Centre
Casablanca
Morocco

Morton Beiser
Professor of Distinction
Department of Psychology
Ryenon University
Professor Emeritus
Cultural Pluralism and Health
University of Toronto
Toronto, Ontario
Canada

Dinesh Bhugra
Professor of Mental Health &
Cultural Diversity
Institute of Psychiatry, King's College
London
London, UK

Kamaldeep Bhui
Professor of Cultural Psychiatry &
Epidemiology
Wolfson Institute of Preventive Medicine
Barts & The London School of Medicine
and Dentistry
Queen Mary University of London
London, UK

Tamsin Black
Consultant Clinical Psychologist
Psychotherapy Department
Mile End Hospital
East London Foundation Trust
London, UK

Miguel Casas
Professor and Head
Servei de Psiquiatria
Hospital Universitari Vall d'Hebron
Universitat Autónoma de Barcelona
Barcelona
Spain

Prabha S. Chandra
Professor of Psychiatry
National Institute of Mental Health and
Neurosciences
Bangalore
India

Andrew Cheng
Distinguished Research Fellow and Professor
Institute of Biomedical Sciences
Academia Sinica
Taipei
Taiwan

Francisco Collazos
Psychiatrist Coordinator, Transcultural
Psychiatry Program
Servei de Psiquiatria
Hospital Universitari Vall d'Hebron
Universitat Autónoma de Barcelona
Barcelona
Spain

Tom K. J. Craig
Professor of Social Psychiatry
Institute of Psychiatry
King's College London
London, UK

Nisha Dogra
Senior Lecturer and Honorary Consultant,
Child & Adolescent Psychiatry
Greenwood Institute
Institute of Child Health
University of Leicester
Leicester, UK

Alexander Friedmann
Assistant Professor and MD
Psychiatric University Clinic Vienna
Vienna
Austria

Susham Gupta
Consultant Psychiatrist
East London NHS Foundation Trust
Assertive Outreach Team – City & Hackney
London, UK

Jannat el Harrak
Intercultural Mediator Transcultural
Psychiatry Program
Servei de Psiquiatria
Hospital Universitari Vall d'Hebron
Barcelona
Spain

David Holzer
MD
Psychiatric University Clinic Vienna
Vienna
Austria

Karen Iley
Lecturer in Nursing
School of Nursing
University of Manchester
Manchester, UK

David Ingleby
Professor of Intercultural Psychology
Department of Interdisciplinary Social
Science
Utrecht University
Utrecht
The Netherlands

Peter B. Jones
Professor of Psychiatry
Herschel Smith Building for Brain & Mind
Sciences
Department of Psychiatry
University of Cambridge
Cambridge, UK

Gurvinder Kalra
Assistant Professor, Department of
Psychiatry
LTMGH & LTMM College
Mumbai, India

Khalid Karim
Senior Lecturer and Honorary Consultant
Child & Adolescent Psychiatry
Greenwood Institute
Institute of Child Health
University of Leicester
Leicester, UK

James B. Kirkbride
Sir Henry Wellcome Research Fellow
Herschel Smith Building for Brain & Mind
Sciences
Department of Psychiatry
University of Cambridge
Cambridge, UK

I-Chao Liu
Assistant Professor
Department of Psychiatry
Cardinal Tien Hospital and School of
Medicine
Fu Jen Catholic University
Taipei County
Taiwan

Carol Maggi
Assistant Professor of Psychiatry
Facultad de Ciencias Médicas
Universidad Nacional de Asunción
Asunción
Paraguay

María del Mar Ramos
Psychiatrist
Servei de Psiquiatria
Hospital Universitari Vall d'Hebron
Barcelona
Spain

Driss Moussaoui
Professor and Chairman
Department of Psychiatry

Ibn Rushd University Psychiatric Centre
Casablanca
Morocco

Priyadarshini Natarajan
CT3 speciality trainee
South London and Maudsley NHS
Foundation Trust
London, UK

James Nazroo
Professor of Sociology
School of Social Sciences
University of Manchester
Manchester, UK

Roger Man Kin Ng
Consultant Psychiatrist
Department of Psychiatry
Kowloon Hospital
Hong Kong

Norman Poole
Locum Consultant in Liaison
Psychiatry
St Bartholomew's Hospital
London, UK

Adil Qureshi
Psychologist Psychotherapy
Coordinator, Transcultural
Psychiatry Program
Servei de Psiquiatria
Hospital Universitari Vall d'Hebron
Barcelona
Spain

Hilda-Wara Revollo
Psychologist
Pre-doctoral intern
Transcultural Psychiatry Program
Servei de Psiquiatria
Hospital Universitari Vall d'Hebron
Universitat Autónoma de Barcelona
Barcelona
Spain

Pablo Ronzoni
Academic Clinical Fellow in
Psychiatry
University of Leicester
Leicester, UK

Pedro Ruiz
Professor and Executive Vice Chair
Department of Psychiatry and Behavioral
Sciences
University of Miami Miller School of
Medicine
Miami, Florida
USA

Ajit Shah
Professor of Ageing, Ethnicity and Mental
Health
International School for Communities,
Rights and Inclusion
University of Central Lancashire
Preston, UK

Laura Simich
Centre for Addiction and Mental Health,
Toronto and Assistant Professor
Departments of Psychiatry
and Anthropology
University of Toronto,
Toronto, Canada

Daya Somasundaram
Professor, Discipline of Psychiatry
Clinical Associate
University of Adelaide Glenside
Campus
Glenside, SA
Australia

Thomas Stompe
Professor and MD
Psychiatric University Clinic Vienna
Vienna
Austria

Rachel Tribe
Professor
School of Psychology
University of East London
London, UK

Stephen Turner
Academic Clinical Fellow in
Psychiatry
Institute of Psychiatry
King's College London
London, UK

Cristina Visiers
Intercultural Mediation Trainer
Transcultural Psychiatry Program
Servei de Psiquiatria

Hospital Universitari
Vall d'Hebron
Barcelona
Spain

Wojteck Wojcik
Academic Clinical Fellow
Department of Psychological Medicine
Institute of Psychiatry
King's College London
London, UK

Anna Yusim
Senior Resident in Psychiatry
New York University School of Medicine
New York, NY
USA

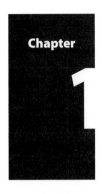

Chapter

1

Introduction: setting the scene

Dinesh Bhugra and Susham Gupta

Introduction

People have migrated from one place to another since the start of human existence, for all kinds of reasons and varying durations. These reasons have included exploration and survival. Although researchers and clinicians have observed responses to migration and studied its impact ever since explorers and merchants started to travel around the world, it is only recently that a sobering assessment of the impact of migration on individuals, taking into account social and economic factors related to globalisation, is being studied closely. According to a United Nations estimate, one-third of the world's population can be defined as a migrant, i.e. they live and/or work in a place away from their region of birth. The International Organisation for Migration (2008) estimates there are about 214 million migrants worldwide, making them 3% of the world's population.

Definitions

Migration can be defined as a change in location of the place of residence of an individual for any length of time. This shift can be across national and cultural boundaries or within the boundaries of the same country, from rural to urban areas or from urban to rural areas. Thus migration can be international or intranational. The factors which influence migration can be described as 'pull' or 'push' factors (Rack, 1982). Pull factors attract the individual for economic betterment or for educational uplift, whereas push factors include political factors which may extrude individuals out of one culture into another. Aspirations on the part of the individual and their family will influence the reasons for and settlement after migration. Changing demographics in the population of western societies, which mean that migrants are required to carry out unpopular jobs, and continuing political turmoil in some regions are likely to encourage people to migrate, either internally or externally.

Effect of migration and factors affecting mental health

The process of migration can be divided into three stages: pre-migration, migration and post-migration. Pre-migration involves the decision to migrate and the preparation for such a move. The second stage, migration itself, is the physical relocation of individuals from one site to another. The third stage, post-migration, is defined as the adjustment of the immigrant to the social, political, economic and cultural framework of the new society. Social and cultural rules of the new culture and new roles related to gender, employment, etc. will have

Migration and Mental Health, ed. Dinesh Bhugra & Susham Gupta. Published by Cambridge University Press. © Cambridge University Press 2011.

to be learnt at this stage. In the initial stages of migration, migrants may have comparatively lower rates of mental illness and health problems than in the latter stages. This may be because of the younger age at the initial stage of migration and subsequent problems with acculturation and the potential discrepancy between attainment of goals and actual achievement in the latter stages (Bhugra *et al.*, 1999). Although three discrete stages have been described there will inevitably be an overlap between stages. For example, preparation for migration may well continue while the migratory process is taking place and also the post-migration adjustment period may carry on for a considerable period after migration. Migration can influence mental health as a result of a number of social, economic, psychological, physical and cultural causes, especially among vulnerable individuals; and in return all these factors can also affect the process and reasons for migration, although the directional nature of this relationship may not always be entirely clear.

The impact of migration on an individual's mental health is multifaceted and affects different aspects of the individual, whether it is biological, social or psychological. It is possible that the three stages of migration will bring specific challenges and stressors with them (Bhugra, 2004).

Pre-migratory factors will include both personal and sociocultural factors. For example, schizotypal personality, pre-existing propensity to mental disorder associated with vulnerability factors, be they biological or sociopsychological (such as perinatal trauma and early childhood adversities), can predispose individuals to mental disorders at a later stage. Alienation from one's own culture may well bring about isolation and will affect an individual's identity. The process of migration can itself add stress and contribute to this process. The planning of the process of migration and degree of disparity between pre-migration and post-migration ethnic, cultural and socio-economic status are important, and the resultant experience can vary widely.

In the post-migration phase, individuals and groups will settle down in different ways. Most migrants are able to adjust well with binational or bicultural identities. Most migrants will make huge contributions to the new culture and economy as well as to the countries or regions of their origin. Migrants worldwide remit back billions of dollars to families, which has a positive impact in these regions and can be a big contributor to the local economy.

Stress – biological

Studies from the Japanese in the USA and the Sudanese in the UK have illustrated that the rates of physical illness change and start to match those of the new country accordingly over a period of time (Lin *et al.*, 1979). (See also Chapter 23 on physical health.)

It is not surprising that, as a result of environmental changes, such as climate and food, biological changes may occur. Furthermore, continuing stress and cumulative life events will affect biological responses. If the theory of entrapment and low self-esteem in the aetiology of depression is explored further, it is inevitable that migrants may feel caught, not only across cultural divides, but they may also feel trapped in their jobs, houses and other settings. Such a feeling will contribute to feeling low and alienated and will lower their self-esteem further.

Physical illnesses can contribute to mental illness and associated stress; therefore it is crucial that psychiatrists are aware of the links and are willing to explore them. Migration and associated stress will influence a whole spectrum of mental health disorders, as illustrated later in this book. There are also important issues around identification of these disorders, especially how cultures affect them and their presentations and care pathways into the healthcare system. There is also the impact or 'burden' on the healthcare system as well as on individuals and those who care for them in the personal or social sector.

Cultural bereavement

Migration involves a series of losses, such as the family and the familiar society; both emotional and structural losses are experienced. There may be a loss of language (especially colloquial and dialect), and changes in attitudes, values, social structures and support networks. Grieving for this loss can be viewed as a healthy reaction and a natural consequence of migration; however, if the symptoms cause significant distress or impairment and last for a specified period of time, psychiatric intervention may be warranted (Wojcik and Bhugra 2010; see also Chapter 11).

The expressions of bereavement are modified by cultural norms – how culture dictates rituals and taboos related to loss and grief. The role of culture in dealing with bereavement and grief is very important. The importance of culturally contextualising these expressions of grief is crucial in differentiating between abnormal and normal reactions to loss.

Normal adaptation occurs mostly in the form of acculturation. However, adaptation is not a simple process: a whole new process of redefining one's identity and place in the new society has to be negotiated and many find themselves maladapted to their surroundings. Factors can both increase risk and protect against this and are often interwoven and vary at both individual and community levels. Cultural identity includes factors such as gender, generation, culture of origin, language proficiency, socio-economic factors, religion, preferred cuisine, lifestyles, intergender relationships, level of sociocentricity, cultural attitudes and values, etc.

Migration and mental disorders

There is little doubt that many factors determine the outcome of migration. Premorbid personality traits will undoubtedly influence the way in which an individual perceives and copes with the process of migration and settlement afterwards. As an individual's own concept of self and their cultural identity changes, a sense of 'self' and the migratory experiences all contribute to coping with the settling down in the new culture and the outcome thereafter. Social support and networks and the attitude of the new society to the migrants and migration will also affect how one fits in. A person's ability to communicate with others from different backgrounds and wider culture, both verbally and non-verbally, will also have an impact on the experience of settling down and a sense of belonging. The migrant's intent, purpose of migration, knowledge about the new culture, openness to new experiences and previous proximity (cultural and geographical) to the new culture will influence the individual's response, as will the new culture's attitudes to the migrant, which can vary from being friendly to ambivalent or antagonistic. There is no doubt that migration itself brings about changes in the socio-economic, vocational, cultural and legal status for the migrant, and discrepancies in aspiration and achievement will further contribute to the stress of settling down.

Associated factors: the role of social and economic inequalities

The relationship between social inequalities and mental health is well known and it is inevitable that if migrants suffer from social and economic inequalities they are also likely to suffer from mental ill-health, though the mediating factors may well vary. Ever since Ödegaard's findings (1932), the link between migration and psychosis has been studied and, in spite of various challenges, cannot be discounted. One of the major findings in Ödegaard's study, that the peak of mental illness occurred 10–12 years after migration, is often ignored. The question that needs to be addressed is – why this gap? Is it social factors which cause the discrepancy between social expectations, personal expectations and achievement? Ethnic disadvantage, racialisation and social inequalities could play a fundamental role in mental ill-health as a component of wider disadvantage. Other than aetiological investigations, epidemiological studies can help to monitor trends and risk factors of diseases. They also assist investigation of inequalities in health and ensure access to appropriate treatment (see also Chapter 8).

Racial disadvantage

Modood *et al.* (1997) reported that in the UK one in eight people of ethnic minority experiences some form of racial harassment in a year. Repeated racial harassment is a common experience, including physical attacks on self or property. In their study, one-fifth reported being refused a job for racial reasons and only a few believed that there was no racial prejudice with employers. One in four whites reported prejudice against Asian people and a fifth against Caribbean people. There is no doubt that these affect an individual's self-esteem and allow the continuing hassle to act as a chronic stressor, which will contribute to poor social functioning. Using the immigration experiences to Britain as an example, Layton-Henry (1992) noted that the public picture of tolerance and friendliness was partly correct but needs to be qualified in a number of ways as there is public discrimination in employment (from employers and unions alike) and housing. Incidents of violence against migrants were reported as far back as 1948. Racist views expressed by politicians further contributed to discrimination, both public and private. Migrant women have made a significant contribution to the economies of countries in western Europe and contribute to offsetting the impact of ageing populations. With the increase in heterogeneity has come an increase in racism and discrimination (Layton-Henry, 1992, page 220).

According to UK studies, those of African-Caribbean descent are three to five times more likely to be admitted to a psychiatric hospital with a first diagnosis of psychosis than white people (see Chapter 2). They have more complex and coercive pathways into care, are more likely to present to hospital services in crisis and to be assessed as dangerous by healthcare workers, and to have compulsory treatment. They are also more likely to remain in long-term contact with services after discharge. However, there are low rates of treatment for depression for African-Caribbeans, indicating that there may be different causative factors and approach strategies. If they were related to cultural bereavement, then rates of depression would be higher, but the rates across different migrant groups are variable, in the UK at least (see Nazroo 1997).

The role of racialised social relationships needs further scrutiny. Racism reflects an ideology of superiority and justification of institutional and individual practices that create and reinforce oppressive systems of race relations and inequality between racial or ethnic groups, thus creating a racialised social order. This is reflected in racist interpersonal behaviour, and institutional policies and formal and informal practices, including everyday 'minor' incidents. This attitude leads to economic and social deprivation, socially inflicted trauma (experienced or witnessed) and negative interactions and mistrust with public agencies and resulting inadequate healthcare. However, sociocultural problems around identity, intergenerational differences, ambivalence towards both the host and originating cultures, and dysfunctional acculturation, complicated by cumulative discrimination and racism (both overt and covert) factors are likely to contribute to stresses experienced by these groups.

Perceived discrimination has been studied as a possible precipitant and stressor for the development of psychosis. Veling *et al.* (2006) found perceived discrimination among ethnic minority groups classified in terms of discrimination to be high in Moroccans, medium in migrants from Netherlands Antilles, Surinam and other non-western countries, low in the Turkish and very low in those from other western/westernised countries. This rate corresponds roughly with the rate of prevalence of psychosis in these communities.

The social defeat hypothesis (Cantor-Graae and Selten, 2005) takes into account various forms of inequalities (social, financial, educational, employment, etc.) in relation to high expectation and low achievement and the possible effect on the dopaminergic system in the mesolimbic pathway, which is seen to play a significant role in the development of schizophrenia. They propose that repetition of such experiences leads to behavioural sensitisation and mental health problems.

A large study looked at the possible effect of migration on psychopathology of psychoses in migrant groups in Austria and in their home countries (see Chapter 9). Independent of their migration status, patients from post-modern/modern countries more frequently report on delusions of grandeur or guilt, while delusions of persecution are more frequent in migrants. Delusions of being loved, of poisoning and visual hallucinations are more frequently reported by patients living in their countries of birth than by migrants. The latter report more auditory hallucinations. Thought insertion and withdrawal are more prevalent in migrants from traditional countries; first rank symptoms and auditory hallucinations in migrants from post-modern/modern countries. Made volition and somatic passivity are most frequent with patients living in post-modern/modern countries.

Even though cannabis and substance misuse has been linked to psychosis, there is little evidence that increased use of illicit substances explains the raised rates of psychoses among immigrant groups. Evidence from both the UK and the Netherlands suggests that the frequency of cannabis consumption in the general population is not raised in the black Caribbean group. Veen and colleagues (2002) have shown that the raised rates of schizophrenia in Moroccan and Surinamese immigrants in the Netherlands are unlikely to be due to substance abuse (not restricted to cannabis).

Depression, anxiety and other common mental disorders

The findings are mixed for differences in prevalence of common mental disorders and rates are not as elevated as for psychosis. Two major UK studies found differences in the prevalence of depression: the ONS National Study of Psychiatric Morbidity did not find any evidence of raised rates in black groups (Jenkins *et al.*, 1997a; b), while the Ethnic Minority Illness Rates in the Community (EMPIRIC) observed a 60% higher prevalence in black compared to the white group (Weich *et al.*, 2004). However, black groups may be less likely to receive a diagnosis of depression from their GP (Gillam *et al.*, 1989). Smaller studies have found a raised rate in Asians with possibly higher somatisation disorders (Commander *et al.*, 1997, 2004).

Suicidal and self-harm behaviour appears to vary by ethnicity and sex. South Asian men have lower rates of suicide in the UK than the white group (Thompson and Bhugra, 2000), while Asian women, particularly younger women, have higher rates although this might be changing (Soni-Raleigh *et al.*, 1990; Thompson and Bhugra, 2000). Many Asian immigrant communities have maintained their cultural identity and traditions even after generations of overseas residence. There is a premium on academic and economic success and a stigma attached to failure. There is also the overriding authority of elders (especially parents and in-laws) and expected unquestioning compliance from younger family members. Pressures are intensified for young Indian women, given their rigidly defined roles in

Indian society: submission and deference to males and elders, arranged marriages, the financial pressures imposed by dowries, and ensuing marital and family conflicts (Soni-Raleigh et al., 1990; Soni-Raleigh and Balarajan, 1992). There is a lower rate of suicide in black Caribbean groups (Soni-Raleigh et al., 1990). Studies have found higher rates of suicide in migrants to Sweden, particularly second-generation groups (Hjern and Allbeck, 2002). Suicide and suicidal behaviour may be related to social stress and acculturation.

Eating disorders: research evidence indicates that rates of eating disorders are elevated in teenagers who have migrated, although these findings are not consistent (Bhugra and Bhui, 2003).

PTSD: most research on post-traumatic stress disorder (PTSD) in migrants in refugee and asylum groups and a review of over 7000 refugees found PTSD to be ten times more likely in these groups than in the general population (Fazel et al., 2005). There may be some overlap with psychosis (15–40%) and a greater risk of other common mental disorders.

Some substance misuse disorders are related to cultural backgrounds. Khat use in the Somalian and Ethiopian migrant communities in some European countries has brought about new challenges. The use of cannabis in some African-Caribbean migrant communities has come under scruting but it is debatable whether this differs significantly from the local populations, although recent evidence indicates that more potent cannabis may be more likely to produce high levels of schizophrenia.

Migration and environment

The impact of migration on the environment is not discussed widely. It is inevitable that mass movement of peoples is likely to influence changes in the environment, which in turn may cause biological changes in the individuals themselves. There are isolated populations that have high rates of consanguinity in two types: primary (ancient tribes with biological equilibrium) and secondary (where a group detaches itself from a larger group) (Neel, 1992). Groups may start as small sized, but may expand slowly. Yanase (1992) divides isolates into four categories, and argues that isolation affects breeding structures, migration patterns and genetic distance. These changes can be seen as an evolutionary process.

Migration of isolates raises some interesting questions about the impact of the process itself on social and biological variations. The study of migrants has included looking at biological markers and seeing whether these are genetically fixed or not (Lasker and Mascie-Taylor, 1988; Baker, 1992). Baker (1992) rightly cautions that in studies related to migration, not all environmental variables can be controlled. Apart from methodological problems alluded to in the conduct of epidemiological studies control of multiple environmental factors adds another dimension.

Migration and special groups

Migration and its effect on child mental health

Various factors may impact on the outcome of migration in children. Their experiences will depend on factors such as whether migration occurs with parents and family, separation from one or both parents (owing either to migration of the parents or of the child), who looks after them and where they migrate to. Migration can include seasonal migration of parents or youngsters for work away from home, serial migration of family members, parental migration without the children, family migration etc. Children can be lone migrants for better education or due to factors related to safety (see Chapter 15).

Not all children can cope equally well with adversities and disruption to their lives. Children may be unable to understand the reason for the separations and may feel abandoned. They may have difficulty forming attachments, coping with losses or reunion with families after a period of time. At times older children may end up looking after younger siblings. Parents themselves may suffer the consequences of separation, e.g. guilt and loss. Children, especially girls who are separated from families, are particularly vulnerable to physical, emotional and sexual abuse as well as exploitation.

Much of the research in this area has originated from the USA and may be hard to generalise to other parts of the world. Vollebergh *et al.*, (2005) and Alati *et al.* (2003) did not find higher rates of mental illness in migrant children in the Netherlands and Australia, respectively. However, in the Dutch study immigrant parents reported more problems in their daughters than non-immigrant parents. Teachers reported lower levels of internalising, social and thought problems but higher externalising problems with girls. Internalising problems could lead to depression, anxiety and mental health problems in later life while externalising problems can lead to behavioural problems. Both could result in secondary problems such as poor academic achievement and substance misuse, but research in this area is limited. Kupersmidt and Martin (1997) assessed the prevalence of psychiatric disorders in children (aged 8–11 years) of Mexican and African-American migrant farm workers in North Carolina. They found elevated levels of pathology, with 59% of the children revealing one or more psychiatric disorders. The most common disorders were anxiety related (50%). These included phobias, separation anxiety and avoidance. Parenting styles could differ among cultures and could be interpreted as maltreatment. Underachievement is not universal. Children of some migrant communities have higher levels of school performance owing to values placed on education. Living in a neighbourhood with a higher concentration of immigrants is associated with less problem behaviour but the reverse is true for non-immigrant children and could be related to lesser discrimination, greater social support in the former and disadvantaged socio-economic status of the latter.

Adapting to a new environment by children can be challenging and needs support from authorities and schools. Various factors mentioned above could affect the adaptation process, including overcoming language barriers, attitudes faced in the community and school, integration attained by the family in general, residency status and intergenerational differences. Access to mental health services may be limited because of lack of awareness and lack of perceived need as well as poor provision. It is important to recognise that migrant children will also have the same range of mental health problems as non-migrants and detection of these problems can be a challenge with communication barriers, expectations and attitudes of all involved. 'Migrant children' form a heterogeneous group and their needs vary widely. There needs to be better consensus regarding terminology to identify mental health and social problems, offer culturally sensitive and appropriate interventions, plan services and for improvement in research designs and measuring outcomes to take place.

Elderly

Migration can affect the elderly in various ways. The reasons and motives for migration can be the same as those of younger migrants or could be because of their dependent status on younger family members who are the primary migrants. There is also an ever-increasing group who had migrated in their working years and have grown older in the host culture. Both these groups face a number of challenges with changes in their social, cultural and economic set-ups. They face multiple jeopardy due to problems faced because of ageism, racism, gender disparities, restricted access to health and welfare services and class struggle (Boneham, 1989; see also Chapter 14).

Communicating distress, especially with language barriers, can be a significant reason in not seeking help and not engaging in therapeutic alliance, no matter what age group is being studied. Many cultures have different idioms for communicating distress and some may even lack comparable terms for clinical concepts of depression and dementia and presentation with more somatic symptoms. Finally, the plight of many elderly people left behind by migrating families needs to be highlighted. At times they may be left with responsibilities of looking after young children and other elderly relatives. Breakdown of the family, of social and financial support, may make them vulnerable. However, many migrant families send money to their elders, who can offset some of the loss of social support but provide much needed financial support. Level of contact and the distance from families may also affect outcomes. The lower prevalence of depression in elderly Thai people left behind by rural–urban migrants compared with elderly rural Thai parents of non-migrants is a possible example (Abas *et al.*, 2009).

LGBT individuals

Lesbian, gay, bisexual and transgendered (LGBT) individuals may migrate either because of their sexual minority status or for other reasons, and discover their sexual identity after migration. The push factors for them will be different, in that homophobia or bi-negativity attitudes in their country of origin will influence the decision to migrate. For transgender individuals, a potential factor may be the availability of medical and surgical interventions which pull them towards the new society (see Chapter 17). Negative attitudes to the sexual minority status in the new country may place them in triple jeopardy – as a result of migrant status, minority or sexual identity which may be further complicated by factors such as age, gender or religion. Thus, further alienation may make it difficult to settle down. Data on the prevalence of psychiatric disorders among these groups are sparse. Clinicians' views on sexual minorities, on religious attitudes to sex and other factors will influence healthcare delivery for this group.

Women and families

Women may be primary migrants or may follow their families, spouses or partners. Their experiences of the act of migration and its consequences will depend upon gender roles and gender role expectations in their culture of origin and in the new society. It is possible that their own culture expects them to have traditional roles and carry traditional values to pass on to the next generation, but that the new culture expects them to have more modern views. With more women migrating and working, it is likely that they will experience more stress and pressure to conform, thereby putting them in a position of conflict between the two cultures (see Chapter 16). When families migrate or come together in the new culture, levels of acculturation in different members will vary, which will affect individual expectations of the new society. Changing structures of the family following migration from more traditional joint or extended families to nuclear families (with altered patterns of social support) will add to the stress being experienced by the individual. These changes will lead to altered social and individual expectations of women and family members.

Needs of refugees

The 1951 Geneva Convention defines a refugee as someone who has 'a well-founded fear of being persecuted for reasons of race, religion, nationality, membership of a particular social group or political opinion, is outside the country of his nationality and is unable or owing to such fear, is unwilling to avail himself of the protection of that country...' A further distinction of 'asylum seeker' is made for people who have left their country of origin, have applied to be recognized as a refugee and are awaiting a decision from the new government. Currently, there are over 20.8 million 'people of concern' to the United Nations, and about 40% of these are refugees. Pakistan and Iran host a fifth of the world's refugee population. According to the United Nations High Commissioner for Refugees, in 2005 there were some 668 000 applications for asylum or refugee status in the industrialised world, the majority to Europe (374 000). The USA is followed by the UK and France with the largest number of asylum applications overall, but numbers are starting to fall (United Nations High Commissioner for Refugees. Basic facts, 2006, available at: http://www.unhcr. org/cgibin/texis/vtx/basics).

Refugees are probably the most vulnerable of all groups of migrants. The individual experiences of refugees and asylum seekers can contribute to elevated rates of psychiatric disorders. Forced migration is usually not planned and is associated with various forms of trauma, uncertain legal and immigration status, loss of social support and resources. These problems can be compounded by the attitudes of the host countries, where they might be at the receiving end of discrimination because of race, politics and religion, unwelcoming response, poor living conditions in deprived and even segregated camps, limited employment and educational opportunities, and rights which limit normal day to day existence. After the initial relief of post-migration arrival in a safe haven it is not uncommon for frustration and disillusionment to develop as new problems emerge. These include language and cultural barriers, concerns about legal status and entitlements, unemployment, homelessness, isolation, lack of access to education and healthcare services, and family separation. There is surprisingly little public acceptance of the importance of tackling these problems.

Refugee children: children of refugees may have been separated from their parents, witnessed members of their family being tortured, or experienced violence or torture themselves. They may be living with just one parent, in fragmented families or with unfamiliar carers. Some will have arrived alone and most, if not all, will have experienced multiple losses. These experiences will eventually emerge in the form of emotional distress and aberrant behaviours. They may appear mature beyond their age in some settings yet immature in others. The most common conditions include anxiety, depression and conduct disorder. It is not known whether there are any unique manifestations of these disorders in refugees over and above what is commonly seen in the general population. Despite their experiences, most refugee children have many strengths and few need specific psychiatric treatment. Where they do, the principles of management are broadly the same – space and time to think about their experiences, help to become part of the local community, to learn and to make friends. Experiences at school are particularly important – an atmosphere of warmth and stability can go a long way towards restoring a sense of security.

The spectrum of mental ill-health among refugees differs in degree and presentation rather than in any absolute way from that of the host population. The most common disorders are those characterised by anxiety and depression, such as PTSD and major depression, reflecting the experience of trauma and loss that these populations experience. There may be anxieties around families left behind or guilt at having migrated. Post-traumatic disorders are often high in those fleeing troubled regions, physical and sexual violence, torture, loss of family members and persecution. A recent meta-analysis concluded that rates of common mental disorders were twice as high in refugee populations as in economic migrants (40% versus 21%) (Lindert *et al.*, 2009).

A heavy-handed response by authorities in new countries can further add to the post-migration trauma. PTSD and common mental disorders in asylum groups increase with length of stay in detention (Laban *et al.*, 2004; Hallas *et al.*, 2007) and with unemployment, absence of family support and complicated asylum processes (Laban *et al.*, 2004). Asylum seekers may be less likely to engage with mental health services as shown in the UK (McCrone *et al.*, 2005) and in the Netherlands (Laban *et al.*, 2007).

Once trauma has been disclosed, the acknowledgement of symptoms of anxiety and PTSD are important but need careful interpretation. There is a risk of pathologising and medicalising an otherwise normal human response to extreme adversity. On the other hand, there is a serious danger in dismissing too easily clinically significant disorders as simply caused by trauma. Services have to be sensitive to the needs and required specialised skills, including training of interpreters.

Refugees in some countries are entitled to clinical services and medical treatment, but access is not always straightforward, requiring at the very least some familiarity with how healthcare is organised. In some western countries there has been the development of specialist refugee health teams connected to primary care. These teams provide information and advice to refugees, facilitate access to healthcare and provide support to frontline services. They often work in loose partnership with a variety of refugee community organisations that deliver immigration advice and assistance with housing and welfare benefits. In low- and middle-income (LAMI) countries such as Pakistan and Iran, which have the highest burden of refugees, there are few provisions for specialist healthcare (especially mental health) and the needs of the refugee population add to the burden of the poorly funded local services and usually lead to further marginalisation of this group.

There is substantial evidence for the efficacy of psychological, psychosocial or 'talking therapies', which are primarily western in origin. Their appropriateness among non-western cultures has been questioned by some, who point out that most asylum seekers come from cultures where talking therapy is quite an alien concept. It can be argued that a more acceptable model for counselling might be one that starts with a background knowledge of the circumstances from which the patient has fled and acknowledges the relevance of practical advice and a more problem-focused (rather than emotion-focused) approach. In the absence of empirical studies testing the efficacy of specific psychotherapeutic approaches in refugee populations, experts concur on the following broad principles. An emphasis on helping to problem-solve and to achieve practical outcomes such as access to employment and education may be of as much benefit, if not more. Victims of torture may have co-morbid medical conditions which may mask psychological problems, and both will require treatment.

Sexual violence is a taboo subject in many cultures and, together with the distress the memories produce, victims of torture may be reluctant to talk about their experiences. The notion of disclosing personal experiences to a relative stranger (therapist, counsellor) is an alien experience for many refugees. Time is needed to build up trust, allowing the trauma story to emerge gently so that it becomes a familiar and comfortable theme rather than something shamefully hidden away. Disclosure is best managed when the social situation is stable and when both patient and healthworker are confident about managing the disclosures and the distress that will emerge.

The main aim of mental health and social services should be to provide psychological support, treatment and other support to the refugee patient to achieve basic goals and some normalcy in the host society such as attaining stability, education and work opportunities, housing etc. This requires multisector collaboration with social workers, refugee organisations, housing and employment agencies, and needs appropriate government and international funding.

Issues in mental health service delivery for migrants and minority communities

There have been recent efforts to integrate current knowledge and information on mental health service delivery for migrants and minority communities. Central issues are access to services and the quality of the services provided to this group.

It is important to provide appropriate information for migrants and ethnic minorities and develop a close working relationship with these communities. Healthcare organisations should develop participatory, collaborative partnerships with communities and utilise a variety of formal and informal mechanisms to facilitate community and patient/consumer involvement in designing and implementing confidential listening and assistance service (CLAS)-related activities. The main barriers are those of language and culture, problems around diagnosis, biased perceptions and (unconscious) assumptions and inadequate cultural competence of service providers.

Good practice in working with migrants when using interpreters

Health services should be inclusive and accessible. The main barrier to care for immigrants can be language, which can only be bridged by good quality interpreter services (for details see Chapter 20). Some countries, like the UK, have tried to incorporate this in policy documents, e.g. the National Service Framework for Mental Health (Department of Health, 1999) and Delivering Race Equality in Mental Health Care – An Action Plan for Reform Inside and Outside Services (Department of Health, 2005), which can provide guidance to other national services. It might be argued that failure to provide language services where there is a known language need is a form of indirect discrimination. There is also the need for appropriate training for clinicians and interpreters to be able to work in close partnership. Translation is an interactive dynamic medium and not just translation. This is particularly true in the case of culture-bound idioms of distress and 'syndromes'. Issues of control, power, triangulation and accountability may arise. It is important to make interpreters and clinicians feel at ease and offer them the best opportunity to use their language skills and cultural understandings, and be a part of the same team there to help the client. Moving from a dyad to a triadic consultation raises a number of issues. According to Tribe (1999), the four modes of interpreting are: (1) psychotherapeutic or constructionist; (2) linguistic; (3) the advocate or adversarial/community; and (4) cultural broker/bicultural. There are differences in the way interpreters interpret and patients expect them to interpret.

Ethical issues of confidentiality, neutrality, respect towards the individual and her or his community, professionality and integrity, precision and totality and cultural competence are essentials, and need to be incorporated in the training process.

Cultural competence and help-seeking

Although in the past decade or two cultural competence has become a fashionable term to use, good clinical practice has always relied at looking at individual patients' social and cultural factors, understanding them and their impact on the illness being experienced. However, for migrants' mental heath needs, cultural awareness becomes a very significant aspect of assessment of their mental state and in planning any therapeutic interactions. Lo and Fung (2003, page 162) define cultural competence as an ability 'to perform and obtain positive clinical outcomes in cross-cultural encounters'. This also includes different levels of competence, for example, generic cultural competence (i.e. principles) and specific cultural competence (related to any given culture). Recognising the differences in the therapeutic encounter, sensitivity to the patients' and their families' explanations and concerns, and awareness of strengths and weaknesses of the individuals and their cultures allow clinicians to engage patients from other cultures, thereby increasing therapeutic adherence. Within any given culture there will be a level of heterogeneity in attitudes and beliefs. Cultures are fluid and evolve in response to a number of factors and the explanatory models of illness will change. It is these explanatory models which tell the clinician why help is being sought, for what condition and the expected outcome. It is necessary that even if clinicians' and patients' explanatory models differ, the clinician is aware of the possibility that decisions to seek help and comply with treatment will be determined by explanatory models.

Alternative medicine and approaches

In cultures where Cartesian mind–body dualism is not a prevalent model, the interaction between somatic symptoms and psychological distress will be significant. Socio-economic and educational status, attitudes, beliefs and knowledge of distress and illness models, past experiences and outcome expectations will all influence from where and when help is sought. A significant proportion of healthcare encounters will occur in personal, folk or social sectors (whatever the illness) and only a small proportion will reach the professional healthcare sector. Healthcare systems from other cultures, e.g. Chinese, Ayurveda, Greek, are built upon complex systems of theory and clinical practice developed over several millennia. Herbal medicine, dietary taboos, dietary supplements and other interventions form part of these approaches. Migrant patients may be using them and unless specifically asked may not offer this information for a number of reasons. Thus, as part of the assessment, the clinician must explore this in a sensitive and appropriate manner. Patients may use explanations related to culture-bound syndromes, although these conditions may be more accurately described as culturally influenced rather than bound.

This volume brings together recent issues related to migrants' health. The heterogeneity of the migratory experience and post-migration settling down mean that clinicians must focus on individual issues rather than bland policies. Policy-makers need to listen to stakeholders to develop appropriate policies which can be translated into good clinical practice, whether that is psychotherapy, pharmacotherapy, a combination of the two and/ or the use of interpreters. It is essential that spiritual values and concepts of the self of migrants are taken into account when delivering psychiatric services. Special needs of groups such as children, unaccompanied adolescents, LGBT individuals or refugees will need to be borne in mind. The problems related to service delivery also include those at the institutional levels, which may be influenced by government policies and available resources.

This volume is not meant to be a complete resource book for dealing with migrants' mental health, but a starting block to lead clinicians and researchers into further exploration of the health needs of migrants and their dependents.

References

Abas, M. A., Punpuing, S., Jirapramukpitak, T. et al. (2009). Rural–urban migration and depression in ageing family members left behind. *British Journal of Psychiatry*, **195**, 54–60.

Alati, R., Najman, J. M., Shuttlewood, G. J., Williams, G. M., Bor, W. (2003). Changes in mental health status amongst children of migrants to Australia: a longitudinal study. *Sociology of Health & Illness*, **25**(7), 866–88.

Baker, T. P. (1992). Migrant studies and their problems. In D. F. Roberts, N. Fujiki, K. Torizuka eds., *Isolation, Migration and Health*. Cambridge: Cambridge University Press, pp. 167–70.

Bhugra, D. (2004). Migration and mental health. *Acta Psychiatrica Scandinavica*, **109**(4), 243–58.

Bhugra, D., Bhui, K. (2003). Eating disorders in teenagers in East London: a survey. *European Eating Disorders Review*, **11**(1), 46–57.

Bhugra, D., Mallett, R., Leff, J. (1999). Schizophrenia and African-Caribbeans: a conceptual model of aetiology. *International Review of Psychiatry*, **11**(2), 145–52.

Boneham, M. (1989). Ageing and ethnicity in Britain: the case of elderly Sikh women in a Midlands town. *New Community*, **15**, 447–59.

Cantor-Graae, E., Selten, J. P. (2005). Schizophrenia and migration: a meta-analysis and review. *American Journal of Psychiatry*, **162**, 12–24.

Commander, M. J., Sashidharan, S. P., Odell, S. M., Surtees, P. G. (1997). Access to mental health care in an inner city health district II: association with demographic factors. *British Journal of Psychiatry*, **170**, 317–20.

Commander, M. J., Odell, S. M., Surtees, P. G., Sashidharan, S. P. (2004). Care pathways for South Asian and white people with depressive and anxiety disorder in the community. *Social Psychiatry and Psychiatric Epidemiology*, **39**, 259–64.

Department of Health. (1999). *National Service Framework for Mental Health*. London: Department of Health.

Department of Health. (2005). *Delivering Race Equality in Mental Health Care*. London: Department of Health.

Fazel, M., Wheeler, J., Danesh, J. (2005). Prevalence of serious mental disorder in 2000 refugees resettled in Western countries – a systematic review. *Lancet*, **365**, 1309–14.

Gillam, S. J., Jarman, B., White, P. et al. (1989). Ethnic differences in consultation rates in urban general practice. *British Medical Journal*, **299**, 953–7.

Hallas, P., Hansen, A., Staehr, M. et al. (2007). Length of stay in asylum centres and mental health in asylum seekers: a retrospective study from Denmark. *BMC Public Health*, **7**(1), 288.

Hjern, A., Allbeck, P. (2002). Suicide in first and second generation immigrants in Sweden: a comparative study. *Social Psychiatry and Psychiatric Epidemiology*, **37**, 423–9.

International Organisation for Migration (2008). *United Nations' Trends in Total Migrant Stock: The 2008 Revision*. http://esa.un.org/migration (accessed 17 June 2010).

Jenkins, R., Bebbington, P., Brugha, T. et al. (1997a). The National Psychiatric Morbidity Surveys of Great Britain – strategy and methods. *Psychological Medicine*, **27**, 765–74.

Jenkins, R., Lewis, G., Bebbington, P. et al. (1997b). The National Psychiatric Morbidity Survey of Great Britain: initial findings from the household survey. *Psychological Medicine*, **27**, 775–89.

Kupersmidt, J. B., Martin, S. L. (1997). Mental health problems of children of migrant and seasonal farm workers: a pilot study. *Journal of the American Academy of Child and Adolescent Psychiatry*, **36**, 224–32.

Laban, C. H., Gernaat, H. B., Komproe, I. H. et al. (2004). Impact of a long asylum procedure on the prevalence of psychiatric disorders in Iraqi asylum seekers in The Netherlands.

Journal of Nervous and Mental Disease, **192**(12), 843–51.

Laban, C. H., Gernaat, H. B., Komproe, I. H. *et al.* (2007). Prevalence and predictors of health service use among Iraqi asylum seekers in The Netherlands. *Social Psychiatry and Psychiatric Epidemiology*, **42**(10), 837–44.

Lasker, G. W., Mascie-Taylor, C. G. N. (1988). The framework of migration studies. In C. G. N. Mascie-Taylor and G. W. Lasker, eds., *Biological Aspects of Human Migration*. Cambridge: Cambridge University Press.

Layton-Henry, Z. (1992). *The Politics of Immigration*. Oxford: Blackwell.

Lin, K.-M., Tazuma, L., Maston, M. (1979). Adaptational problems of Vietnamese refugees I: health and mental health issues. *Archives of General Psychiatry*, **36**, 955–61.

Lindert, J., von Ehrenstein, O. S., Priebe, S., Mielek, A., Brahler, E. (2009). Depression and anxiety in labour migrants and refugees: a systematic review and meta-analysis. *Social Science and Medicine*, **69**, 246–57.

Lo, H.-T., Fung, K. P. (2003). Culturally competent psychotherapy. *Canadian Journal of Psychiatry*, **48**, 161–70.

McCrone, P., Bhui, K. S., Craig, T. *et al.* (2005). Mental health needs, service use and costs among Somali refugees in the UK. *Acta Psychiatrica Scandinavica*, **111**(5), 351–7.

Modood, T., Berthoud, R., Lahey, J. *et al.* (1997). *Ethnic Minorities in Britain: Diversity and Disadvantage*. London: PSI.

Nazroo, J. (1997). *Ethnicity and Mental Health*. London: PSI.

Neel, J. V. (1992). The distinction between primary and secondary isolates. In D. F. Roberts, N. Fujiki, K. Torizuka, eds., *Isolation, Migration and Health*. Cambridge: Cambridge University Press, pp. 17–22.

Ödegaard, O. (1932). Emigration and insanity. *Acta Psychiatrica et Neurologica*, (Suppl. 4), 1–206.

Rack, P. (1982). *Race, Culture and Mental Disorder*. London: Tavistock.

Soni-Raleigh, V., Balarajan, R. (1992). Suicide and self burning among Indians and West Indians in England and Wales. *British Journal of Psychiatry*, **161**, 365–8.

Soni-Raleigh, V., Bulusu, R., Balarajan, R. (1990). Suicides among immigrants from the Indian subcontinent. *British Journal of Psychiatry*, **156**, 46–50.

Thompson, N., Bhugra, D. (2000). Rates of deliberate self harm in Asians: findings and models. *International Review of Psychiatry*, **12**(3): 37–43.

Tribe, R. (1999). Therapeutic work with refugees living in exile: observations on clinical practice. *Counselling Psychology Quarterly*, **12**, 233–43.

United Nations High Commissioner for Refugees. Basic facts, 2006, available at: http://www.unhcr.org/cgibin/texis/vtx/basics

Veen, N., Selten, J. P., Hoek, H. W. *et al.* (2002). Use of illicit substances in a psychosis incidence cohort: a comparison among different ethnic groups in the Netherlands. *Acta Psychiatrica Scandinavica*, **105**(6), 440–3.

Veling, W., Selten, J. P., Veen, N. *et al.* (2006). Incidence of schizophrenia among ethnic minorities in the Netherlands: a four-year first-contact study. *Schizophrenia Research*, **86**, 189–93.

Vollebergh, W. A., ten Have, M., Dekovic, M. *et al.* (2005). Mental health in immigrant children in The Netherlands. *Social Psychiatry and Psychiatric Epidemiology*, **40**, 489–96.

Weich, S., Nazroo, J., Sproston, K. *et al.* (2004). Common mental disorders and ethnicity in England: the EMPIRIC study. *Psychological Medicine*, **34**, 1543–51.

Wojcik, W., Bhugra, D. (2010). Loss and cultural bereavement. In D. Bhugra, T. Craig and K. S. Bhui, eds., *Mental Health of Refugees and Asylum Seekers*. Oxford: Oxford University Press.

Yanase, T. (1992). Time trends in the break-up of isolates. In D. F. Roberts, N. Fujiki and K. Torizuka, eds., *Isolation, Migration and Health*. Cambridge: Cambridge University Press, pp. 23–8.

Epidemiological aspects of migration and mental illness

James B. Kirkbride and Peter B. Jones

Editors' introduction

In some countries, some groups of migrants appear to have increased rates of psychiatric disorders. Over the past three-quarters of a century, it has been demonstrated that migrant groups show higher levels of psychotic disorders. Most of the research has been done with schizophrenia and in the West. From Norwegian migrants to the USA to the African-Caribbean migrants to the UK, a two-fold to 14-fold increase has been demonstrated compared with the local populations. In this chapter, James Kirkbride and Peter Jones set the scene and, using the data from a recent multicentred study in the UK, illustrate that these rates are not artificial. Various hypotheses, including predisposition to migrate, high rates in countries of origin, misdiagnosis, post-migration and socio-economic differences, are examined and discussed. As they conclude, it is important to have an awareness of such differences, even if the causes of the variation are overlapping, so that preventative strategies can be put into place. In due course, epidemiological studies may allow researchers to explore aetiological factors in some detail, which will enable medical, social and psychological interventions to be developed.

Introduction

This chapter focuses on the epidemiological study of major psychiatric illnesses among migrant groups and their offspring. The main focus is on psychotic disorders, for which there is most evidence of elevated rates in immigrant groups and their offspring. However, the evidence with regard to other psychiatric outcomes – common mental disorders, suicide and post-traumatic stress disorder (PTSD) – is also considered. The scope of the review is international, although policy recommendations are likely to be national or provincial in application, given that the social context of migration is likely to be a crucial contributory factor that will vary by time and place. The chapter is divided into four parts. The first three comprise a critical review of the epidemiological literature on migration and psychotic disorders (Part 1), common mental disorders and PTSD (Part 2), and suicide and suicidal behaviour (Part 3), respectively. The main historical and contemporary hypotheses posited to explain the raised (or otherwise) rates of mental illness in immigrant groups and their offspring, and the degree of support for each are also summarised. Finally, in Part 4 potential policy recommendations are proposed to address the excess morbidity of mental illness in some immigrant and black and minority ethnic (BME) groups in the UK, with this intended to be a heuristic exercise for other nations.

Migration and Mental Health, ed. Dinesh Bhugra & Susham Gupta. Published by Cambridge University Press. © Cambridge University Press 2011.

Migration takes place for many different social, economic, political and cultural reasons, some positive, some negative. Migration also takes place at many different levels (cities, regions, countries), spanning different time periods (days, weeks, months, years). Given the complexities surrounding the epidemiological study of mental illness, including the absolute rarity of disorders, some of these subtleties have no doubt remained elusive within the field. Permanent, economic migrants have been the focus of much of the research on psychosis, common mental disorders and suicide in developed countries. The prevalence and severity of common mental disorders and PTSD have also been studied amongst refugee populations and asylum seekers in both the developed and developing world, while there is a growing, methodologically robust epidemiological literature on the mental health of short-term and rural–urban migrants and those left behind in developing countries.

The meaning and context of migration has no doubt changed since the earliest studies of migration and mental health in the 1930s. For much of the twentieth century, migration may have been a once-in-a-lifetime commitment, conducted at considerable expense, associated with prohibitively large geographical and communication barriers with one's country of origin. With the advent of globalisation, improved communication links over large geographical areas and the commodification and commercialisation of global air travel, the context and propensity to migrate has become an increasingly accessible and viable opportunity for a larger proportion of people. This has altered the meaning and context of migration and whether such changes will have an effect on the mental health of migrants will require further elucidation.

This chapter attempts to provide an inclusive, unbiased and critical review of the available literature on migration and mental illness. It is not, however, a formal systematic review. We have not explored the grey or unpublished literature, performed structured searches or meta-analytical techniques. Readers interested in such reviews are referred to excellent, recent systematic reviews on schizophrenia and other psychotic disorders (Cantor-Graae and Selten, 2005; McGrath et al., 2004) and common mental disorders (Lindert et al., 2008, 2009). Rather, we have attempted to present a comprehensive, representative, critical reading of the current evidence to inform policy decisions.

Part 1 Psychotic disorders

Introduction

Elevated rates of psychoses emerge in various immigrant populations

The first research suggesting that schizophrenia was elevated in migrant populations was published in 1932 by a Norwegian psychiatrist, Ørnulv Ødegaard. He reported that the hospitalised rate of insanity in Norwegian emigrants to Minnesota in the USA was twice that of either the Norwegian population in Norway or native-born Americans (Ødegaard, 1932). Later work conducted by Malzberg in New York (1964, 1969) also found raised rates of schizophrenia among immigrants, independent of differences with the host population in age structure and level of urbanisation. More recently, historical studies have attempted to determine whether elevated rates of psychosis were evident in immigrant populations in the early twentieth century by looking back at archived care records. Smith and colleagues (2006), for example, analysed clinical records between 1902 and 1913 for all psychiatric admissions to hospital in British Columbia, Canada. The authors were able to diagnose patients according to the current *Diagnostic and Statistical Manual* (4th edition) (DSM-IV) classification. They found that the rate of schizophrenia in immigrants from Britain and Continental Europe was 54% higher than in the Canadian-born population at the time.

The earliest reports of elevated rates of psychotic disorders in the UK occurred in the 1960s (Hemsi, 1967), following a period of substantial postwar immigration to fill labour shortages in many of the lowest paid sectors of the economy. In 1967, Hemsi reported significantly higher rates of psychotic illness in black Caribbean immigrants to south London than in the background population of the UK. This finding was confirmed in several later studies in the UK over the next two decades (Bhugra *et al.*, 1997; Castle *et al.*, 1991; Cochrane, 1977; Coid *et al.*, 2008; Fearon *et al.*, 2006; Harrison *et al.*, 1988; 1996; 1997; King *et al.*, 1994; Kirkbride *et al.*, 2008; Littlewood and Lipsedge, 1981; van Os *et al.*, 1996; Wessely *et al.*, 1991; 1992; Sugarman and Crauford, 1994; Thomas *et al.*, 1993; McGovern and Cope, 1987). For example, Cochrane (1977) reported higher rates in this group in England and Wales, independent of the age structure of the population. Littlewood and Lipsedge (1981) reported higher rates of schizophrenia in inpatient care in the black Caribbean and West African population in London.

Refinement of incidence rates – methodological advances

A handful of important studies had, by the mid 1980s, reported higher rates of schizophrenia in immigrants to both North American and European countries, but methodological constraints made bias and confounding difficult to exclude as possible explanations for the phenomenon. Predominantly, these difficulties could be separated into completeness of both the numerator (i.e. case), including potential misdiagnosis of psychotic disorders in migrants (Hickling *et al.*, 1999), and denominator (i.e. population at risk), and the separate issue of whether confounding factors explained the association between migration and schizophrenia. In 1988, Harrison and colleagues (1988) published a study which would become a benchmark for future studies in this field. They employed a robust methodology including a prospective, case-finding design and standardised diagnoses in a well defined catchment area. This overcame many, though not all, of the problems associated with ensuring complete case ascertainment and obtaining an accurate estimate of the denominator population. They observed that the incidence of schizophrenia was between 8 and 16 times greater in black Caribbean groups in their study than in the general population of Nottingham (Harrison *et al.*, 1988).

The 1991 UK Census published data by age, sex and ethnicity, so made it possible at last to obtain accurate estimates of the denominator population by ethnicity. Subsequent studies used improved methodology including the adjustment of effects for age and sex which may have explained the raised rates in BME populations. Nevertheless, they continued to report significantly elevated rates of schizophrenia in the black Caribbean population in the UK, although effects were somewhat more modest than in previous results; in the order of three- to eight-fold the rate in the white group (Castle *et al.*, 1991; King *et al.*, 1994; van Os *et al.*, 1996; Thomas *et al.*, 1993; Wessely *et al.*, 1991). Comparably raised rates of schizophrenia were also observed for black African groups in Great Britain (van Os *et al.*, 1996).

While the literature thus far had established that immigrant groups showed higher rates of schizophrenia than the host population in which they lived, one outstanding issue was whether these elevated rates were attributable to a tendency to over-diagnosis of immigrants with schizophrenia. In the mid 1990s the Aetiology and Ethnicity in Schizophrenia and Other Psychoses [ÆSOP] study (Kirkbride *et al.*, 2006) was designed, in part to establish whether immigrant groups and their offspring had elevated rates across the spectrum of psychotic disorders. The ÆSOP study was conducted over 2 years (1997–99) in three British cities – London, Nottingham and Bristol – and employed a robust case-finding design based on the WHO 10-country study, including a leakage study to identify cases potentially missed by the initial screening process. Standardised diagnoses using ICD-10 and DSM-IV were made by consensus, by a multiethnic panel of clinicians following presentation of a case vignette from the clinician responsible for each subject. Although the clinicians who compiled these vignettes were not blind, this study went further than any research before or since to minimise possible rater bias, by blinding the panel of clinicians to the ethnicity of the subject. Inter-rater reliability was high, from 1.0 for any psychosis, to 0.6–0.8 for specific disorders. The population at risk was estimated from the 2001 census, which for the first time separated white British from other white groups to allow for a more accurate comparison of incidence rates between host and migrant groups. In this sample, Fearon *et al.* (2006) were able to confirm that rates of schizophrenia were significantly raised in black Caribbean (relative risk [RR]: 9.1; 95% Confidence interval [CI]: 6.6–12.6) and black African (RR: 5.8; 95% CI: 3.9–8.4) populations compared with the white British group. Notably, these groups also had elevated rates of other psychotic disorders (Fearon *et al.*, 2006; Lloyd *et al.*, 2005). For example, rates of bipolar disorder for black Caribbean (RR: 8.0; 95% CI: 4.3–14.8) and African (RR: 6.2; 95% CI: 3.1–12.1) groups were also elevated. Rates of depressive psychoses were also raised for black Caribbean (RR: 3.2; 95% CI: 1.5–6.1) and black African (RR: 2.1; 95% CI: 0.9–5.0) groups compared with the white British group, though not to the extent as for schizophrenia and bipolar disorder. All these differences remained apparent when men and women were studied separately.

A recent meta-analysis found mixed evidence for elevated rates of mood disorders in immigrants and their offspring (Swinnen and Selten, 2007). Raised rates were significant in the black Caribbean group, but this finding did not extend to other BME groups. However, the study did not differentiate between disorders with and without psychosis and may have concealed heterogeneity in rates by treating all immigrants as a single group (with the exception of the black Caribbean group).

Broadening our understanding of risk in immigrant groups and their offspring

Establishing that rates of psychotic disorders were raised for some immigrant groups provided a primary direction in the search for socioenvironmental causes of mental illness. Early studies were well positioned to combine methodological ingenuity with natural opportunities to study migrant groups, either in large numbers (i.e. Malzberg, 1964; Ødegaard, 1932) or where the excess risk turned out to be extremely large in comparison with the host population (i.e. Fearon *et al.*, 2006; Harrison *et al.*, 1988; van Os *et al.*, 1996). However, many important questions remained, including, but not limited to: whether rates were raised in the offspring of migrants, i.e. so-called second generation immigrants; whether other immigrant groups, in settings outside of the UK and USA, were at increased risk; and whether other confounding factors (beyond age and sex) could explain the elevated rates in immigrant groups.

In 1987, McGovern and Cope investigated whether elevated rates of schizophrenia extended to second generation immigrants in Birmingham, UK. Using hospitalised admissions, they found that rates of schizophrenia, as well as other psychotic disorders, were raised for both first and second generation black Caribbean groups. This finding was subsequently replicated by other studies in the UK (Harrison *et al.*, 1988, 1996; Sugarman and Crauford, 1994), although no study was directly able to obtain accurate estimates of the population at risk by generational status, because such statistics were not routinely collated in the Census until 2001. Instead, these studies relied on inferential estimates and other less accurate sources of the denominator population (Harrison *et al.*, 1988; McGovern and Cape, 1987). The East London First Episode Psychosis (ELFEP) study overcame this problem (Coid *et al.*, 2008). Designed using the methodology of the WHO 10-country study (Jablensky *et al.*, 1992) and the ÆSOP study (Kirkbride *et al.*, 2006), ELFEP identified all subjects with a first episode psychosis presenting to services in three East London boroughs between 1996 and 1999. Population at risk estimates were obtained from the 2001 Census, to estimate incidence rates of various psychotic disorders by generation status and ethnicity. The study confirmed that both first (non-affective RR: 2.3; 95% CI: 1.2–4.3) and second generation (non-affective RR: 4.9; 95% CI: 3.5–6.9) black Caribbean immigrants were at elevated risk of psychotic disorders after adjustment stratified by age and sex. This finding was also observed for first generation black African and non-British white migrants and their offspring (see Figure 2.1). In a further analysis from the same study, Kirkbride *et al.* (2008) addressed the rates of psychoses in the mixed ethnicity group in more detail; a possible marker of 'third generation' migrant groups. They found that the mixed white and black Caribbean group had significantly increased rates of psychotic disorders, most notably for the affective psychoses (RR: 10.9; 95% CI: 4.5–26.3).

For Asian groups, usually treated as a homogenous group, despite considerable differences in terms of culture, religion, migratory experiences and country of origin (Bhopal *et al.*, 1991), conflicting findings with regard to elevated rates of psychoses have been observed (Bhugra *et al.*, 1997; Fearon *et al.*, 2006; King *et al.*, 1994). The ELFEP study (Kirkbride *et al.*, 2008)

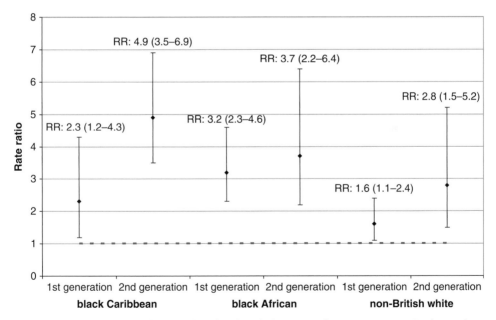

Figure 2.1 Rate ratios adjusted for age and sex for selected ethnic groups by generation status. Baseline is white British group. Values in parentheses are 95% confidence intervals. Adapted from Coid *et al.*, 2008.

analysed data from these three groups, independently, and found evidence that rates of schizophrenia were significantly raised. There was some evidence that effect was restricted to women: the rate of schizophrenia in Pakistani (RR: 4.9; 95% CI: 1.9–13.0) and Bangladeshi women (RR: 4.4; 95% CI: 2.8–8.9) was over four times greater than for white British women. Indian women were at elevated risk of other non-affective psychoses (RR: 2.7; 95% CI: 1.2–5.9). No Asian group appeared to have elevated rates of affective psychoses. Interestingly, further analysis of the sample suggested raised rates in Asian women were present for both first (RR: 3.6; 95% CI: 2.1–6.4) and second generation (RR: 2.3; 95% CI: 1.0–5.3) groups (Coid *et al.*, 2008). The authors of the ELFEP study were also able to adjust for potential differences between the white British and BME groups in terms of socio-economic status but this did not alter the interpretation of their findings, despite some attenuation of excess risk (Kirkbride *et al.*, 2008).

Increased rates of psychotic disorders have been observed in immigrants to several countries, and also in their offspring. Thus, both first and second generation Moroccan and Surinamese immigrants to the Netherlands have been shown to have elevated rates of all psychotic disorders (Selten *et al.*, 2001; Veling *et al.*, 2006), including schizophrenia, ranging from between two and ten times the rate in the native white Dutch group. Second generation Turkish immigrants to the Netherlands may also face an increased risk of schizophrenia and other psychotic disorders (Veling *et al.*, 2006). In a landmark Danish study of over 10 000 cases of schizophrenia, Cantor-Graae and colleagues (2003) demonstrated that first generation migrants to Denmark from nearly every part of the world were at increased risk of disorder after adjustment for age and sex. Compared with the native white Danish group, rates ranged from being twice as high for people born elsewhere in Scandinavia to around four times greater in people born in Australia, Africa and the Middle East. Second generation immigrants in Denmark were also found to have elevated rates of schizophrenia (RR: 1.92; 95% CI: 1.7–2.1) (Cantor-Graae *et al.*, 2003). In Sweden, three studies have shown immigrants to be at elevated risk of schizophrenia (Hjern *et al.*, 2004; Leao *et al.*, 2006; Zolkowska *et al.*, 2001). Two of these inspected rates by generation status (Hjern *et al.*, 2004; Leao *et al.*, 2006), finding raised rates in first and second generation migrant groups.

Outside Scandinavia, the Netherlands and the UK, relatively little epidemiological research on migration and psychosis has been conducted until recently. Two recent studies have investigated rates of psychotic disorder in migrants to Israel, a country with a different immigration pattern from that of Western European countries. Weiser *et al.* (2008) used data from over 660 000 consecutive adolescents given physical and mental health screens at age 16/17 for potential conscription to the Israeli Army. Subjects were then followed up for a mean of 7.7 years and data on hospitalisation for a first episode of any non-affective psychosis (F20–29) was then linked using the Israeli Psychiatric Hospitalization Case Registry. The study demonstrated that both first (hazard ratio [HR]: 1.6; 95% CI: 1.2–2.2) and second generation (HR: 1.4; 95% CI: 1.0–2.0) immigrants in Israel had elevated rates of schizophrenic disorders compared with native-born Israelis. In particular, Ethiopian immigrants and their offspring appeared to have particularly elevated rates of psychotic disorders (RR: 3.0; 95% CI: 1.9–4.7). However, a second Israeli study using data on nearly 100 000 people (case *n* = 637) from the Jerusalem Perinatal Cohort (Corcoran *et al.*, 2009), found no evidence that rates were elevated for second generation immigrants (they did not look at first generation migrants). This negative finding contrasts with the majority of the literature and only one previous study – an Australian case-control study (McGrath *et al.*, 2001) – did not observe increased risk in first or second generation migrant groups. An even earlier

Australian study did, however, observe elevated risk in German, Italian and Polish migrants (Krupinski and Cochrane, 1980). Some negative studies will, inevitably, be attributable to statistical chance but others may reflect genuinely different migratory and postmigratory experiences in some contexts (see Section 2).

Despite research on immigration and mental illness from the USA up until the 1960s (Malzberg, 1964, 1969; Ødegaard, 1932), until recently there has been relatively little evidence from North America on this subject; in part reflecting historical cultural tensions along ethnic and racial dimensions, but also because mass migration to Europe following World War 2 made it easier to study the effect of migration on mental illness elsewhere. A recent population-based birth cohort study in the USA (Bresnahan *et al.*, 2007) has shown that the rate of schizophrenia was three times greater in African-American groups compared with white Americans. Interestingly, a recent study of lifetime psychiatric hospitalisation in the USA (Snowden *et al.*, 2009) also found that both African-American (odds ratio [OR]: 2.5; 95% CI: 1.9–3.3) and black Caribbean (OR: 2.7; 95% CI: 2.0–3.8) groups faced elevated risk when compared with their white counterparts. Further investigation of the Caribbean group suggested this excess risk was restricted to second generation immigrants (OR: 5.5; 95% CI: 3.6–8.3). One further study conducted in New York in the late 1990s reported much increased prevalence of psychotic symptoms in older Caribbean migrants (especially French Caribbeans from Haiti), compared with the whites and blacks born in the US (Cohen *et al.*, 2004).

Main hypotheses

Several hypotheses have been raised to explain elevated rates of psychotic disorders in immigrant groups and their offspring (for example see Bhugra, 2000, 2004; Sharpley *et al.*, 2001). Table 2.1 provides an overview of the main hypotheses in this regard, with a summary of the evidence for and against each. Here, we briefly review each hypothesis in turn (the code presented after each hypothesis corresponds to the code in Table 2.1).

Psychoses predispose people to migrate (H1)

The 'selection' hypothesis – that people with psychoses were more likely to migrate – was first proposed by Ødergaard (1932) who observed that Norwegian immigrants in Minnesota appeared to have poor social adaptation in Norway and, he reasoned, would have gone on to develop psychoses had they not emigrated. Using an innovative study design Selten *et al.* (2002) were able to test this idea on a quasi-hypothetical dataset of Surinamese immigrants to the Netherlands. During the 1970s, more than one-third of the Surinamese population migrated to the Netherlands following political instability around the time of the former country's independence from the latter. In a study of the Dutch psychiatric registry, these immigrants were later found to have roughly four to five times the rate of schizophrenia compared with the Dutch-born group (Selten *et al.*, 2001). Selten and colleagues:

> imagined that the entire population of Surinam had emigrated to the Netherlands and that all the hypothetical additional migrants, consisting of those who in reality had stayed behind, contributed to the Netherlands no new cases of schizophrenia. We repeated the study of the Dutch psychiatric registry and enlarged the denominator for the Surinamese-born population by adding the entire age-correspondent resident population of Surinam during the years in question. We reasoned that the selection hypothesis could be rejected if the risk of schizophrenia for Surinamese-born people remained significantly higher, because this enlargement precluded any possibility of selection (2002, page 670).

Table 2.1 Overview of the main hypotheses, by year, proposed to explain the raised rates of psychosis in immigrants and their offspring

	Hypothesis title	Hypothesis description	Type of hypothesis[a]	Proposed by (year)	Evidence for	Evidence against	Strength (out of 5)[b]	Notes
H1	Predisposition to migrate	People with genetic disposition to psychosis were more likely to migrate	Reverse causality	Ødegaard (1932)	Initial observations of Ødegaard (1932)	Selten et al's (2002) natural experiment rejected hypothesis. Raised rates in second (& later? i.e. Kirkbride et al, 2008) generation groups (i.e. Coid et al, 2008; Harrison et al, 1988; McGovern and Cope, 1987; Veling et al, 2006). Migration highly complex task for people predisposed to psychosis (Jones et al, 1994)	1	
H2	High rates in sending country	Elevated rates in country of origin would explain higher rates in immigrants	Reverse causality	Cochrane and Bal (1987)	None	Incidence rates of schizophrenia in the Caribbean comparable to those in host UK and Dutch population (Bhugra et al, 1996; Hickling and Rodgers-Johnson, 1995; Mahy et al, 1999; Hanoeman et al, 2002). Hospitalised	2	Few comparative studies have been conducted other than the UK versus Caribbean studies noted. Irish comparative study (Cochrane and Bal, 1987) only based on hospitalised rates. Other studies would be informative, i.e.

	Hypothesis	Description	Category	Source	Evidence	Counter-evidence	No.	Findings
						rates in Ireland higher than those for Irish migrants to UK (Cochrane and Bal, 1987)		rates in Morocco versus Moroccans in the Netherlands
H3	Sociodemographic differences	Age, sex, marital status and socio-economic status differences between host and immigrant groups explain differences	Confounding	Cochrane and Bal (1987)	Young, male groups over-represented in initial migrant groups. Also known to be at increased risk of psychosis (Hefner et al., 1993)	Control for age and sex (Coid et al., 2008; Harrison et al., 1988, 1996; van Os et al., 1996; Veling et al., 2006; Cantor-Graae et al., 2003; Zolkowka et al., 2001), latterly SES (Kirkbride et al., 2008; Weiser et al., 2008; Bresnahan et al., 2007). Marital status a consequence, not cause of psychosis (Cochrane and Bal, 1987)	1	
H4	Misdiagnosis of psychotic symptoms	Psychiatrists in host country may misdiagnose psychotic symptoms in migrant groups, unfamiliar with their sociocultural norms, or tendency to over-diagnosis of migrants with schizophrenia versus other psychotic disorders	Bias	Cochrane & Bal (1987)	Early evidence of institutionalised racism in mental health services (Lewis et al., 1990), particularly with regard to pathways to care (Morgan et al., 2005). Psychotic symptoms may be more prevalent in Caribbean migrants (Johns et al., 2002).	Standardised diagnoses used in research, often quasi-blind to ethnicity of subject (Kirkbride et al., 2006). Raised rates of psychotic disorders not limited to schizophrenia (Coid et al., 2008; Fearon et al., 2006; van Os et al., 1996).	2	Rates of psychotic disorders in migrants persisted despite improved study designs and standardised diagnoses. Separate to the problem of institutionalised racism – see Singh and Burns (2006) for controversies surrounding this area. Cultural variation in symptom

Table 2.1 (cont.)

Hypothesis title	Hypothesis description	Type of hypothesis[a]	Proposed by (year)	Evidence for	Evidence against	Strength (out of 5)[b]	Notes
				Poor inter-rater reliability between English and Jamaican psychiatrist (Hickling et al., 1999)	Inter-rater reliability was poor but not racially biased (Hickling et al., 1999)		interpretation needs further research
H5	Migratory and postmigratory factors	Several, but involving negative consequences of migration, acculturation and postmigratory living as relevant. Stress/vulnerability is posited as potential biological mechanism	Confounding	Cochrane and Bal (1987); Bhugra (2000, 2004), Jones and Fung (2005)	Ethnic density effect implicates social support as protective (Boydell et al., 2001; Kirkbride et al., 2008; Veling et al., 2008). Higher rates of psychosis in BME groups which experience greater discrimination (Veling et al., 2007). Neighbourhoods with more ethnic fragmentation have higher rates of psychosis (Kirkbride et al., 2007). Social adversity confounds relationship between psychosis and	Other purportedly stress-induced disorders not raised for immigrants (i.e. depression; Sharpley et al., 2001; Cochrane and Bal, 1987). Immigrants experience similar levels of stress but variation in rates of psychosis is marked (Cochrane and Bal, 1987)	4	Cochrane and Bal's (1987) assertion that experience of migratory factors is similar across all immigrants is unlikely to hold now given likely genetic variation in stress vulnerability and differential experiences of migration along other sociodemographic and sociocultural dimensions (i.e. family structure, social support networks)

				migrancy (Hjern et al., 2004). Greater impact of social disadvantage in black Caribbean migrants than white British (Morgan et al., 2008)		Evidence is mixed, depending on type of risk factor and period of life course. Further research required
H6	Life course factors and neurodevelopment	Factors across the life course, including prenatally perinatally, and through childhood have greater impact in migrants. Includes vitamin D hypothesis: a change in maternal vitamin D exposure after migration alters offspring neurodevelopment	Confounding	Eagles (1991); McGrath (1999); Jones and Fung (2005)	Separation from parents during childhood has greater impact in black Caribbean migrants than white British (Morgan et al., 2007). Prenatal hypovitaminosis D associated with schizophrenia risk in general (McGrath et al., 2004)	No evidence that prenatal perinatal problems have greater role in migrant than native groups (Sharpley et al., 2001). No current evidence directly linking migration, hypovitaminosis and psychosis	3
H7	Substance abuse	Greater substance misuse in migrants accounts for higher rates	Confounding	Jones and Fung (2005)	None	Little evidence cannabis used more in black Caribbean than white patients (McGuire et al., 1995) or general population (i.e. Coulthard et al., 2002; Sandwijk et al., 1995; Sharp and Budd, 2003).	1	Putative link between cannabis and schizophrenia (Moore et al., 2007) combined with misconception that cannabis consumption was more prevalent in black Caribbean fuelled 'hypothesis'

Table 2.1 (cont.)

	Hypothesis title	Hypothesis description	Type of hypothesis[a]	Proposed by (year)	Evidence for	Evidence against	Strength (out of 5)[b]	Notes
						or substance use more generally (Veen et al., 2002)		
H8	Psychological hypotheses	Interpretation of life events have greater impact on psychosis in migrant groups	Mediating factor	Jones and Fung (2005)	Tendency to attribute life events to an external locus may lead to onset of paranoid symptoms in some migrant groups. Evidence is weak (Sharpley and Peters, 1999)	No differences in number of life events experienced by UK white versus black Caribbean migrants (Gilvarry et al., 1999)	3	Difficult to exclude this hypothesis and may mediate or have some overlap with other hypotheses (i.e. H5, H6, H10)
H9	Genetic predisposition	Genetic factors explain higher rates in migrant groups	Genetic confounding	Jones and Fung (2005)	None	Morbid risk is similar for offspring of both black Caribbean migrants and white group in (Sugarman and Craufurd, 1994; Hutchinson et al., 1996). Larger morbid risk in second generation migrants suggests environmental, not genetic pressures alone. Rates of psychosis in Caribbean comparable to	1	Genetic factors alone are unlikely to explain differences in rates between migrants and host population but genetic susceptibility in combination with environmental exposures (i.e. interaction – see Hypothesis 10 might be important)

		those in host UK population (Bhugra et al, 1996; Hickling and Rodgers-Johnson, 1995; Mahy et al, 1999)			Little explicit evidence either way	? (5)	Promising avenue for future research. More studies required
H10	Gene–environment interactions and epigenetic processes	People with underlying susceptibility genes for psychosis at increased risk if exposed to stressful environmental factors, i.e. migration and other postmigratory factors. May be regulated epigenetically, i.e. changes to gene expression following changes to environmental stimuli after migration	Rutter (2002); Broome et al. (2005); Dealberto (2007)	Interaction	Little explicit evidence either way. Ethnic density effect is proxy for interaction between individual phenotype (i.e. BME status) and exposure to environmental stressors (i.e. Boydell et al, 2001; Kirkbride et al, 2008; Veling et al, 2008). No direct study of genes versus environment in psychosis and migrants, but studies are under way (EU-GEI, 2008)		

[a] In accounting for raised rates in immigrant groups and their offspring, the excess risk must be attributable to other factors. Here, we classify these alternative explanations as attributable to one of the following: reverse causality, confounding (i.e. alternative explanation), bias, genetic confounding, mediating factor or interaction effects. Chance, the other facet of epidemiological research, is extremely unlikely to account for the higher rates given the number of studies to report positive associations (Cantor-Graae and Selten, 2005).

[b] Strength of support for each hypothesis out of five, based on our interpretation of current evidence available to support or reject it. There is insufficient evidence available to rate hypothesis 10, though a speculative rating may be attributed.

Duly, they showed that the rate of schizophrenia in Surinamese immigrants remained elevated compared with that of the Dutch-born population, thus arguing against Ødergaard's selection hypothesis. Migration is also a complex undertaking, especially for people who later develop psychosis, since they often have cognitive impairment (Jones *et al.*, 1994). Further, rates appear to be raised in the descendants of first generation immigrants (Harrison *et al.*, 1988, and Crauford 1996; McGovern and Cope, 1987; Sugarman 1994), which doesn't readily fit with this hypothesis.

Higher rates in the immigrants' country of origin (H2)

Three studies have been conducted in the Caribbean (Jamaica, Barbados and Trinidad) to estimate the local incidence of psychoses and compare it with rates in first generation black Caribbean immigrants and the native-born white population in the UK (Bhugra *et al.*, 1996; Hickling and Rodgers-Johnson, 1995; Mahy *et al.*, 1999). Each study found that the incidence of schizophrenia in the Caribbean was comparable to that of the white population in the UK. Therefore, higher rates of schizophrenia in immigrants from the Caribbean are not simply because of higher rates in their countries of origin. Few other comparative studies have been conducted for migrants from countries outside of the Caribbean, but such studies would shed light on other migrant groups, such as Moroccans to the Netherlands (Veling *et al.*, 2006).

Sociodemographic differences account for higher rates (H3)

This hypothesis was originally proposed by Cochrane and Bal in 1987. As shown earlier, most studies thereafter adjusted for age and sex as a matter of course, with evidence that elevated rates remained present in immigrant groups (Cantor-Graae and Selten, 2005). Recently, studies have considered whether socio-economic status (SES) is an alternative explanation for (i.e. confounds) the association between psychosis and immigration. Two Swedish studies (Hjern *et al.*, 2004; Leao *et al.*, 2006) have found that a raised incidence of psychoses persisted in immigrants to Sweden after adjustment for individual level SES, despite some attenuation. This finding has recently been replicated in the ELFEP study in the UK (Kirkbride *et al.*, 2008) and in an Israeli study (Weiser *et al.*, 2008).

Misdiagnosis of psychotic disorders in immigrants (H4)

This hypothesis continues to court controversy (Lewis *et al.*, 1990; Singh, 2009; Singh and Burns, 2006). Several commentators have posited that psychotic symptoms may be more common and more frequently reported in BME populations (Bhugra, 2000, 2004; Sharpley *et al.*, 2001); there is some support for this (Johns *et al.*, 2002). Misdiagnosis of cultural beliefs as psychotic experiences in BME populations by psychiatrists unfamiliar with non-western cultural mores has been put forward to explain the excess rates in migrants (Littlewood and Lipsedge, 1981). One study suggested that inter-rater reliability between a Jamaican and UK psychiatrist for diagnosing schizophrenia was low (Hickling *et al.*, 1999), but there was no evidence of a racist diagnosis – both psychiatrists diagnosed a similar proportion of the black Caribbean group with schizophrenia (52% versus 55%). Furthermore, modern epidemiological studies, such as ÆSOP (Kirkbride *et al.*, 2006) or ELFEP (Coid *et al.*, 2008), which enforce standardised diagnostic criteria show that the incidence of psychosis is raised across a range of psychotic disorders, not limited to schizophrenia (Fearon *et al.*, 2006; Kirkbride *et al.*, 2008), supporting earlier work in this field showing that black Caribbean and other BME groups experienced elevated rates of mania (Leff *et al.*, 1976; van Os *et al.*, 1996) and bipolar disorder

(Lloyd *et al.*, 2005). This issue is quite separate from the notion of institutionalised racism in health and other public services whereby BME populations do not receive culturally, religiously and ethnically sensitive services in the same way as the majority population (Lewis *et al.*, 1990; Singh, 2009; Singh and Burns, 2006) (also see Pathways to Care below).

Migration or postmigratory factors (H5)

This hypothesis was initially dismissed (Cochrane and Bal, 1987) because it was thought that all immigrants would face similar migratory and postmigratory experiences. If such experiences had a homogeneous effect across all black and minority ethnic or immigrant groups, as was assumed, it followed that variation in the rates of psychotic disorder between these groups could not be attributed to such factors. Research since then has demonstrated that while several immigrant groups are at elevated rates of psychosis, there is considerable heterogeneity in the magnitude of these rates. Furthermore, migratory and postmigratory experiences differ vastly across and within different immigrant groups and their offspring. This hypothesis is, once again, attracting considerable attention, in combination with the possible effects of genetic susceptibility, via gene–environment interactions (see H10, below).

Migration itself is a relatively major life event and may place considerable stress upon the individual. This is likely to be compounded by postmigratory experiences, including attempts to secure housing and employment, experiences of discrimination, developing social relationships and networks, and understanding the norms, rules and customs of the host culture (acculturation). In a general population sample, Johns *et al.* (2004) found that, although the prevalence of psychotic symptoms was greater in BME groups, this risk was mostly explained by discrimination and stressful life events. While the prevalence of stressful life events has been shown to be similar across ethnic groups, there is evidence that these experiences are interpreted more negatively in ethnic minorities (Gilvarry *et al.*, 1999).

Three studies, conducted in two different settings (Boydell *et al.*, 2001; Kirkbride *et al.*, 2008; Veling *et al.*, 2006), have now shown that the risk for BME individuals increases as they live in areas with a smaller proportion of BME residents. Additionally, it has been reported that BME populations who face greater degrees of discrimination (Veling *et al.*, 2007), or who have darker skin colour (Cantor-Graae and Selten, 2005), have greater rates of psychoses. In south-east London, Kirkbride *et al.* (2007) have shown that the incidence of psychoses is lower in neighbourhoods where BME groups live in more close-knit communities, lending support to the hypothesis that social cohesion may be protective – in general and for specific BME groups – against the onset of psychoses. In the UK, markers of individual social disadvantage have also been associated with increased risk of psychosis for both black Caribbean groups and the white British population (Morgan *et al.*, 2008). However, the prevalence of social disadvantage was significantly greater among both black Caribbean cases and controls than their white British counterparts, suggesting such factors have a greater impact in some migrant populations. In addition, Hjern and colleagues (2004) have found that markers of social adversity directly confounded the association between psychosis risk and migrant status in a large Swedish sample.

Neurodevelopment and factors across the life course (H6)

A number of physical problems affecting the developing fetus or child have been proposed as possible causes of schizophrenia (see Cannon *et al.*, 2002 for a review). Originally considered as candidate explanations for raised rates of schizophrenia in BME groups, empirical evidence has not supported this view, rather suggesting psychosocial models. Obstetric complications are unlikely to explain elevated rates of schizophrenia in BME populations: in the UK, Hutchinson *et al.* (1997) found these to be twice as common in the white group compared with black Caribbean migrants. Prenatal maternal infection (for example, influenza during the first trimester) increases the risk of schizophrenia (Brown *et al.*, 2004), but it is not known whether this risk is increased for BME populations.

Prenatal hypovitaminosis D is associated with later increased risk of psychosis (McGrath *et al.*, 2004); it is posited via altered neurodevelopment of the fetus (McGrath, 1999). McGrath has proposed that this mechanism would be a candidate to explain the excess rates of psychotic disorders in darker skinned immigrants (Cantor-Graae and Selten, 2005) who move from hotter to colder climates with less hours of sunlight. However, this hypothesis has not yet been explicitly tested.

Childhood life events may be important in the genesis of psychoses in immigrant and BME groups. In a study of childhood parental separation and loss in the ÆSOP study, Morgan *et al.* (2007) showed that the effect size linking schizophrenia and aberrant separation from, or death of, a parent was similar for the white British, black Caribbean and black African groups. However, parental separation events were almost twice as prevalent in the black Caribbean group, suggesting that this risk factor may have a greater overall impact in this population. This risk factor may be a marker for a range of other traumatic life events during childhood that may also be important.

Substance abuse (H7)

There is little evidence that increased use of illicit substances, including cannabis, explains the raised rates of psychoses amongst immigrant and BME groups. In a small study of cases of schizophrenia, cannabis use was not more common among black Caribbean groups than the white group (McGuire *et al.*, 1995). Evidence from both the UK and the Netherlands (Coulthard *et al.*, 2002; Sandwijk *et al.*, 1995; Sharp and Budd, 2003) suggests that the frequency of cannabis consumption in the general population is not raised in the black Caribbean group. Veen and colleagues (2002) have shown that the raised rates of schizophrenia in Moroccan and Surinamese immigrants in the Netherlands are unlikely to be caused by substance abuse (not restricted to cannabis). Note that this is distinct from the question as to whether cannabis and other drugs may increase risk for schizophrenia, in general, with the current consensus suggesting that there is a causal link (Moore *et al.*, 2007), but not a differential association with respect to ethnicity.

Psychological hypotheses (H8)

It has been suggested that a range of psychological hypotheses may explain raised rates of psychosis in immigrant groups and their offspring (Jones and Fung, 2005). Such hypotheses include potential differences between the migrant and host populations in terms of how stressful life events are interpreted. While there is no evidence that migrants experience more life events than the host population (Gilvarry *et al.*, 1999), it is possible that these are perceived more negatively by migrant groups or that they are more likely to attribute such events externally. It is possible that such behaviour may, for some individuals, foster paranoid and other psychotic-like symptoms. We suggest that such psychological hypotheses are probably implicated in the onset of psychosis in migrants, but only in combination with other processes, such as raised social adversity faced by immigrant groups (see H5) (Hjern *et al.*, 2004) and/or in combination with genetic susceptibility for some individuals (i.e. H10). Psychological responses to potentially risky environmental factors may mediate the relationship between the social environment and the onset of psychotic symptoms. Further studies of immigrant and ethnic minority populations will need to consider such models more closely, for example, by comparing rates of psychosis in migrants from and to egocentric and collectivist societies and individual attributional styles within these settings.

Genetic predisposition (H9)

Migrants and their offspring are unlikely to have a greater genetic predisposition to psychosis per se. The evidence reviewed above demonstrated that black Caribbean groups in the Caribbean (Bhugra et al., 1996; Hickling and Rodgers-Johnson, 1995; Mahy et al., 1999) and white Norwegians in Norway (Ødegaard, 1932) did not have elevated rates of psychosis compared with their counterparts who migrated, and we also know that people with psychosis are not more likely to migrate. Further, the morbid risk for second generation black Caribbean immigrants has been shown to be higher than for the first generation (Hutchinson et al., 1996; Sugarman and Craufurd, 1994) suggesting that genetic differences alone are insufficient to explain excess risk in migrant groups. This is separate to the issue of gene–environment interactions, whereby underlying genetic variability between immigrant and host populations in combination with additional environmental stressors may lead to a greater risk of developing psychosis.

Gene–environment interactions and epigenetic processes (H10)

Our reading of the literature suggests that the most convincing evidence for raised rates of psychosis in immigrants and their offspring is found for hypothesis 5 (migratory and postmigratory factors), hypothesis 6 (life course factors and neurodevelopment) and hypothesis 8 (psychological hypotheses). However, any hypothesis would need to explain why and how exposure to such factors resulted in a raised rate of psychosis for immigrant groups, given that non-migrant (i.e. native) groups are also exposed to some of these risk factors (i.e. life course events, discrimination, social isolation). Moreover, any hypothesis would need to be capable of explaining why only a fraction of the people exposed to such factors, immigrants or otherwise, went on to develop psychosis. One possibility is that the development of psychotic symptoms is dependent not only on exposure to detrimental environmental stimuli, but the additional presence of underlying genetic vulnerability. Hypotheses on such gene–environment interactions are relatively recent and few studies have been conducted with regard to psychosis (Caspi et al., 2005); none with regard to the risk of psychosis in immigrants. Nevertheless, there is evidence to suggest this is a promising direction for future research. In a non-migrant birth cohort sample from Dunedin, New Zealand, Caspi et al. (2005) observed that the risk of schizophreniform disorder at age 26 associated with adolescent cannabis use increased with the additional presence of the valine allele on the catechol-O-methyltransferase [COMT] gene at codon 158. Such an interaction may impact via dopaminergic pathways which are also postulated to explain why social stressors, including those faced by immigrants and their offspring, are associated with psychosis (Howes and Kapur, 2009; Kapur et al., 2005; Selten and Cantor-Graae, 2005). Explicit studies are currently being designed to test this hypothesis (EU-GEI, 2009), though, given the difficulty of replicating gene–environment interactions, considerable care and thought will be required in their formulation (Risch et al., 2009).

A further piece of evidence of the importance of gene–environment interactions in the onset of psychosis is taken from the person–environment interaction observed by Boydell *et al.* (2001) and others (Kirkbride *et al.*, 2008; Veling *et al.*, 2008) regarding ethnic density: the risk of psychosis appears to decline for black and minority ethnic individuals as they lived in neighbourhoods where BME groups make up a larger proportion of the total population. Speculatively, this suggests an interaction between individual genetic vulnerability and an interaction with neighbourhood-level socioenvironmental stressors, for which there is some protection when BME individuals live in less fragmented (Kirkbride *et al.*, 2007), more ethnically dense (Kirkbride *et al.*, 2008) neighbourhoods.

A final additional component to this hypothesis is the potential role of epigenetics on the risk of psychosis in immigrants and their offspring (Dealberto, 2007). Epigenetic processes are heritable changes in gene expression which do not alter the DNA sequence itself. Such processes may be important in our understanding of how exposure to different environments is coded at the molecular level. Social environments may be epigenetically coded (Szyf *et al.*, 2008), meaning it will be important to look at such processes as a potential contributing factor to the excess risk of psychosis faced by immigrant groups and their offspring (Peedicayil, 2009).

If found to be important, this final hypothesis may link many of the distal hypotheses mentioned above (migratory stressors, psychological factors, life course events) into a broader common pathway for how exposure to socioenvironmental factors leads to the onset of psychotic symptoms in some, genetically vulnerable, individuals.

Pathways to care

Pathways to care for BME populations have been observed to differ from those of the white British group. Findings from the ÆSOP study suggest that black Caribbean and black African populations are three times more likely to be compulsorily admitted than their white British counterparts (Morgan *et al.*, 2005). Two further studies (Bebbington *et al.*, 1994; Bhui *et al.*, 2003) have observed similar results. However, the ÆSOP study found no evidence that non-British white groups were more or less likely to be compulsorily admitted than their white British counterparts. Mode of referral did not differ significantly between the non-British white and white British groups, although the 'Count Me In' census has suggested the former may be less likely to present via general practitioners (Inspection CfHAa, 2007). Little research has been conducted on pathways to care for other BME groups, though one study (Burnett *et al.*, 1999) found little evidence of differences in terms of compulsory admission between the white and Asian groups, a finding replicated more recently (Inspection CfHAa, 2007).

Part 2 Common mental disorders (depression and anxiety) and post-traumatic stress disorder

The evidence for an association between common mental disorders (CMD) and immigrant and BME status is less clear than for psychotic disorders (Lloyd, 2006). Two major studies of depression have been conducted in the UK, reporting equivocal findings (Jenkins and Meltzer, 1995; Nazroo, 1997). These two studies were the Office for National Statistics National Survey of Psychiatric Morbidity (Jenkins and Meltzer, 1995) and the Ethnic

Minority Psychiatric Illness Rates in the Community (EMPIRIC) study (Nazroo, 1997). The National Psychiatric Morbidity Study found no evidence of a difference in the prevalence of CMD between black Caribbean and white groups in the UK (Jenkins *et al.*, 1997), although Sharpley *et al.* (2001) have suggested that their sample may have been too small. In contrast, the EMPIRIC study observed a 60% increase in prevalence of depression in the black Caribbean group compared with the white group in a community sample in the UK (Nazroo, 1997; Weich *et al.*, 2004). In addition, the National Psychiatric Comorbidity Study found small but significant increases in the prevalence of CMD for 35–54-year-old white Irish (RR: 2.09; 95% CI: 1.16–2.95), Pakistani (RR: 2.38; 95% CI: 1.25–3.53) men compared with their white British counterparts, after adjustment for socio-economic status (Weich *et al.*, 2004). In the same sample, Indian and Pakistani women aged 55–74 years old had higher prevalence rates of CMD than their white British counterparts.

Rates of CMD may be elevated for some BME groups in the UK and lower for others (i.e. Bangladeshi women); (Weich *et al.*, 2004), but the magnitude of this risk, in comparison with psychosis, appears to be smaller. Differences may partly be a reflection of the size of these surveys and partly a reflection of the population from which they are drawn. Often these surveys have been based on general practitioner (GP) surgeries where one would expect higher rates of CMD. Other studies have also been conducted in the UK. Gillam *et al.* (1989) found that the black Caribbean population was much less likely than other ethnic groups to receive a diagnosis of depression or anxiety from their GP than other ethnic groups. Commander *et al.* (1997) observed higher rates of depression in the Asian population compared with white or black groups in Birmingham. Studies have also suggested that Asian migrants may be more likely to somatise their mental health issues as physical illness (Ritsner *et al.*, 2000), but, as Lloyd notes, this is a complex sociocultural issue which may reflect differential cultural approaches to understanding how the mind and body interconnect and the provision of services available to BME groups in their locality (Lloyd, 2006).

A Swedish study (Blomstedt *et al.*, 2007) highlighted the possible need for recent adult age immigrants from Eastern Europe, who were twice as likely as the Swedish group to report psychiatric illness and psychosomatic complaints, adjusted for age, sex, marital status and a range of other socioenvironmental variables. This research has potential implications across Western Europe, including the UK, in terms of health service planning, given large waves of emigration from Eastern Europe following EU expansion since 2004.

There is a growing literature on the prevalence of CMD in both migrants and those left behind following rural to urban migration in developing countries. In China, rural to urban migrants were not found to have poorer mental health than existing urban residents (Li *et al.*, 2007), while studies of Mexican immigrants to the US have found no differences in their prevalence of depression compared with either Mexican citizens or US residents (Grant *et al.*, 2004; Vega *et al.*, 1998). In a population-based sample of over 1100 parents over 60 years, Abas *et al.* (2009) found a lower prevalence of depression amongst parents in rural Thailand for whom all children had migrated away from the area, compared with those parents for whom children had remained nearby. These differences remained statistically significant after adjustment for potential confounding by markers of social support, health, wealth and parental characteristics. The authors concluded by suggesting that the remittances sent back from children may allow such families greater prestige and social standing while elevating them away from poverty (Abas *et al.*, 2009).

Less research has been done regarding the possible explanations for higher rates of CMD in BME and immigrant groups (Lindert *et al.*, 2008), but there is some evidence that postmigratory factors might be important in the onset of depression (Thapa *et al.*, 2007). In a case-control study of Irish immigrants in London, Ryan and colleagues found that poorly planned migration was one risk factor for depression (Ryan *et al.*, 2006). Evidence also suggests acculturated individuals are more likely to experience depression (Haasen *et al.*, 2008; Han *et al.*, 2007; Miller *et al.*, 2006), and a study in the USA found the risk of depression increased in Mexican immigrants with length of stay (Hernandez and Chamey, 1998). One possible explanation for this is that acculturation stress acts on the hypothalamic-pituitary-adrenal axis to increase the risk of depression (Haasen *et al.*, 2008). A recent cross-sectional study of school children in the USA ($n = 5147$) found that perceived racial and ethnic discrimination was associated with greater symptomatology for depression, attention deficit hyperactivity disorder and conduct disorder (Coker *et al.*, 2009). Further evidence from the EMPIRIC study in the UK (Bhui *et al.*, 2005) found that an increased risk of CMD in BME was associated with reports of unfair treatment (OR: 2.0; 95% CI: 1.2–3.2) or racial insults (OR: 2.3; 95% CI: 1.4–3.6), particularly amongst black Caribbean, Indian, Bangladeshi and white Irish groups. This suggests that common environmental exposures, such as discrimination, might be risk factors for a suite of psychiatric disorders, with underlying genetic susceptibility perhaps differentiating the exact biological mechanisms and manifestation of clinical disorder involved.

A recent meta-analysis has found that the prevalence of CMD was roughly twice as high in refugees as in other economic migrants, with estimates placed at around 40% (Lindert *et al.*, 2009). Unsurprisingly, refugees are also at significantly raised rates of post-traumatic stress disorder (PTSD). A recent review (Fazel *et al.*, 2005) of 7000 refugees to western countries found that they were up to 10 times more likely to experience PTSD than the general population. Such PTSD may be the primary reason for presentation to services, or may complicate the picture when refugees present with other mental and physical health complaints. For children, there is evidence that unaccompanied minors arriving in the UK have poorer engagement with services and different pathways to care than children arriving with one or more primary caregivers (Michelson and Sclare, 2009). Both groups had similar levels of post-migration stress but the former group was more likely to exhibit PTSD symptoms and less likely to remain in contact with services. Similar findings have also been observed in the Netherlands (Pinto Wiese and Burhorst, 2007). Importantly, there may be substantial comorbidity between PTSD and other psychiatric disorders. One cross-sectional study of Croatian war veterans estimated that 80% of the sample met criteria for the diagnosis of an Axis 1 psychiatric disorder (Ivezic *et al.*, 2000). In refugee groups there may be some phenomenological overlap between PTSD and psychosis (Pepper and Agius, 2009), with comorbidity estimates varying from 15% to 40% (David *et al.*, 1999; Kozaric-Kovacic and Borovecki, 2005), although this phenomenological overlap may remain largely undetected in clinical settings (Seedat *et al.*, 2003).

There is some evidence that for asylum seekers a longer length of asylum increases (doubles) the risk of CMD (Hallas *et al.*, 2007; Laban *et al.*, 2004), with the risk of poor psychopathology most strongly associated with issues surrounding unemployment, the family and the asylum procedure itself (Laban *et al.*, 2005). A recent systematic review (Robjant *et al.*, 2009) of the mental health effect of detaining asylum seekers found that those detained presented with considerable psychopathology in terms of CMD, PTSD and suicide and suicidal ideation. The review reaffirmed the above finding that length of detention increased severity of symptoms (Porter and Haslam, 2005), and concluded by stating that some of this adverse psychopathology might be attributable to the effects of detention itself (Robjant et al., 2009). In the Netherlands, at least, there is some evidence that asylum seekers are unlikely to engage with mental health services (Laban et al., 2007), something that has also been reported in the UK (McCrone et al., 2005).

Part 3 Suicide and suicidal behaviour

The risk of suicide in BME groups appears to vary by sex and ethnicity. In the UK, Asian men generally have lower rates of suicide than the host population (Thompson and Bhugra, 2000), but there is some evidence that rates may be elevated for Asian women (Bhugra et al., 1999a, b; Soni Raleigh, 1996; Soni Raleigh et al., 1990; Thompson and Bhugra, 2000). Among Asian women in the UK, perceived causes of suicide include violence by the husband and being trapped in an unhappy family situation and depression (Hicks and Bhugra, 2003). Ahmed and colleagues have stressed the importance of understanding how cultural factors, including acculturation, cultural conflicts, stigma and interpersonal relationships, may mediate the pathway between self-harm and resilience and distress (Ahmed et al., 2007). The black Caribbean population in the UK appears to have lower rates of suicide than the white British group (Soni Raleigh, 1996), though in contrast one Dutch study found elevated rates of suicide for male Surinamese immigrants (Garssen et al., 2007), while another found higher rates of attempted (though not completed) suicide amongst female Surinamese immigrants in the Hague (Burger et al., 2009). Further research in the Netherlands has shown that the risk of suicide in the children of Moroccan and Turkish immigrants is over three times greater than white Dutch children (de Jong, 1994), while another study reported elevated prevalence of suicidal ideation amongst Turkish adolescents in Utrecht (van Bergen et al., 2008). A study from the USA reported elevated rates of suicidal attempts and substance use in second generation Latino groups compared with their first generation counterparts (Peña et al., 2008) a finding that became even more pronounced for subsequent generations, and independent of several confounders. This finding complements another study of Mexican immigrants and their offspring in the USA, which has shown that both first (OR: 1.84; 95% CI: 1.09–3.09) and later generation (OR: 1.56; 95% CI: 1.03–2.38) Mexican immigrants had an elevated risk of suicidal ideation than Caucasian Americans (Borges et al., 2009).

Eastern European immigrants to Sweden appear to have higher rates of suicide than the Swedish born population. Rates may be particularly elevated in second generation groups (Hjern and Allebeck, 2002). In Canada, the risk of suicide appears to be lower in most immigrant groups than in Canadian-born groups (Malenfant, 2004). For immigrants there appears to be some relationship between deliberate self-harm (DSH) and ethnic density, as for schizophrenia. Thus, Neeleman et al. (2001) observed that rates of DSH for Asian and black Caribbean groups tended to decrease as the ethnic density of these populations increased. This trend was, however, also found to be non-linear, suggesting other neighbourhood level factors may influence the incidence of DSH for immigrant groups.

Part 4 Policy recommendations

Formulating policy recommendations with a view to reducing the burden of psychotic disorders in black and minority ethnic and immigrant groups presents one of the greatest challenges to public mental health. In part, any recommendations will depend on synthesising the available evidence, presented in this chapter and elsewhere, incorporating many psychiatric perspectives not limited to epidemiology but extending to public health, health services research and health economics. A better understanding of the epidemiology of mental illness among migrant groups forms only one part of the mental health matrix in this regard, and it is difficult to establish policy recommendations from this domain alone. For psychosis, elevated rates in BME groups vary by ethnic group, generation and sex, making generic policy recommendations of limited utility. Rather, targeted policies for particular groups may be more effective. However, as reviewed above, there is as yet no clear emergent consensus as to what factors contribute to the increased risk of psychosis in immigrants and their offspring; making it difficult to devise effective prevention strategies. For other psychiatric disorders, such as depression, it is unclear as to whether rates are elevated, and any strategies for prevention would require careful formulation. There is better evidence for PTSD amongst refugees and asylum seekers, potentially allowing services to be tailored to these groups, although an increasing awareness of phenomenological overlap with other psychiatric disorders will be vital. For suicide, rates appear to be elevated for some BME groups and it may be possible to establish targeted policy recommendations here. Any policy formulation will clearly be specific to a given locality, be it nationally, regionally or locally, given the emergent evidence that the risk of some psychiatric disorders is dependent on the context within which it is embedded.

Given the above complexities we are hesitant to promote any specific policy recommendations until the epidemiological evidence presented here has been synthesised with other findings. Nevertheless, we have previously been commissioned, as part of the Foresight project (www.foresight.gov.uk) by the Government Office for Science in the UK, to write a discussion paper to consider putative interventions for psychosis and other mental disorders (Kirkbride and Jones, 2008). Although the scope and outlook of this report was primarily centred on the UK, it may be a useful starting point to conceptualise policy recommendations in this area, while highlighting some of the associated complexities involved.

References

Abas, M. A., Punpuing, S., Jirapramukpitak, T. et al. (2009). Rural–urban migration and depression in ageing family members left behind. British Journal of Psychiatry, 195(1), 54–60.

Ahmed, K., Mohan, R. A., Bhugra, D. (2007). Self-harm in South Asian women: a literature review informed approach to assessment and formulation. American Journal of Psychotherapy, 61(1), 71–81.

Bebbington, P. E., Feeney, S. T., Flannigan, C. B. et al. (1994). Inner London collaborative audit of admissions in two health districts. II: Ethnicity and the use of the Mental Health Act. British Journal of Psychiatry, 165(6), 743–9, 759.

Bhopal, R. S., Phillimore, P., Kohli, H. S. (1991). Inappropriate use of the term 'Asian': an obstacle to ethnicity and health research. Journal of Public Health Medicine, 13(4), 244–6.

Bhugra, D. (2000). Migration and schizophrenia. Acta Psychiatrica Scandinavica, 102, 68–73.

Bhugra, D. (2004). Migration and mental health. Acta Psychiatric Scandinavica, 109(4), 243–58.

Bhugra, D., Hilwig, M., Hossein, B. et al. (1996). First-contact incidence rates of schizophrenia in Trinidad and one-year follow-up. British Journal of Psychiatry, 169(5), 587–92.

Bhugra, D., Leff, J., Mallett, R., et al. (1997). Incidence and outcome of schizophrenia in Whites, African-Caribbeans and Asians in London. Psychological Medicine, 27(4), 791–8.

Bhugra, D., Baldwin, D. S., Desai, M. et al. (1999a). Attempted suicide in west London, II. Inter-group comparisons. Psychological Medicine, 29(5), 1131–9.

Bhugra, D., Desai, M., Baldwin, D. S. (1999b). Attempted suicide in west London, I. Rates across ethnic communities. *Psychological Medicine*, **29**(5), 1125–30.

Bhui, K., Stansfeld, S., Hull, S., *et al.* (2003). Ethnic variations in pathways to and use of specialist mental health services in the UK. Systematic review. *British Journal of Psychiatry*, **182**, 105–16.

Bhui, K., Stansfeld, S., McKenzie, K. *et al.* (2005). Racial/ethnic discrimination and common mental disorders among workers: findings from the EMPIRIC study of ethnic minority groups in the United Kingdom. *American Journal of Public Health*, **95**(3), 496–501.

Blomstedt, Y., Johansson, S. E., Sundquist, J. (2007). Mental health of immigrants from the former Soviet Bloc: a future problem for primary health care in the enlarged European Union? A cross-sectional study. *BMC Public Health*, 7, 27.

Borges, G., Breslau, J., Su, M. *et al.* (2009). Immigration and suicidal behavior among Mexicans and Mexican Americans. *American Journal of Public Health*, **99**(4), 728–33.

Boydell, J., van Os, J., McKenzie, K. *et al.* (2001). Incidence of schizophrenia in ethnic minorities in London: ecological study into interactions with environment. *British Medical Journal*, **323**(7325), 1336–8.

Bresnahan, M., Begg, M. D., Brown, A. *et al.* (2007). Race and risk of schizophrenia in a US birth cohort: another example of health disparity? *International Journal of Epidemiology*, p. dym041.

Broome, M. R., Woolley, J. B., Tabraham, P. *et al.* (2005). What causes the onset of psychosis? *Schizophrenia Research*, **79**(1), 23–34.

Brown, A. S., Begg, M. D., Gravenstein, S. *et al.* (2004). Serologic evidence of prenatal influenza in the etiology of schizophrenia. *Archives of General Psychiatry*, **61**(8), 774–80.

Burger, I., van Hemert, A. M., Schudel, W. J. *et al.* (2009). Suicidal behavior in four ethnic groups in the Hague, 2002–2004. *Crisis*, **30**(2), 63–7.

Burnett, R., Mallett, R., Bhugra, D. *et al.* (1999). The first contact of patients with schizophrenia with psychiatric services: social factors and pathways to care in a multi-ethnic population. *Psychological Medicine*, **29**(2), 475–83.

Cannon, M., Jones, P. B., Murray, R. M. (2002). Obstetric complications and schizophrenia: historical and meta-analytic review. *American Journal of Psychiatry*, **159**(7), 1080–92.

Cantor-Graae, E. and Selten, J.-P. (2005). Schizophrenia and migration: a meta-analysis and review. *American Journal of Psychiatry*, **162**(1), 12–24.

Cantor-Graae, E., Pedersen, C. B., McNeil, T. F. *et al.* (2003). Migration as a risk factor for schizophrenia: a Danish population-based cohort study. *British Journal of Psychiatry*, **182**, 117–22.

Caspi, A., Moffitt, T. E., Cannon, M. *et al.* (2005). Moderation of the effect of adolescent-onset cannabis use on adult psychosis by a functional polymorphism in the catechol-O-methyltransferase gene: longitudinal evidence of a gene X environment interaction. *Biological Psychiatry*, **57**(10), 1117–27.

Castle, D., Wessely, S., Der, G. *et al.* (1991). The incidence of operationally defined schizophrenia in Camberwell, 1965–84. *British Journal of Psychiatry*, **159**, 790–4.

Cochrane, R. (1977). Mental-illness in immigrants to England and Wales – analysis of mental-hospital admissions, 1971. *Social Psychiatry*, **12**(1), 25–35.

Cochrane, R. and Bal, S. S. (1987). Migration and schizophrenia: an examination of five hypotheses. *Social Psychiatry*, **22**(4), 181–91.

Cohen, C. I., Magai, C., Yaffee, R. *et al.* (2004). Racial differences in paranoid ideation and psychoses in an older urban population. *American Journal of Psychiatry*, **161**(5), 864–71.

Coid, J. W., Kirkbride, J. B., Barker, D. *et al.* (2008). Raised incidence rates of all psychoses among migrant groups: findings from the East London first episode psychosis study. *Archives of General Psychiatry*, **65**(11), 1250–8.

Coker, T. R., Elliott, M. N., Kanouse, D. E. *et al.* (2009). Perceived racial/ethnic discrimination among fifth-grade students and its association with mental health. *American Journal of Public Health*, **99**(5), 878–84.

Commander, M. J., Dharan, S. P., Odell, S. M. *et al.* (1997). Access to mental health care in an inner-city health district. II: Association with demographic factors. *British Journal of Psychiatry*, **170**, 317–20.

Corcoran, C., Perrin, M., Harlap, S. *et al.* (2009). Incidence of schizophrenia among second-generation immigrants in the Jerusalem perinatal cohort. *Schizophrenia Bulletin*, **35**(3), 596–602.

Coulthard, M., Farrell, M., Singleton, N. *et al.* (2002). *Tobacco, Alcohol and Drug Use and Mental Health*. London: HMSO.

David, D., Kutcher, G. S., Jackson, E. I. *et al.* (1999). Psychotic symptoms in combat-related posttraumatic stress disorder. *Journal of Clinical Psychiatry*, **60**(1), 29–32.

Dealberto, M. J. (2007). Why are immigrants at increased risk for psychosis? Vitamin D insufficiency, epigenetic mechanisms, or both? *Medical Hypotheses*, **68**(2), 259–67.

de Jong, J. T. V. M. (1994). Ambulatory mental health care for migrants in the Netherlands. *Curare*, **17**(1), 25–34.

Eagles, J. M. (1991). The relationship between schizophrenia and immigration: are there alternatives to psychosocial hypotheses? *British Journal of Psychiatry*, **159**, 783–9.

EU-GEI. (2008). Schizophrenia aetiology: do gene–environment interactions hold the key? *Schizophrenia Research*, **102**(1–3), 21–6.

EU-GEI. (2009). Genetic Epidemiology + Genome Wide Association = GEWIS: gene–environment-wide interaction studies in psychiatry. *American Journal of Psychiatry*, **166**(9), 964–6.

Fazel, M., Wheeler, J., Danesh, J. (2005). Prevalence of serious mental disorder in 7000 refugees resettled in western countries: a systematic review. *Lancet*, **365**(9467), 1309–14.

Fearon, P., Kirkbride, J. B., Morgan, C. *et al.* (2006). Incidence of schizophrenia and other psychoses in ethnic minority groups:

results from the MRC AESOP Study. *Psychological Medicine*, **36**(11), 1541–50.

Garssen, M. J., Hoogenboezem, J., Kerkhof, A. J. (2007). [Suicide among Surinamese migrants in the Netherlands by ethnicity]. *Tijdschrift voor Psychiatrie*, **49**(6), 373–81.

Gillam, S. J., Jarman, B., White, P. *et al.* (1989). Ethnic differences in consultation rates in urban general practice. *British Medical Journal*, **299**(6705), 953–7.

Gilvarry, C. M., Walsh, E., Samele, C. *et al.* (1999). Life events, ethnicity and perceptions of discrimination in patients with severe mental illness. *Social Psychiatry and Psychiatric Epidemiology*, **34**(11), 600–8.

Grant, B. F., Stinson, F. S., Hasin, D. S. *et al.* (2004). Immigration and lifetime prevalence of DSM-IV psychiatric disorders among Mexican Americans and non-Hispanic whites in the United States: results from the National Epidemiologic Survey on Alcohol and Related Conditions. *Archives of General Psychiatry*, **61**(12), 1226–33.

Haasen, C., Demiralay, C., Reimer, J. (2008). Acculturation and mental distress among Russian and Iranian migrants in Germany. *European Psychiatry*, **23**(Suppl. 1), 10–13.

Hafner, H., Maurer, K., Loffler, W. *et al.* (1993). The influence of age and sex on the onset and early course of schizophrenia. *British Journal of Psychiatry*, **162**, 80–6.

Hallas, P., Hansen, A., Staehr, M. *et al.* (2007). Length of stay in asylum centres and mental health in asylum seekers: a retrospective study from Denmark. *BMC Public Health*, **7**(1), 288.

Han, H. R., Kim, M., Lee, H. B. *et al.* (2007). Correlates of depression in the Korean American elderly: focusing on personal resources of social support. *Journal of Cross Cultural Gerontology*, **22**(1), 115–27.

Hanoeman, M., Selten, J.-P., Kahn, R. S. (2002). Incidence of schizophrenia in Surinam. *Schizophrenia Research*, **54**(3), 219–21.

Harrison, G., Owens, D., Holton, A. *et al.* (1988). A prospective study of severe mental disorder in Afro-Caribbean patients. *Psychological Medicine*, **18**(3), 643–57.

Harrison, G., Brewin, J., Cantwell, R. *et al.* (1996). The increased risk of psychosis in African-Caribbean migrants to the UK: a replication. *Schizophrenia Research*, **18**(2–3), 102.

Harrison, G., Glazebrook, C., Brewin, J. *et al.* (1997). Increased incidence of psychotic disorders in migrants from the Caribbean to the United Kingdom. *Psychological Medicine*, **27**(4), 799–806.

Hemsi, L. K. (1967). Psychiatric morbidity of West Indian immigrants. *Social Psychiatry*, **2**, 95–100.

Hernandez, D. and Charney, E. (1998). *The Health and Well-being of Children in Immigrants Families*. Washington: National Academy Press.

Hickling, F. W. and Rodgers-Johnson, P. (1995). The incidence of first contact schizophrenia in Jamaica. *British Journal of Psychiatry*, **167**(2), 193–6.

Hickling, F. W., McKenzie, K., Mullen, R. *et al.* (1999). A Jamaican psychiatrist evaluates diagnoses at a London psychiatric hospital. *British Journal of Psychiatry*, **175**, 283–5.

Hicks, M. H. and Bhugra, D. (2003). Perceived causes of suicide attempts by U.K. South Asian women. *American Journal of Orthopsychiatry*, **73**(4), 455–62.

Hjern, A. and Allebeck, P. (2002). Suicide in first- and second-generation immigrants in Sweden: a comparative study. *Social Psychiatry and Psychiatric Epidemiology*, **37**(9), 423–9.

Hjern, A., Wicks, S., Dalman, C. (2004). Social adversity contributes to high morbidity in psychoses in immigrants – a national cohort study of two generations of Swedish residents. *Psychological Medicine*, **34**, 1025–33.

Howes, O. D. and Kapur, S. (2009). The dopamine hypothesis of schizophrenia: version III–the final common pathway. *Schizophrenia Bulletin*, sbp006.

Hutchinson, G., Takei, N., Fahy, T. A. *et al.* (1996). Morbid risk of schizophrenia in first-degree relatives of white and African-Caribbean patients with psychosis. *British Journal of Psychiatry*, **169**(6), 776–80.

Hutchinson, G., Takei, N., Bhugra, D. *et al.* (1997). Increased rate of psychosis among African-Caribbeans in Britain is not due to an excess of pregnancy and birth complications. *British Journal of Psychiatry*, **171**, 145–7.

Inspection, CfHAa. (2007). *Count Me In*. London: Commission for Healthcare Audit and Inspection.

Ivezic, S., Bagaric, A., Oruc, L. *et al.* (2000). Psychotic symptoms and comorbid psychiatric disorders in Croatian combat-related posttraumatic stress disorder patients. *Croatian Medical Journal*, **41**(2), 179–83.

Jablensky, A., Sartorius, N., Ernberg, G. *et al.* (1992). Schizophrenia: manifestations, incidence and course in different cultures. A World Health Organization ten-country study. *Psychological Medicine Monograph Supplement*, **20**, 1–97.

Jenkins, R. and Meltzer, H. (1995). The national survey of psychiatric morbidity in Great Britain. *Social Psychiatry and Psychiatric Epidemiology*, **30**(1), 1–4.

Jenkins, R., Lewis, G., Bebbington, P. *et al.* (1997). The National Psychiatric Morbidity surveys of Great Britain – initial findings from the household survey. *Psychological Medicine*, **27**(4), 775–89.

Johns, L. C., Nazroo, J. Y., Bebbington, P. *et al.* (2002). Occurrence of hallucinatory experiences in a community sample and ethnic variations. *British Journal of Psychiatry*, **180**, 174–8.

Johns, L. C., Cannon, M., Singleton, N. *et al.* (2004). Prevalence and correlates of self-reported psychotic symptoms in the British population. *British Journal of Psychiatry*, **185**, 298–305.

Jones, P. B. and Fung, W. L. A. (2005). Ethnicity and mental health: the example of Schizophrenia in the African Caribbean population in Europe. In M. Rutter, M. Tienda, eds. *Ethnicity and Causal Mechanisms*. Cambridge: Cambridge University Press.

Jones, P., Rodgers, B., Murray, R. *et al.* (1994). Child development risk factors for adult schizophrenia in the British 1946 birth cohort. *Lancet*, **344**(8934), 1398–402.

Kapur, S., Mizrahi, R., Li, M. (2005). From dopamine to salience to psychosis – linking biology, pharmacology and phenomenology of psychosis. *Schizophrenia Research*, **79**(1), 59–68.

King, M., Coker, E., Leavey, G. *et al.* (1994). Incidence of psychotic illness in London: comparison of ethnic groups. *British Medical Journal*, **309**(6962), 1115–19.

Kirkbride, J. B. and Jones, P. B. (2008). *Putative Prevention Strategies to Reduce Serious Mental Illness in Migrant and Black and Minority Ethnic Groups*. Foresight Mental Capital and Wellbeing: Discussion Paper 12. London: Her Majesty's Stationary Office. http://www.foresight.gov.uk/Mental%20Capital/ListOfDiscussionPapers.pdf

Kirkbride, J. B., Fearon, P., Morgan, C. *et al.* (2006). Heterogeneity in incidence rates of schizophrenia and other psychotic syndromes: findings from the 3-center ÆSOP study. *Archives of General Psychiatry*, **63**(3), 250–8.

Kirkbride, J. B., Morgan, C., Fearon, P. *et al.* (2007). Neighbourhood-level effects on psychoses: re-examining the role of context. *Psychological Medicine*, **37**(10), 1413–25.

Kirkbride, J., Boydell, J., Ploubidis, G. *et al.* (2008a). Testing the association between the incidence of schizophrenia and social capital in an urban area. *Psychological Medicine*, **38**(8), 1083–94.

Kirkbride, J. B., Coid, J. W., Barker, D. *et al.* (2008b). Psychoses, ethnicity and socio-economic status. *British Journal of Psychiatry*, **193**(1), 18–24.

Kozaric-Kovacic, D. and Borovecki, A. (2005). Prevalence of psychotic comorbidity in combat-related post-traumatic stress disorder. *Military Medicine*, **170**(3), 223–6.

Krupinski, J. and Cochrane, R. (1980). Migration and mental health – a comparative study. *Journal of Intercultural Studies*, **1**, 49–57.

Laban, C. J., Gernaat, H. B., Komproe, I. H. *et al.* (2004). Impact of a long asylum procedure on the prevalence of psychiatric disorders in Iraqi asylum seekers in The Netherlands.

Journal of Nervous and Mental Disease, **192**(12), 843–51.

Laban, C. J., Gernaat, H. B., Komproe, I. H. *et al.* (2005). Postmigration living problems and common psychiatric disorders in Iraqi asylum seekers in the Netherlands. *Journal of Nervous Mental Disease*, **193**(12), 825–32.

Laban, C., Gernaat, H., Komproe, I. *et al.* (2007). Prevalence and predictors of health service use among Iraqi asylum seekers in the Netherlands. *Social Psychiatry and Psychiatric Epidemiology*, **42**(10), 837–44.

Leao, T. S., Sundquist, J., Frank, G. *et al.* (2006). Incidence of schizophrenia or other psychoses in first- and second-generation immigrants: a national cohort study. *Journal of Nervous and Mental Disease*, **194**(1), 27–33.

Leff, J. P., Fischer, M., Bertelsen, A. (1976). A cross-national epidemiological study of mania. *British Journal of Psychiatry*, **129**, 428–42.

Lewis, G., Croft-Jeffreys, C., David, A. (1990). Are British psychiatrists racist? *British Journal of Psychiatry*, **157**, 410–15.

Li, L., Wang, H.-M., Ye, X.-J. *et al.* (2007). The mental health status of Chinese rural–urban migrant workers. *Social Psychiatry and Psychiatric Epidemiology*, **42**(9), 716–22.

Lindert, J., Schouler-Ocak, M., Heinz, A. *et al.* (2008). Mental health, health care utilisation of migrants in Europe. *European Psychiatry*, **23**(Suppl. 1), 14–20.

Lindert, J., Ehrenstein, O. S. V., Priebe, S. *et al.* (2009). Depression and anxiety in labor migrants and refugees – a systematic review and meta-analysis. *Social Science & Medicine*, **69**(2), 246–57.

Littlewood, R. and Lipsedge, M. (1981). Some social and phenomenological characteristics of psychotic immigrants. *Psychological Medicine*, **11**(2), 289–302.

Lloyd, K. (2006). Common mental disorders among black and minority ethnic groups in the UK. *Psychiatry*, **5**(11), 388–91.

Lloyd, T., Kennedy, N., Fearon, P. *et al.* (2005). Incidence of bipolar affective disorder in three UK cities: results from the ÆSOP study. *British Journal of Psychiatry*, **186**(2), 126–31.

Mahy, G. E., Mallett, R., Leff, J. *et al.* (1999). First-contact incidence rate of schizophrenia on Barbados. *British Journal of Psychiatry*, **175**, 28–33.

Malenfant, E. C. (2004). Suicide in Canada's immigrant population. *Health Reports*, **15**(2), 9–17.

Malzberg, B. (1964). Mental disease among native and foreign-born whites in New York State, 1949–1951. *Mental Hygiene*, **48**, 478–99.

Malzberg, B. (1969). Are immigrants psychologically disturbed? in S. Plog and R. Edgerton, eds. *Changing Perspectives in Mental Illness.* New York: Holt, Rinehart and Winston, p. 395–421.

McCrone, P., Bhui, K., Craig, T. *et al.* (2005). Mental health needs, service use and costs among Somali refugees in the UK. *Acta Psychiatrica Scandinavica*, **111**(5), 351–7.

McGovern, D. and Cope, R. V. (1987). First psychiatric admission rates of first and second generation Afro Caribbeans. *Social Psychiatry*, **22**(3), 139–49.

McGrath, J. (1999). Hypothesis: is low prenatal vitamin D a risk-modifying factor for schizophrenia? *Schizophrenia Research*, **40**(3), 173–7.

McGrath, J., El-Saadi, O., Cardy, S. *et al.* (2001). Urban birth and migrant status as risk factors for psychosis: an Australian case-control study. *Social Psychiatry and Psychiatric Epidemiology*, **36**(11), 533–6.

McGrath, J., Saari, K., Hakko, H. *et al.* (2004a). Vitamin D supplementation during the first year of life and risk of schizophrenia: a Finnish birth cohort study. *Schizophrenia Research*, **67**(2–3), 237–45.

McGrath, J., Saha, S., Welham, J. *et al.* (2004b). A systematic review of the incidence of schizophrenia: the distribution of rates and the influence of sex, urbanicity, migrant status and methodology. *BMC Medicine*, **2**(13).

McGuire, P. K., Jones, P., Harvey, I. *et al.* (1995). Morbid risk of schizophrenia for relatives of patients with cannabis-associated psychosis. *Schizophrenia Research*, **15**(3), 277–81.

Michelson, D. and Sclare, I. (2009). Psychological needs, service utilization and provision of care in a specialist mental health clinic for young refugees: a comparative study. *Clinical Child Psychology and Psychiatry*, **14**(2), 273–96.

Miller, A. M., Sorokin, O., Wang, E. *et al.* (2006). Acculturation, social alienation, and depressed mood in midlife women from the former Soviet Union. *Research in Nursing & Health*, **29**(2), 134–46.

Moore, T. H. M., Zammit, S., Lingford-Hughes, A. *et al.* (2007). Cannabis use and risk of psychotic or affective mental health outcomes: a systematic review. *Lancet*, **370**(9584), 319–28.

Morgan, C., Mallett, M. R., Hutchinson, G. *et al.* (2005). Pathways to care and ethnicity I. Sample characteristics and compulsory admission: report from the ÆSOP study. *British Journal of Psychiatry*, **186**(4), 281–9.

Morgan, C., Kirkbride, J. B., Leff, J. *et al.* (2007). Parental separation, loss and psychosis in different ethnic groups: a case-control study. *Psychological Medicine*, **37**(4), 495–503.

Morgan, C., Kirkbride, J., Hutchinson, G. *et al.* (2008). Cumulative social disadvantage, ethnicity and first-episode psychosis: a case-control study. *Psychological Medicine*, **38**, 1701–15.

Nazroo, J. (1997). *Ethnicity and Mental Health.* London: Policy Studies Institute.

Neeleman, J., Wilson-Jones, C., Wessely, S. (2001). Ethnic density and deliberate self harm; a small area study in south east London. *Journal of Epidemiology and Community Health*, **55**(2), 85–90.

Ødegaard, Ø. (1932). Emigration and insanity. *Acta Psychiatrica Neurologica*, Suppl. 4, 1–206.

Peedicayil, J. (2009). The role of epigenetics in the raised incidence rates of psychoses among migrant groups. *Archives of General Psychiatry*, **66**(5), 564.

Peña, J., Wyman, P., Brown, C. *et al.* (2008). Immigration generation status and its association with suicide attempts, substance use, and depressive symptoms among Latino adolescents in the USA. *Prevention Science*, **9**(4), 299–310.

Pepper, H. and Agius, M. (2009). Phenomenology of PTSD and psychotic symptoms. *Psychiatria Danubina*, 21(1), 82–4.

Pinto Wiese, E. B. and Burhorst, I. (2007). The mental health of asylum-seeking and refugee children and adolescents attending a clinic in the Netherlands. *Transcultural Psychiatry*, 44(4), 596–613.

Porter, M. and Haslam, N. (2005). Predisplacement and postdisplacement factors associated with mental health of refugees and internally displaced persons: a meta-analysis. *Journal of the American Medical Association*, 294(5), 602–12.

Risch, N., Herrell, R., Lehner, T. *et al.* (2009). Interaction between the serotonin transporter gene (5-HTTLPR), stressful life events, and risk of depression: a meta-analysis. *Journal of the American Medical Association*, 301(23), 2462–71.

Ritsner, M., Ponizovsky, A., Kurs, R. *et al.* (2000). Somatization in an immigrant population in Israel: a community survey of prevalence, risk factors, and help-seeking behavior. *American Journal of Psychiatry*, 157(3), 385–92.

Robjant, K., Hassan, R., Katona, C. (2009). Mental health implications of detaining asylum seekers: systematic review. *British Journal of Psychiatry*, 194(4), 306–12.

Rutter, M. (2002). The interplay of nature, nurture, and developmental influences: the challenge ahead for mental health. *Archives of General Psychiatry*, 59(11), 996–1000.

Ryan, L., Leavey, G., Golden, A. *et al.* (2006). Depression in Irish migrants living in London: case-control study. *British Journal of Psychiatry*, 188(6), 560–6.

Sandwijk, J. P., Cohen, P. D., Musterd, S. *et al.* (1995). *Licit and Illicit Drug Use in Amsterdam. Report of a Household Survey in 1994 on the Prevalence of Drug Use among the Population of 12 years and over*. Amsterdam: University of Amsterdam.

Seedat, S., Stein, M. B., Oosthuizen, P. P. *et al.* (2003). Linking posttraumatic stress disorder and psychosis: a look at epidemiology, phenomenology, and treatment. *Journal of Nervous and Mental Disease*, 191(10), 675–81.

Selten, J. P. and Cantor-Graae, E. (2005). Social defeat: risk factor for schizophrenia? *British Journal of Psychiatry*, 187(2), 101–2.

Selten, J. P., Veen, N., Feller, W. *et al.* (2001). Incidence of psychotic disorders in immigrant groups to The Netherlands. *British Journal of Psychiatry*, 178, 367–72.

Selten, J.-P., Cantor-Graae, E., Slaets, J. *et al.* (2002). Odegaard's selection hypothesis revisited: schizophrenia in surinamese immigrants to the Netherlands. *American Journal of Psychiatry*, 159(4), 669–71.

Sharp, C. and Budd, T. (2003). *Minority Ethnic Groups and Crime: Findings From the Offending Crime Survey, 2003*. Home Office Online Report 33/05 2003 [cited 2 September, 2008].

Sharpley, M. S. and Peters, E. R. (1999). Ethnicity, class and schizotypy. *Social Psychiatry and Psychiatric Epidemiology*, 34(10), 507–12.

Sharpley, M., Hutchinson, G., McKenzie, K. *et al.* (2001). Understanding the excess of psychosis among the African-Caribbean population in England. Review of current hypotheses. *Br J Psychiatry Suppl*, 40, S60–8.

Singh, S. P. (2009). Shooting the messenger: the science and politics of ethnicity research. *British Journal of Psychiatry*, 195(1), 1–2.

Singh, S. P. and Burns, T. (2006). Race and mental health: there is more to race than racism. *British Medical Journal*, 333(7569), 648–51.

Smith, G. N., Boydell, J., Murray, R. M. *et al.* (2006). The incidence of schizophrenia in European immigrants to Canada. *Schizophrenia Research*, 87(1–3), 205–11.

Snowden, L. R., Hastings, J. F., Alvidrez, J. (2009). Overrepresentation of black Americans in psychiatric inpatient care. *Psychiatric Services*, 60(6), 779–85.

Soni Raleigh, V. (1996). Suicide patterns and trends in people of Indian subcontinent and Caribbean origin in England and Wales. *Ethnic Health*, 1(1), 55–63.

Soni Raleigh, V., Bulusu, L., Balarajan, R. (1990). Suicides among immigrants from the Indian subcontinent. *British Journal of Psychiatry*, 156, 46–50.

Sugarman, P. A. and Craufurd, D. (1994). Schizophrenia in the Afro-Caribbean community. *British Journal of Psychiatry*, **164**(4), 474–80.

Swinnen, S. G. H. A. and Selten, J. P. (2007). Mood disorders and migration: meta-analysis. *British Journal of Psychiatry*, **190**(1), 6–10.

Szyf, M., McGowan, P., Meaney, M. J. (2008). The social environment and the epigenome. *Environmental and Molecular Mutagenesis*, **49**(1).

Thapa, S. B., Dalgard, O. S., Claussen, B. R. *et al.* (2007). Psychological distress among immigrants from high- and low-income countries: findings from the Oslo Health Study. *Nordic Journal of Psychiatry*, **61**(6), 459–65.

Thomas, C. S., Stone, K., Osborn, M. *et al.* (1993). Psychiatric morbidity and compulsory admission among UK-born Europeans, Afro-Caribbeans and Asians in central Manchester. *British Journal of Psychiatry*, **163**, 91–9.

Thompson, N. and Bhugra, D. (2000). Rates of deliberate self-harm in Asians: findings and models. *International Review of Psychiatry*, **12**(1), 37–43.

van Bergen, D. D., Smit, J. H., van Balkom, A. J. *et al.* (2008). Suicidal ideation in ethnic minority and majority adolescents in Utrecht, the Netherlands. *Crisis*, **29**(4), 202–8.

van Os, J., Castle, D. J., Takei, N. *et al.* (1996). Psychotic illness in ethnic minorities: clarification from the 1991 census. *Psychological Medicine*, **26**(1), 203–8.

van Os, J., Takei, N., Castle, D. J. *et al.* (1996). The incidence of mania: time trends in relation to gender and ethnicity. *Social Psychiatry and Psychiatric Epidemiology*, **31**(3–4), 129–36.

Veen, N., Selten, J. P., Hoek, H. W. *et al.* (2002). Use of illicit substances in a psychosis incidence cohort: a comparison among different ethnic groups in the Netherlands.

Acta Psychiatrica Scandinavica, **105**(6), 440–3.

Vega, W. A., Kolody, B., Aguilar-Gaxiola, S. *et al.* (1998). Lifetime prevalence of DSM-III-R psychiatric disorders among urban and rural Mexican Americans in California. *Archives of General Psychiatry*, **55**(9), 771–8.

Veling, W., Selten, J. P., Veen, N. *et al.* (2006). Incidence of schizophrenia among ethnic minorities in the Netherlands: a four-year first-contact study. *Schizophrenia Research*, **86**(1–3), 189–93.

Veling, W., Selten, J.-P., Susser, E. *et al.* (2007). Discrimination and the incidence of psychotic disorders among ethnic minorities in The Netherlands. *International Journal of Epidemiology*, **36**(4), 761–8.

Veling, W., Susser, E., van Os, J. *et al.* (2008). Ethnic density of neighborhoods and incidence of psychotic disorders among immigrants. *American Journal of Psychiatry*, **165**(1), 66–73.

Weich, S., Nazroo, J., Sproston, K. *et al.* (2004). Common mental disorders and ethnicity in England. *Psychological Medicine*, **34**(8), 1543–51.

Weiser, M., Werbeloff, N., Vishna, T. *et al.* (2008). Elaboration on immigration and risk for schizophrenia. *Psychological Medicine*, **38**(08), 1113–19.

Wessely, S., Castle, D., Der, G. *et al.* (1991). Schizophrenia and Afro-Caribbeans – a case-control study. *British Journal of Psychiatry*, **159**, 795–801.

Wessely, S., Castle, D., Murray, R. (1992). A case control study of schizophrenia and ethnicity – 1964–1984. *Schizophrenia Research*, **6**(2), 103.

Zolkowska, K., Cantor-Graae, E., McNeil, T. F. (2001). Increased rates of psychosis among immigrants to Sweden: is migration a risk factor for psychosis? *Psychological Medicine*, **31**(4), 669–78.

Chapter

3

Migration and mental illness: an epidemiological perspective*

I-Chao Liu and Andrew T. A. Cheng

Editors' introduction

Epidemiological studies related to the field of migration have demonstrated that rates of psychotic disorders among some migrant groups are higher than expected. In Chapter 2, Kirkbride and Jones illustrated this by proposing hypotheses to explain such variation and assessing each hypothesis. Liu and Cheng focus on some of the methodological issues related to research design, time of assessment, cross-sectional nature of these studies and other factors. Issues related to refugees and asylum seekers are somewhat different because of the trauma they may suffer and the application of the stress-diathesis model here. As expected, post-traumatic stress disorders will show a higher prevalence among refugees and asylum seekers. Methodological, especially sampling, problems in these groups raise issues about the implications of such studies.

Liu and Cheng also explore the factors related to returning migrants and internal migration. They conclude that both social and genetic factors need to be understood in explaining the variation in rates, and early life experiences may determine the outcome of mental illness in the new settings. Using a number of factors in identifying aetiology will also enable clinicians to develop appropriate management plans.

Introduction

One of the major aspects of social changes following rapid globalisation from the second half of the last century is migration. According to the International Organization for Migration, there are now about 192 million people living outside their place of birth, which is about 3% of the world's population (http://www.iom.int/jahia/Jahia/about-migration). This means that roughly one of every 35 persons in the world is a migrant. The number includes 26 million internally displaced persons, and 16 million cross-national refugees and asylum seekers (UN High Commission for Refugees, 2008). In other words, at least one out of every 400 people alive in the world today is a refugee. The rapidly growing number of immigrants has brought about an increase in research about their physical and mental health.

By definition, migration refers to the change in the location of residency by individuals and/or their families. There have been various socio-economic, political, cultural and

---

* Revised from a paper presented at the XIXth Congress of the World Association for Social Psychiatry, Prague, 21–24, October 2007.

Migration and Mental Health, ed. Dinesh Bhugra & Susham Gupta. Published by Cambridge University Press. © Cambridge University Press 2011.

religious reasons for migration, including fleeing persecution, pursuing a better education or economic environment, and seeking political or religious freedom (Bhugra, 2004; Cheng and Chang, 1999).

Migration has often been classified as voluntary or involuntary, internal (within a nation) or international. Three categories of migrants that have received most attention in research are refugees, asylum seekers and economic immigrants (including temporary labour migrants). In general, refugees and asylum seekers tend to have more traumatic exposures, whereas economic migrants might have better resources and preparation for migration.

Migration involves a complex process, starting from pre-migration to migration and then to post-migration stages, including substages of overcompensation, decompensation and acculturation. Migration has been regarded as having a substantial impact on people's mental health, either as a precipitating or as an aggravating factor. Each stage of migration could involve certain risk factors for mental health, including individual personality and traumatic experiences (such as violence and war during pre-migration); duration of waiting period; degrees of exhaustion; types of trauma during the migration process; social adversity; racial discrimination; living conditions and legal status post-migration.

Methodological issues

Research design

Most studies used a cross-sectional design and assessed short-term and/or long-term effects of migration on mental health retrospectively. Three kinds of comparative strategy have been used in previous studies, including comparisons between immigrants and people in their original country; between foreign-born immigrants and their descendents born in the new country; and between native people and immigrants, either the first or the second generations.

The first type of comparison can investigate genetic and social selection factors leading to migration and their effects on mental health. The second type can study post-migration social and acculturative effects on mental health among immigrants across generations. The third type can assess genetic and environmental effects on mental health across different ethnic groups and generations.

Time and assessment

The time of investigation is a key issue in assessing the impact of migration on mental health. A proportion of immigrants may remit from mental illness precipitated by migration over time. Conversely, detrimental post-migration environments may influence the course of such morbidity, or precipitate a new mental illness. There have been a few follow-up and intergeneration studies, which are particularly invaluable in bringing novel insights into the genetic and environmental risk factors for specific mental disorders.

The use of the same cross-culturally valid and reliable instruments in different language versions among the comparison groups is a fundamental requirement in the study of migration and mental health. One recent study pointed out the potential benefit and the need of using additional probes and decision rules based on cultural formulation as making diagnoses of psychotic disorders among immigrants (Zandi et al., 2008). Definitions in ethnicity, race, nationality and place of birth in subject recruitment need to be consistent across studies (Minas, 2001; Vega et al., 1998).

With these methodological considerations in mind, the main findings in previous studies are summarised, and their implications for prevention and the mental health service are discussed.

Migration and psychotic disorders

Earlier studies among immigrants suggested a negative migration effect on people who were in the early incipient stage of illness, notably schizophrenia, prior to migration. The classical study by Ødegaard (1932) revealed a higher rate of hospitalisation of severe psychotic disorders among Norwegian immigrants in Minnesota, USA than among the native-born population, and an even higher rate among migrants who returned to Norway (Ødegaard, 1932). Ødegaard explained the phenomena in terms of a selective tendency for vulnerable and insecure individuals who have failed in interpersonal relationships in their home country to migrate.

Several studies have then reported an increased incidence of schizophrenia and all psychotic disorders in selected immigrant groups, including both the first and second generation African-Caribbean immigrants in the UK (Bhugra et al., 1997; Harrison et al., 1988, 1997; Mortensen et al., 1997; Selten et al., 1997). The finding has remained robust after controlling for potential confounding factors, including different demographic character-istics of immigrant populations; diagnostic bias and misclassification in ethnic minorities; differential thresholds for admission (selective referral); use of prevalence or incidence as the morbidity index, with or without age standardisation; use of cannabis and other illicit drugs, genetic risk for schizophrenia in immigrants and local inhabitants; and methods of calculat-ing the population at risk.

As shown in Table 3.1, a number of recent studies in some European countries and Israel have replicated the finding of an excess in schizophrenia and other non-affective psychosis among the first and second generation African-Caribbean, Moroccan, Surinamese, Finnish and East and South European immigrants.

Ethnic density of neighbourhoods had been found to be associated with the incidence of psychotic disorders among immigrants in a Dutch study. An elevated incidence rate was found for immigrants in low-ethnic-density neighbourhoods, but not in high-ethnic-density neighbourhoods. The authors proposed two possible mechanisms behind high ethnic dens-ity: to mitigate the effect of discrimination and to increase social access to normalise function (Veling et al., 2008).

The increased genetic risk for schizophrenia and all non-affective psychoses among Caribbean migrants was found in the first generation and in siblings of the second gen-eration, but not in parents of the second generation (Harrison et al., 1997). This suggests that the increased incidence in immigrants is not solely because of a higher genetic predispos-ition. Recently, there has been an increasing interest in the impact of social stressors on brain functioning and on the pathogenesis of schizophrenia (Selten et al., 2007). Both biological (e.g. prenatal and childhood infections) and social (e.g. life events and social adversity) environmental factors arising from the experience of migration may precipitate psychotic disorders in those who are genetically vulnerable and contribute to the increase in the incidence of psychoses in certain ethnic groups (Harrison et al., 1997; Selten et al., 1997).

In a recent review of this issue, Broome et al. (2005) have put forth the following comment: 'A plausible model of the onset of psychosis needs to draw not only on neuro-sciences, but also on the insights of social psychiatry and cognitive psychology'. He also

Table 3.1 Risks of psychoses among first and second generation immigrants in recent studies

| Authors | Date | Country | Immigrants | Relative risk | |
				First generation	Second generation
Harrison et al.[a]	1988	England	Caribbean	6.8	11.6
Selten et al.[b]	2001	Netherlands	Moroccan	4.5	8.0
			Surinamese	3.2	5.5
Hjern et al.[c]	2004	Sweden	Finnish	1.6–2.6	2.0–2.5
			European (East and South)	1.9–3.1	1.7–2.2
Cantor-Graae et al.[d]	2005	Sweden	Black and white	2.9–4.0	1.4–2.0
Leao et al.[e]	2006	Sweden	Finnish	1.6–2.5	2.3–2.3 (SCH)
				2.3–2.3	2.2–2.3 (NAP)
Weiser et al.[f]	2008	Israel	Mixed	1.62	1.41–1.49
Coid et al.[g]	2008	England	Caribbean	2.3	4.9 (non-affective)
				3.2	4.2 (affective)

[a] ICD-9 schizophrenia; [b] DSM-IV schizophrenia, schizophreniform and schizoaffective; [c] ICD-9 and ICD-10 schizophrenia and other psychosis; [d] DSM-IV schizophrenia (SCH) and other non-affective psychosis (NAP); [e] ICD-9 and ICD-10 schizophrenia and other non-affective psychosis; [f] ICD-9 and ICD-10 schizophrenia; [g] DSM-IV non-affective and affective psychoses

mentioned that social adversity, like migration and social isolation, can result in the onset of psychosis. More studies are required to clarify the exact environmental factors and their interaction with genetic vulnerability to generate the excess of psychosis among certain immigrant groups.

Involuntary migration: refugees and asylum seekers

Since the second half of the last century, the majority of involuntary migration has come from developing countries and East Europe. Hospital and population-based studies among refugees and asylum seekers have repeatedly observed high rates of a wide range of psychiatric disorders. A significantly higher morbidity was reported in asylum seekers compared to refugees (Gerritsen et al., 2006).

The high morbidity has been attributed to loss and traumatic events before or during the migration process, and post-migration stresses involving traumas, asylum procedures, detention, readjustment in family, job, housing, socio-economic living conditions and social isolation (poor social support and discrimination) (Gerritsen et al., 2006; Keller et al., 2003; Laban et al., 2005; Robjant et al., 2009). Laban et al. (2005) have thus suggested that the government should consider shortening the asylum procedures, allowing the refugees to work, and giving preference to family reunion.

A meta-analysis involving 22 221 refugees and 45 073 non-refugee controls from 59 studies has reported a poorer mental health condition among refugees, associated with certain predisplacement refugee characteristics and postdisplacement factors. The former included an older age (65 or above), a higher education, a female gender, being displaced from rural areas, and a higher predisplacement socio-economic status. Postdisplacement factors included living in institutional accommodation, experiencing restricted economic opportunity, being displaced internally within their own country, being repatriated to a country they had previously fled, or having unresolved initiating conflict (Porter and Haslam, 2005). A recent systematic review and meta-analysis among 24 051 migrants also showed high prevalence rates of depression and anxiety in refugees. The prevalence rates in refugees are found to be almost two-fold higher than in labour migrants (44% versus 20% for depression; 40% versus 21% for anxiety) (Lindert et al., 2009).

Few studies investigated the long-term effect of migration trauma among refugees resettled in the host country. One study among Vietnamese refugees in Australia ($n = 1161$) revealed a fall of the risk of mental illness across time and a higher risk (OR = 4.7) of chronic morbidity among those exposed to more than three traumatic events during migration more than 10 years ago (Steel et al., 2002). The other study, among Cambodian refugees in the USA ($n = 596$) after 20 years of resettlement, found 70% reported exposure to violence after migration, high rates of post-traumatic stress disorder (PTSD) (62%) and major depression (51%), and low rates of alcohol use disorder (4%). Risk factors for PTSD and major depression included pre-migration and post-migration traumas and older age (Marshall et al., 2005).

A much higher level of psychiatric morbidity among refugee children, especially PTSD, depression and anxiety disorders, has consistently been reported in previous studies (Fazel and Stein, 2002), with a total rate around 40–50% (Hodes, 1998). Factors contributing to this may include direct experience of or witnessing violence, loss of parents and family, and being looked after by parents who themselves have psychopathology and cannot cope with the children's demands (Garmezy, 1991). A recent study indicated that Middle Eastern refugee children in Denmark are susceptible to the effects of pre-migration trauma, but certain risk and protective factors at the individual, family and community level can mediate the long-term effects on mental health. It has been found that a stressful social life such as discrimination in the new country predicted subsequent psychological problems eight or nine years after arrival, more than pre-migration traumatic experiences (Montgomery and Foldspang, 2008).

Studies among general immigrants

A large number of studies did not differentiate refugees from voluntary immigrants in their study samples. Findings from them regarding the magnitude of mental illness, in particular common non-psychotic mental disorder, have been rather inconsistent. Some reported higher rates of anxiety and mood disorders among adult immigrants (Mirsky et al., 2008) and both internalising and externalising problem behaviours among immigrant children (Vollebergh et al., 2005); some did not find any difference; and some conversely observed lower rates among immigrants (Angold et al., 2002; Grant et al., 2004). Such disparity may have several explanations, including differences in sample recruitment, in case definition and case identification methods, in time of study along the migration process and in heterogeneity of the study immigrants.

In the past two decades, large scale studies conducted in the USA have consistently found a lower lifetime prevalence of anxiety, mood and substance use disorders among Mexican (Burnam *et al.*, 1987), Hispanic (Ortega *et al.*, 2000), Asian (Takeuchi *et al.*, 2007) and non-Hispanic white immigrants (Grant *et al.*, 2004) than among US-born natives of the same national origin. Such lower rates were further observed only in the first foreign-born generation in the early years of migration (Breslau *et al.*, 2007; Vega *et al.*, 1998), including a comparison between them and the residents in their country of origin by Vega and his colleagues (1998). This study used both English and Spanish versions of the Composite International Diagnostic Interview (CIDI) in a community sample recruited from Fresno County, California, USA. Numbers of study subjects were comparable across different comparing groups. While the overall lifetime prevalence rate among foreign-born Mexican immigrants (24.9%) was much lower than those among US-born Mexican Americans (48.7%), rates were similar between Mexican immigrants and Mexican citizens (23.4%), and between Mexican Americans and the national population (48.6%). A further analysis found that Mexican immigrants with less than 13 years of residence had a lower rate (18.4%) than Mexican citizens, and the rate was higher for those with more than 13 years of residence (32.3%) (Breslau *et al.*, 2007).

These findings might be interpreted to show that Mexican immigrants are better off in the initial years after immigration in comparison with their counterparts in Mexico, possibly because of a positive selective migration (healthy migration) of the mentally fit (Burnam *et al.*, 1987; Grant *et al.*, 2004; Fennelly, 2007). This advantage reverses over time, possibly as a result of acculturation stress (Ortega *et al.*, 2000; Rogler *et al.*, 1991), or difficulties in adaptation to the host society and culture, including poor housing, poverty or downward socio-economic status, barriers to healthcare and social services, discrimination, and adaptation to smoking, substance use and unhealthy American diet (Fennelly, 2007).

One of the major limitations of the US migration studies concerns the representativeness of the migrant samples. The National Comorbidity Study (NCS) and NCS Replication Study only interview English-speaking migrants in the USA, excluding those who can only speak their mother tongues. Furthermore, as the subjects were recruited exclusively from American civilians, illegal immigrants were not included. History of refugee status and asylum seeking were not taken. These immigrants are very likely to have different risks for psychiatric morbidity than immigrant American civilians.

All the studies employed cross-sectional and retrospective cohort design. The recall bias certainly cannot be avoided, particularly with lifetime prevalence estimation. The best strategy to overcome these shortcomings is to adopt the longitudinal cohort study design, preferably with frequent assessments in the first few years after migration.

Returned immigrants: what have they learnt?

One recent study among Mexican citizens (*n* = 5826) found that respondents who had a history of migration to the USA or had family members who migrated in the USA were more likely to develop substance use disorder and to have a current substance use disorder than were other Mexicans. The authors speculated that international migration may play a role in transforming substance use norms and pathology in Mexico (Borges *et al.*, 2007). The study may serve as an example showing how acculturative influence can be detrimental to the immigrants and those that remain at home.

In a recent report, a group of returnee refugees from the former Yugoslavia, Iraq and Turkey were compared with refugees who decided to stay in Germany (von Lersner *et al.*, 2008).

Using the German version of the Mini International Neuropsychiatric Interview for diagnostic interview, a prevalence rate of 44% for psychiatric disorders in the group of returnees and a rate of 78% in the group of stayers was found, remarkably higher than in the average population in western countries. The authors indicated that pre-migration traumatic experience during war and refuge has predisposed refugees to poor coping with post-migration stressors in exile.

Internal migration: selective migration?

The main difference between international migration and voluntary migration within the same country is that the stress associated with the latter is much less complicated and largely involves subcultural adaptation (such as urban–rural) without language barrier or traumas such as detention. Rural–urban migration is a common social mobility in developing countries, where loss of economic viability of rural industries and the concentration of wealth and jobs in cities has resulted in massive rural-to-urban migrations (Minas, 2001).

One community study conducted in Taiwan found lower rates of depression symptoms in migrant urban young women (0.4%) than in native rural counterparts (9.8%) (Cheng, 1989). Both the adverse rural social environment with more chronic adversities (53% in rural and 25% in urban young female cases) and a positive selective migration to the cities were proposed to explain the difference. Urbanisation may act as a moderator over the effect of selective migration. The motivation for migration among the rural Taiwanese young women to the cities is not confined to economic reasons. Other psychosocial reasons include the escape from chronic adversities, such as in-law conflict and unequal status between husband and wife in rural Taiwan.

A study in China did not find a significant difference in mental health status (measured by SF-36) between migrant and native urban workers in Hangzhou city. Migrants' upward economic status and better job opportunities, as well as higher social capital in the cities, were proposed to explain the findings (Li et al., 2007). Another study has examined the association between two common problem behaviours, illicit drug use and hazardous/harmful drinking, and rural–urban migration among young Thai people. Findings indicated that rural–urban migration was not associated with illicit drug use, whereas hazardous/harmful drinking was related to being late migrants. The authors hypothesised that alcohol was probably consumed to establish friendships with peers or to deal with job-related stress or unemployment frustration in late migrants (Jirapramukpitak et al., 2008).

One specific aspect of migration that has often been neglected is the migration of aboriginal peoples from their reserved lands to the cities in countries like the USA, Canada, Australia and New Zealand, China, Taiwan, Japan and some countries in South America. Few studies have investigated the impact of such migration on physical and mental health related to acculturative stress hitherto. For example, such stress may have precipitated or aggravated alcohol and substance use disorders and mood disorders among aboriginal immigrants living in the host society, or those returned to their reserved lands, probably in a frustrated retreat. Further studies are warranted.

Migration and suicide

Suicide rates have been consistently observed to be higher among immigrants. Studies among immigrants from 15 countries in Sweden (Ferrada-Noli, 1997) and from seven countries in Australia (Burvill, 1998) reported predominantly higher suicide rates than that in their countries of origin (with a similar rank order in the countries of origin) and in Sweden.

Suicide risk was generally higher among foreign migrants compared with the native population in Denmark, and the risk was highest among Nordic-born migrants (Sundaram *et al.*, 2006). The study in Stockholm County reported the highest suicide rate among immigrants living in low income areas with poor psychiatric care (Ferrada-Noli and Asberg, 1997). These seem to suggest a negative selective migration.

The relation of time of residence in a new country to suicide rates is still inconclusive. However, a recent US study revealed an increased suicide risk among immigrants and an inverse relationship between a shorter duration of residence and a higher suicide risk, suggesting that suicide prevention should focus on more recent immigrants (Kposowa *et al.*, 2008).

How can we explain the controversial findings between common mental disorders and suicide related to migration? Perhaps the heterogeneity of immigrant populations implies that there is a small subgroup among them with a particularly higher risk for suicide (e.g. those suffering from severe depression before or after migration, and/or having experienced severe traumas which may or may not come from involuntary migration). On the other hand, a substantial proportion of immigrants, particularly those in internal migration, might belong to the positive migration category (healthy migrants).

Use of mental health service among immigrants

The enquiry into the magnitude of mental disorders and the risk factors associated with migration is useful for primary prevention. However, studies regarding the use of mental health services among immigrants and the evaluation of their effects are equally important for secondary and tertiary prevention.

Previous studies suggest that, comparing to native peoples, non-European immigrants to Canada and the USA tend to under-use mental health services (Abe-Kim *et al.*, 2007; Chen and Kazanjian, 2005; Huang and Spurgeon, 2006). The lower rate of use by immigrants could not be explained by differences in sociodemographics, somatic or psychological symptoms, length of stay in the host country or use of alternative sources of help. Possible explanations for this discrepancy include cultural and linguistic barriers (Kirmayer *et al.*, 2007), inappropriate practise of physicians, beliefs in non-medical interventions (God and traditional folk medicine) (Whitley *et al.*, 2006) and illness causes (Minas *et al.*, 2007).

A recent review indicated that, in some countries, migrants without legal documents are not eligible for healthcare services; therefore access to mental health services is limited by both the social frame and legal status of the host country (Lindert *et al.*, 2008). Help-seeking patterns of migrants also contribute to the consumption of mental health services. A different pattern of utilisation of mental healthcare by migrants was found in the literature. All non-western immigrants to the Netherlands tend to come into contact with psychiatric emergency services, compared with the natives (Mulder *et al.*, 2006). However, rehabilitation and psychotherapy are, in general, less used by migrants than by natives (Lindert *et al.*, 2008).

Suggestions for future research

Future studies on migration and mental health need to consider the use of cross-culturally valid and reliable standardised psychiatric interviews and culturally valid measurement for acculturation; the inclusion of representative samples from the immigrant population with clearly defined ethnicity; more detailed collection of pre-migration information (clinical, social, cultural); the enquiry of a clear history of the migration process (voluntary or involuntary); and the use of sibling-pair or longitudinal cohort study design.

Conclusions

Influenced by both biological and psychological factors, cultural and social changes arising from migration may put vulnerable migrants at risk for developing mental problems. On the other hand, social support has consistently been viewed as a protective factor in the relationship between migration and mental disorders. A plausible hypothesis is that early life experience and culturally bound life attitudes in immigrants determines the outcome of mental health in the new country. The relationship is, however, mediated by the process of migration and is moderated by the experiences operative in the destination country. International collaborative research will lead to integration of research findings and improvement in hypothesis generation and mental health services.

References

Abe-Kim, J., Takeuchi, D. T., Hong, S. et al. (2007). Use of mental health-related services among immigrant and US-born Asian Americans: results from the National Latino and Asian American Study. *American Journal of Public Health*, **97**, 91–8.

Angold, A., Erkanli, A., Farmer, E. M. et al. (2002). Psychiatric disorder, impairment, and service use in rural African American and white youth. *Archives of General Psychiatry*, **59**, 893–901.

Bhugra, D. (2004). Migration and mental health. *Acta Psychiatrica Scandinavica*, **109**, 243–58.

Bhugra, D., Leff, J., Mallett, R. et al. (1997). Incidence and outcome of schizophrenia in Whites, African-Caribbeans and Asians in London. *Psychological Medicine*, **27**(4), 791–8.

Borges, G., Medina-Mora, M. E., Breslau, J., Aguilar-Gaxiola, S. (2007). The effect of migration to the United States on substance use disorders among returned Mexican migrants and families of migrants. *American Journal of Public Health*, **97**, 1847–51.

Breslau, J., Aguilar-Gaxiola, S., Borges, G. et al. (2007). Risk for psychiatric disorder among immigrants and their US-born descendants: evidence from the National Comorbidity Survey Replication. *Journal of Nervous and Mental Disease*, **195**, 189–95.

Broome, M. R., Woolley, J. B., Tabraham, P. et al. (2005). What causes the onset of psychosis? *Schizophrenia Research*, **79**, 23–34.

Burnam, M. A., Hough, R. L., Escobar, J. I. et al. (1987). Six-month prevalence of specific psychiatric disorders among Mexican Americans and non-Hispanic whites in Los Angeles. *Archives General Psychiatry*, **44**, 687–94.

Burvill, P. W. (1998). Migrant suicide rates in Australia and in country of birth. *Psychological Medicine*, **28**, 201–8.

Cantor-Graae, E., Zolkowska, K., McNeil, T. F. (2005). Increased risk of psychotic disorder among immigrants in Malmo: a 3-year first-contact study. *Psychological Medicine*, **35**, 1155–63.

Chen, A. W. and Kazanjian, A. (2005). Rate of mental health service utilization by Chinese immigrants in British Columbia. *Canadian Journal of Public Health*, **96**, 49–51.

Cheng, T. A. (1989). Urbanisation and minor psychiatric morbidity. A community study in Taiwan. *Social Psychiatry and Psychiatric Epidemiology*, **24**, 309–16.

Cheng, A. T. A. and Chang, J. C. (1999). Mental health aspects of culture and migration (Editorial Review). *Current Opinion in Psychiatry*, **12**, 217–22.

Coid, J. W., Kirkbride, J. B., Barker, D. et al. (2008). Raised incidence rates of all psychoses among migrant groups: findings from the East London first episode psychosis study. *Archives of General Psychiatry*, **65**, 1250–8.

Fazel, M. and Stein, A. (2002). The mental health of refugee children. *Archives of Disease in Childhood*, **87**, 366–70.

Fennelly, K. (2007). The "healthy migrant" effect. *Minnesota Medicine*, **90**, 51–3.

Ferrada-Noli, M. (1997). A cross-cultural breakdown of Swedish suicide. *Acta Psychiatrica Scandinavica*, **96**, 108–16.

Ferrada-Noli, M. and Asberg, M. (1997). Psychiatric health, ethnicity and socio-economic factors among suicides in Stockholm. *Psychological Reports*, **81**, 323–32.

Garmezy, N. (1991). Resilience in children's adaptation to negative life events and stressed environments. *Pediatric Annals*, **20**, 459–60, 463–6.

Gerritsen, A. A., Bramsen, I., Deville, W. *et al.* (2006). Physical and mental health of Afghan, Iranian and Somali asylum seekers and refugees living in the Netherlands. *Social Psychiatry and Psychiatric Epidemiology*, **41**, 18–26.

Grant, B. F., Stinson, F. S., Hasin, D. S. *et al.* (2004). Immigration and lifetime prevalence of DSM-IV psychiatric disorders among Mexican Americans and non-Hispanic whites in the United States: results from the National Epidemiologic Survey on Alcohol and Related Conditions. *Archives of General Psychiatry*, **61**, 1226–33.

Harrison, G., Owens, D., Holton, A., Neilson, D., Boot, D. (1988). A prospective study of severe mental disorder in Afro-Caribbean patients. *Psychological Medicine*, **18**, 643–57.

Harrison, G., Glazebrook, C., Brewin, J. *et al.* (1997). Increased incidence of psychotic disorders in migrants from the Caribbean to the United Kingdom. *Psychological Medicine*, **27**, 799–806.

Hjern, A., Wicks, S., Dalman, C. (2004). Social adversity contributes to high morbidity in psychoses in immigrants – a national cohort study in two generations of Swedish residents. *Psychological Medicine*, **34**, 1025–33.

Hodes, M. (1998). Refugee children. *British Medical Journal*, **316**, 793–4.

Huang, S. L. and Spurgeon, A. (2006). The mental health of Chinese immigrants in Birmingham, UK. *Ethnic Health*, **11**, 365–87.

Jirapramukpitak, T., Prince, M., Harpham, T. (2008). Rural–urban migration, illicit drug use and hazardous/harmful drinking in the young Thai population. *Addiction*, **103**, 91–100.

Keller, A. S., Rosenfeld, B., Trinh-Shevrin, C. *et al.* (2003). Mental health of detained asylum seekers. *Lancet*, **362**, 1721–3.

Kirmayer, L. J., Weinfeld, M., Burgos, G. *et al.* (2007). Use of health care services for psychological distress by immigrants in an urban multicultural milieu. *Canadian Journal of Psychiatry*, **52**, 295–304.

Kposowa, A. J., McElvain, J. P., Breault, K. D. (2008). Immigration and suicide: the role of marital status, duration of residence, and social integration. *Archives of Suicide Research*, **12**, 82–92.

Laban, C. J., Gernaat, H. B., Komproe, I. H., van der Tweel, I., De Jong, J. T. (2005). Postmigration living problems and common psychiatric disorders in Iraqi asylum seekers in the Netherlands. *Journal of Nervous Mental Disease*, **193**, 825–32.

Leao, T. S., Sundquist, J., Frank, G. *et al.* (2006). Incidence of schizophrenia or other psychoses in first- and second-generation immigrants: a national cohort study. *Journal of Nervous Mental Disease*, **194**, 27–33.

Li, L., Wang, H. M., Ye, X. J. *et al.* (2007). The mental health status of Chinese rural-urban migrant workers: comparison with permanent urban and rural dwellers. *Social Psychiatry and Psychiatric Epidemiology*, **42**, 716–22.

Lindert, J., Schouler-Ocak, M., Heinz, A., Priebe, S. (2008). Mental health, health care utilisation of migrants in Europe. *European Psychiatry*, **23**(Suppl 1), 14–20.

Lindert, J., Ehrenstein, O. S., Priebe, S., Mielck, A., Brahler, E. (2009). Depression and anxiety in labor migrants and refugees – a systematic review and meta-analysis. *Social Science and Medicine*, **69**, 246–57.

Marshall, G. N., Schell, T. L., Elliott, M. N., Berthold, S. M., Chun, C. A. (2005). Mental health of Cambodian refugees 2 decades after resettlement in the United States. *Journal of the American Medical Association*, **294**, 571–9.

Minas, H. (2001). Migration, equity and health. In: M. McKee, P. Garner, R. Stott, eds. *International Co-operation in Health*. Oxford: Oxford University Press, pp. 151–74.

Minas, H., Klimidis, S., Tuncer, C. (2007). Illness causal beliefs in Turkish immigrants. *BMC Psychiatry*, **7**, 34.

Mirsky, J., Kohn, R., Levav, I., Grinshpoon, A., Ponizovsky, A. M. (2008). Psychological distress and common mental disorders among immigrants: results from the Israeli-based component of the world mental health survey. *Journal of Clinical Psychiatry*, **69**, 1715–20.

Montgomery, E., Foldspang, A. (2008). Discrimination, mental problems and social adaptation in young refugees. *European Journal of Public Health*, **18**, 156–61.

Mortensen, P. B., Cantor-Graae, E., McNeil, T. F. (1997). Increased rates of schizophrenia among immigrants: some methodological concerns raised by Danish findings. *Psychological Medicine*, **27**, 813–20.

Mulder, C. L., Koopmans, G. T., Selten, J. P. (2006). Emergency psychiatry, compulsory admissions and clinical presentation among immigrants to the Netherlands. *British Journal of Psychiatry*, **188**, 386–91.

Ødegaard, Ø. (1932). Emigration and insanity. *Acta Psychiatrica et Neurologica* Suppl. **4**, 1–206.

Ortega, A. N., Rosenheck, R., Alegria, M., Desai, R. A. (2000). Acculturation and the lifetime risk of psychiatric and substance use disorders among Hispanics. *Journal of Nervous Mental Disease*, **188**, 728–35.

Porter, M., Haslam, N. (2005). Predisplacement and postdisplacement factors associated with mental health of refugees and internally displaced persons: a meta-analysis. *Journal of the American Medical Association*, **294**, 602–12.

Robjant, K., Hassan, R., Katona, C. (2009). Mental health implications of detaining asylum seekers: systematic review. *British Journal of Psychiatry*, **194**, 306–12.

Rogler, L. H., Cortes, D. E., Malgady, R. G. (1991). Acculturation and mental health status among Hispanics. Convergence and new directions for research. *American Psychologist*, **46**, 585–97.

Selten, J. P., Slaets, J. P., Kahn, R. S. (1997). Schizophrenia in Surinamese and Dutch Antillean immigrants to The Netherlands: evidence of an increased incidence. *Psychological Medicine*, **27**, 807–11.

Selten, J. P., Veen, N., Feller, W. *et al.* (2001). Incidence of psychotic disorders in immigrant groups to The Netherlands. *British Journal of Psychiatry*, **178**, 367–72.

Selten, J. P., Cantor-Graae, E., Kahn, R. S. (2007). Migration and schizophrenia. *Current Opinion in Psychiatry*, **20**, 111–15.

Steel, Z., Silove, D., Phan, T., Bauman, A. (2002). Long-term effect of psychological trauma on the mental health of Vietnamese refugees resettled in Australia: a population-based study. *Lancet*, **360**, 1056–62.

Sundaram, V., Qin, P., Zollner, L. (2006). Suicide risk among persons with foreign background in Denmark. *Suicide and Life-Threatening Behavior*, **36**, 481–9.

Takeuchi, D. T., Zane, N., Hong, S. *et al.* (2007). Immigration-related factors and mental disorders among Asian Americans. *American Journal of Public Health*, **97**, 84–90.

UN (United Nations) High Commission for Refugees. (2008). *United Nations High Commissioner for Refugees' 2008 Global Trends: Refugees, Asylum-seekers, Returnees, Internally Displaced and Stateless Persons*, 2008. http://www.unhcr.org/statistics.

Vega, W. A., Kolody, B., Aguilar-Gaxiola, S. *et al.* (1998). Lifetime prevalence of DSM-III-R psychiatric disorders among urban and rural Mexican Americans in California. *Archives of General Psychiatry*, **55**, 771–8.

Veling, W., Susser, E., van Os, J. *et al.* (2008). Ethnic density of neighborhoods and incidence of psychotic disorders among immigrants. *American Journal of Psychiatry*, **165**, 66–73.

Vollebergh, W. A., ten Have, M., Dekovic, M. *et al.* (2005). Mental health in immigrant children in the Netherlands. *Social Psychiatry and Psychiatric Epidemiology*, **40**, 489–96.

von Lersner, U., Wiens, U., Elbert, T., Neuner, F. (2008). Mental health of returnees: refugees in Germany prior to their state-sponsored repatriation. *BMC International Health and Human Rights*, **8**, 8.

Weiser, M., Werbeloff, N., Vishna, T. *et al.* (2008). Elaboration on immigration and

risk for schizophrenia. *Psychological Medicine*, **38**, 1113–19.

Whitley, R., Kirmayer, L. J., Groleau, D. (2006). Understanding immigrants' reluctance to use mental health services: a qualitative study from Montreal. *Canadian Journal of Psychiatry*, **51**, 205–9.

Zandi, T., Havenaar, J. M., Limburg-Okken, A. G. *et al.* (2008). The need for culture sensitive diagnostic procedures: a study among psychotic patients in Morocco. *Social Psychiatry and Psychiatric Epidemiology*, **43**, 244–50.

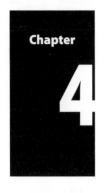

Globalisation: internal borders and external boundaries

Dinesh Bhugra and Susham Gupta

Editors' introduction

Although globalisation by itself is a recent concept and has led to a number of major publications, for centuries there has always been some degree of interconnectedness among nation states, though sometimes such connections were relatively weak and distant. Along with this interconnectedness, which has become closer due to the internet and better, quicker means of communication, the movement of goods and people has become more prominent. Some countries provide the resources for the manufacture of consumer goods which are produced in other countries and are consumed totally and partially elsewhere. Thus, traditional boundaries between cultures, societies and countries are becoming relatively pervious. In this chapter, Bhugra and Gupta argue that the processes of globalisation influence market, political and social forces; on the one hand, there is a push for westernisation and some kind of homogenisation and on the other a return to traditional values. Although people become acculturated, so do cultures, which are always dynamic. The process of globalisation has both positive and negative aspects, and clinicians must remain alert to such changes in cultures to which they themselves belong and from which their patients may come. Understanding the impact of globalisation on the individual and on society is helpful in making sense of factors faced by migrants.

Introduction

Migration across nations and within a nation, for example from rural to urban centres, is an inevitable consequence of globalisation. Even though migration has been occurring for millennia, the reasons for such large movements of people, resources and products are a twentieth-century phenomenon. That is not to say that the raw materials and finished products did not move across nations in earlier times; they did, but the extent and the volume are unprecedented. The three angles of the triangle of globalisation can be understood as interconnectedness of people, raw materials and products. The impact of movement of materials and products will affect the mental state of people – those who are migrating, those they leave behind and those who are struggling to move.

Globalisation is more than increased global interconnectedness. Movement of resources, trade products and people form a part of this process. Changes in communication systems have led to previously unheard of levels of movement of ideas and availability. Over the past centuries, the world has become increasingly smaller. From a reduction in travel times to changes in communication from letters to email, it is inevitable that there will be a contraction

Migration and Mental Health, ed. Dinesh Bhugra & Susham Gupta. Published by Cambridge University Press. © Cambridge University Press 2011.

both in time and space. It is also likely that with such increasing closeness, traditional boundaries between societies and cultures and also between individuals will diminish and may even disappear. Consequently, there are several possible outcomes. Both at individual and cultural levels, the change may lead to deculturation, assimilation, acculturation or an overwhelming response returning to the roots of the culture which feels threatened.

Gupta and Bhugra (2009) suggest that various manifestations of globalisation include rapid communication, cheap modes of travel, increasing deregulation in economic matters and international political organisations. As Okasha (2005) indicates, this invariably leads to cross-cultural communication. The driver for a rapid march of globalisation has been the need for developed countries to buy goods at low prices and their ability to dictate to markets to deliver these goods. Consequently, the relationships between three groups of players in the drama of globalisation become extremely important. These include consumers, producers and those who provide the raw materials (but who may or may not be the producers). However, all groups are consumers to varying degrees, but only rich consumers are able to dictate the demands of production, and in this case these are developed nations. Nobel Prize winner Stiglitz (2002) argues that market deregulation will favour the dominant strong economies of the west. He criticises that such deregulation fails to provide emerging economies and low-income countries the wherewithal to strengthen their infrastructure. He worries that such an approach will lead to further poverty, inequality and social injustice.

The processes of globalisation influence not only the market forces but also political and social forces. There will be social, political and economic expectations and aspirations on the part both of the individual and the culture. If these are not met, then it is quite likely that such a discrepancy will lower both the individual's self-esteem and those of the culture. Complicating this further is the possibility that the discrepancies within the culture add to an increasing sense of disaffection and alienation. These changes are often rapid and it is crucial that service providers are able to deliver services that are acceptable. We know that both poverty and lack of education mediate and influence rates of mental disorders. As noted earlier, it is inevitable that globalisation will influence concepts of time and place in people's social functioning, which will influence relationships in turn. The cultural dynamics shift in any culture over the years. Some of these are related to economic changes, rapid urbanisation and industrialisation and others change by exposure to other cultures through the expansion of the media – written and visual – through the internet, television, newspapers, magazines and journals. Political aspects of globalisation need to be borne in mind too. The exposure of the public to political imperatives both internal and external will bring about changes in structures which will in turn influence individuals and kinships. Another possible impact of globalisation is acculturative, where language, dress codes, dietary habits, etc. may change. The meanings of language and communication will also be influenced.

People move across cultures, societies, nations and cities for all types of reasons. Migration has been defined as a process of social change where an individual, either alone or with others, leaves one geographical area for another for a number of reasons (Bhugra, 2004a, c). Migration can be in either direction from rural to urban areas.

Definitions: the process of migration is defined on a number of parameters, such as purpose, whether it is a response to push or pull factors, occupation per se (such as diplomats moving regularly) or other reasons. It may be primary or secondary. Motivation for migration will also play a role in the process, and the actual length of the process by which people decide, plan and organise the process and then carry out such a process are all important factors.

The response to the process of migration will depend upon a number of factors, such as the age at which this occurs, the gender of the individual, whether they are primary or secondary migrants, their socio-economic and educational status, whether the process was voluntary or forced, whether there was time and support available to prepare or the physical distances involved in such a process. Thus a picture starts to emerge that there is no homogeneity in the experiences of the migrants or in the process of migration itself. The responses to the idea of migration will vary from over-enthusiastic acceptance to a dejected acceptance. It is also likely that different ethnic groups will respond to the same process in completely different ways (see Sashidharan, 1993).

Social inequalities, whether in housing or income, as well as status have led to an increase in mental health disorders. Income inequality and prevalence of mental disorders have a positive linear relation in developed countries (Pickett *et al.*, 2006). These have been attributed to different levels of social trust and cohesion (Wilkinson, 2005), negative view of self-status and -worth (Charlesworth *et al.*, 2004) and a perceived lack of control over one's work and life (Marmot, 2004). (See Gupta and Bhugra, 2009 for further discussion.)

Another complicating factor in the social inequality is the role of gender. As societies become closer, the awareness of equality or lack thereof by populations adds another dimension. Gender roles and gender role expectations will add to a further sense of power-lessness, thereby affecting self-esteem and its role in mental illness. With more women migrating and supporting families elsewhere, there is an urgent need to explore areas of gender role expectations (see Chapter 16).

A recent review in the UK (Marmot, 2010) recommends that every child be given the best start in life. Every child, adolescent and adult should be enabled to maximise their capabilities. Creating fair employment with a healthy standard of living for all, along with creating and developing healthy communities and preventive strategies, are some of the other recommendations (Hunter *et al.*, 2010). Globalisation and migration brings additional pressures to do with housing, education of migrant children, problematic employment and isolation and alienation. Hunter *et al.* (2010), and Hertzman *et al.* (2010) suggest that early support for children and healthy early childhood development (including physical, social, emotional and language cognitive development) are necessary. However, this has to be across the globe in this day and age with shrinking of distances and increased connectedness.

Reasons for migration

Reasons for migration are many and have been covered elsewhere in this volume (see Chapter 13). However, in the context of globalisation several issues start to emerge; these include changes in the society to which people move and also in the society that is left behind.

Education and economic factors are more likely to add to the possibility of movement, particularly within the same environment and intranational migration. More importantly, the movement within the country to seek jobs and increasing urbanisation brings with it separate types of stressors and also changes in family structures. It is worth exploring these issues at some length here (see Figure 4.1).

As noted above, economic factors add to the likelihood of developing psychiatric disorders and these are likely to be caused by industrialisation and urbanisation as illustrated in Figure 4.1.

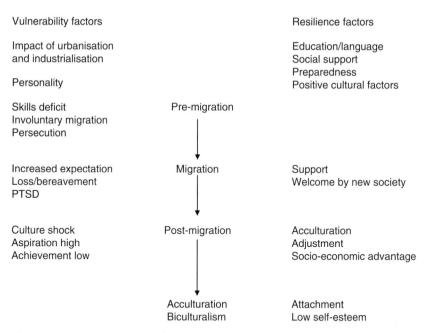

Vulnerability factors

Impact of urbanisation
and industrialisation

Personality

Skills deficit
Involuntary migration
Persecution

Pre-migration

Increased expectation
Loss/bereavement
PTSD

Migration

Culture shock
Aspiration high
Achievement low

Post-migration

Acculturation
Biculturalism

Resilience factors

Education/language
Social support
Preparedness
Positive cultural factors

Support
Welcome by new society

Acculturation
Adjustment
Socio-economic advantage

Attachment
Low self-esteem

Figure 4.1 Migration, globalisation factors and mental illness (after Bhugra, 2004c).

Perception change of mental disorders

There is no doubt that with an increasing connectedness and closer communication, attitudes towards mental illness and explanatory models of distress will change. It is inevitable that as societies undergo changes through globalisation and industrialisation, they will become more technical and perhaps less traditional. As Tseng (2004) has highlighted, it is possible that, with industrialisation, explanatory models of mental illness may move from supranatural or natural to more medical, social or psychological ones. Although this theoretical approach indicates a more western model, it has clear advantages in the context of market-driven economies. Cultural shifts related to exposure to the internet, television and other media will increase the likelihood of changes in perception of mental illness. As traditional sociocentric societies change towards egocentric or nuclear family settings, it is possible that a shift from an external locus of control model of mental illness (i.e. illness is caused by external factors such as evil eye, diet or star constellations) to an internal locus of control (i.e. caused by the self) will also occur. These changes will also place the individual in direct conflict with older generations. Some cultures may have to adapt to deal with the increasing stress by changing their attitudes and styles of dealing with individuals. These changes will produce further tension and anxiety on the cultures in transition. Thus at a macro level the society will need to deal with these by changing the laws (for example, pressure on governments to change laws on homosexual behaviour), economic strategies or political approaches. Another key factor in changing explanatory models and idioms of distress will be changes related to healthcare delivery and healthcare systems. With globalisation and movement of people, especially healthcare professionals, another important issue is raised. For example, Patel et al. (2006) have argued about the Great Brain Robbery, where healthcare professionals from low-income countries migrate to richer countries. Consequently, those trainees who are coming through the system may wish to train in western models of care so that they can migrate in due course. Inequality in healthcare systems in low-income countries will be more obvious as public systems are ill equipped and private healthcare systems may be expensive and uncontrolled. Therefore, a multitude of factors will play a role in creating an impact on healthcare delivery. Unregulated growth in private healthcare and medical schools will exploit high expectations both of the providers and the consumers. Dominance of western cultural values has already been shown to lead to development of eating disorders in cultures which previously did not have these disorders following introduction of television (Becker, 2004). Increasing levels of obesity, hypertension and diabetes mellitus in some cultures can be linked with changes in dietary systems and lifestyles.

The advent of the internet and increased access, along with multiple social networking sites, have led to the development of multiple identities which may change the way individuals look at themselves and at others (see Jones *et al.*, 2010 for further discussion). The interaction between personal internal identity and the external global identity will lead to identity confusion (Arnett, 2002) and conflict. Where the local culture remains traditional and expects traditional values, the individual may deal with this in a cognitively dissonant way. Furthermore, when one set of identity relationships interact with each other, then tension and distress may arise, especially if the roles and role expectations are not clear both to the culture and to the individual. There may be resistance to these changes again both at personal and social levels, creating further problems. Social exclusion leads to increased levels of psychiatric morbidity. Therefore a complex relationship between globalisation at micro and at macro levels starts to emerge.

Additional problems in the mental health of women and the elderly may emerge as the individual male migrates, leaving elderly dependants and female partners behind or, as noted elsewhere, female migrants may face other problems if they migrate by themselves. Children and adolescents are also vulnerable, with increased peer pressure and consumerism, changing parental expectations to academic achievements and changing parental roles playing an important role. Migrant children themselves may find it difficult to adjust to the new society owing to cultural values and problems with language, among other factors.

Feelings of exploitation in migrant workers and perhaps associated powerlessness and lack of control may contribute to a sense of frustration, anger and poor mental health. This may be channelled through to violent response or radicalisation (Ghodse, 2003). On the other hand, increased connectedness can influence political change and bring about better support, consensus and aid quickly. Migration of people is an integral part of the process of globalisation.

Migration is a process which can be broadly divided into pre-migration, migration and post-migration phases. That is not to say that these are discrete phases; inevitably there will be an overlap and, equally, changes that an individual goes through will not occur in isolation either but in varying phases and paces. In the pre-migration phase, migrants identify reasons for leaving one's own land and have expectations of the post-migration life based of individual needs for safety, financial security, personal or political freedom. Preparations are usually a part of this phase and include identifying resources needed for migration and survival, modes of travel needed and contacts in the new place. In the case of forced migration this preparation may not be possible and inadequate preparation can add to psychological problems, e.g. adjustment disorders. The experience of the actual process of migration can differ vastly. Those with little support or migrating under coercion or illegal circumstances can experience various trauma and exploitations, including physical, psychological and financial.

The post-migration experiences on arrival can be the first tryst with reality (they may differ vastly from expectations), leading to feelings of isolation and inadequacy. Language skills, financial status and support from community members all play a significant part. The varying attitude of the receiving culture and its people also affect this experience. Over a period of time the migrant can weigh his achievements with his or her initial aspirations. The level of cultural adjustment and acculturation will again differ according to personal and external factors. The aspiration–achievement gap has recently been identified as a possible contributor to subsequent mental health problems after migration (Bhugra *et al.*, 1999). Hence, quality of experiences at all stages contributes to the overall mental health impact on the migrant.

Sociological theories

Rex (1987) draws a distinction between colonial societies (which rely to a large degree on coercive sanctions deployed by the ruling group) and advanced metropolitan industrial societies which have lesser coercive sanctions (page 87). Colonial societies rely on these coercive sanctions and also have higher levels of racism and racialism. Rex (1987) suggests that metropolitan societies have a greater tendency towards cultural unity, value consensus and the use of normative sanctions, but inbuilt is the likelihood of developing race relations problems. This adds a further dimension in relation to the post-migration experiences of migrants who, by virtue of their race, skin colour, religion or other factors, may face racism and bullying. There is no doubt that even metropolitan societies are multilayered complex organisations with several factors at interplay.

The politics related to immigration have changed public expectations and attitudes. From pre-Second World War to post-Idi Amin, migration to Britain has led to a sense of cognitive dissonance. A grudging welcome and acceptance of migrants was granted when they were needed to provide basic services for which an adequate local workforce was not available. However, these attitudes changed further after expansion of the European Union. Migrants seeking help and jobs in the 1990s are perceived to place real pressures on housing and property. One of the most striking features of postwar migration has been the diversity of geographical areas from whence the migrants came (Layton-Henry, 1992). However, different European countries have developed different ways of dealing with migrants and expectations of how governments make decisions. Migrant workers have made a major contribution to the economies of Western European countries (Layton-Henry, 1992). However, the same can be applied to the USA and Australia. The pressures on governments to shut the doors to migrants are often acutely embarrassing and xenophobic, and yet the consumers want cheap products and are unwilling to do low status jobs. Trapped in unskilled jobs with racist attitudes and behaviours has produced a generation of migrants who feel trapped.

Another interesting and useful notion of the rise of the therapeutic culture of the self linked with more general political transformation has been described by Rose (1996). This approach will be useful in understanding the social and political context within which concepts of the self appear and form. Relationships of the self with others around are the key to personal happiness and social efficacy, Rose concurs. The re-creation of the self in response to changed political, social and economic environments as experienced by migrants raises serious issues in management and discovery of the inner resources. Rose (1996) suggests that self-hood and attributes of the self, feelings, intentions and the like are understood as properties of conversations – i.e., those of social interaction. Hence the identity and the notions of self are both cultural and social and should be seen together rather than in isolation. Thus concepts of the self will change and shift as a result of global movement of people and as a potential consequence of increasing interconnectedness of countries and their people.

Adjustment to new cultures can be complex. There are individual factors such as the personality and the grittiness of the migrant. People moving from a sociocentric to an egocentric culture, or the other way round, can find adjusting to the new social order difficult. It is important to remember that not all members of a sociocentric or egocentric culture would share these societal traits and may adjust without much difficulty. But with most there could be an early and ongoing sense of lack of support or intrusion according to the predominant cultural traits of those around them (see also Chapter 11).

The process of cultural adjustment is from both sides. Migrants also influence the host culture. The growth in migration has now led to many multicultural societies all over the world leading to enriching of existing cultures as well as causing considerable conflicts.

Elsewhere in this volume, processes of acculturation and its varying types are described (see Chapter 11). Here we focus on the impact of such processes on cultures rather than individuals.

Berry (2007) highlights the relationship between acculturation and identity. The cultural identity can be seen at both an individual and group level. Under these circumstances when two cultures come into close contact, changes are likely to occur in both cultures and these changes depend upon the strength of each culture and whether these are majority/minority or not. The contact between two cultures may be caused by close proximity, invasion or migration. It may also be because of learning about one culture through an indirect contact through media and exchange of information through visitors.

Assimilation: as Berry (2007) points out, at the cultural level, the two groups in contact (whether dominant or non-dominant) have some knowledge of the history, the contact and potential consequences of such a contact. The interactions between two cultures are also related to whether one or both cultures in close contact wish to maintain their respective identities or whether one wishes to change more than the other. It is inevitable that some of these changes will be influenced by the majority nature of one culture. The relationship between the individuals and cultures can lead to integration, assimilation, separation or marginalisation. Berry (2007) provides an extremely helpful observation which indicates that maintenance of heritage, culture and identity on one axis and relationships on the second axis will produce strategies valid for both majority and minority societies. It is inevitable that often with such contact the majority culture may respond by multiculturalism, melting pot approach, segregation or exclusion.

As a result of two cultures coming in contact – directly or indirectly – there may be acculturative stress both at the individual level and at the group level. Berry (1992) conceptualises such acculturative stress in three ways. The first is behavioural shift (where individual behaviours change) – sometimes this may be forced, selective or accidental. Using behavioural shifts individuals may adjust to the new culture – behaviours are easier to change than attitudes. The second type of acculturative stress is when events change the individual in a stressful way. Individuals may decide that behavioural change may not help them to cope and this leads to stress, especially when they feel bewildered by the new culture. The third approach of coping is through psychopathology, which may result from abnormal coping and abnormal psychology. Berry (2007) recommends using the term 'acculturative stress' rather than 'culture shock'. He suggests that the term 'shock' has more negative connotations and also that the phenomenon is intercultural. Berry (1997) points out that behavioural shifts can lead to separation and marginalisation. Such coping strategies can lead to changes in cultural values, relationships, settling down and subsequently policy changes.

Biculturalism is often seen in the children of those who have migrated and are brought up in the new culture. Some may find it easier navigating in both cultures, though some generational or cultural conflict may emerge. The intergenerational conflict between 'traditional' and 'less traditional' views can lead to tensions in the family and has been shown to be associated with psychiatric illness (Bhugra 2004b). Awareness of one's own culture, cultural identity and differences with the other culture will influence one's cognitive and emotional responses. However, unless carefully nurtured, identity development may lead to a sense of confusion and changes in emotion, cognition and body, and cultural values will all play a role in this. Migrants often describe personal sacrifices to help their families and others dependent upon them (see Ghuman, 1994). Ghuman (1994, page 32) notes that as the family (especially in sociocentric cultures) exerts a major influence on the identity development of adolescents, the differences across cultures become more intriguing to explore. It is obvious that the structure of the family and the family's own development both as individual members and as a cohesive group will also play a role in the way children grow up. Stopes-Roe and Cochrane (1991) also point out the changes that children of migrant parents are likely to go through. The behavioural changes in trying to conform to the larger new society are more likely to occur sooner than attitudinal ones.

Social structures will also change in each culture and when the two cultures come in contact. Societies vary in how they are structured or organised and these structures are important in the social control employed (Segall *et al.*, 1990). As these authors note, class and caste are some of the structures and when they change as a response to acculturation the social responses will also change. They also vary in complexity and, with cultures being egocentric or sociocentric or masculine or feminine, further dimensions are added (Hofstede, 1980/2001).

At population level both ecological and sociopolitical contexts are important and both of these lead to biological and cultural adaptations which will then go on to affect individuals through sociological influences, acculturation and genetic and cultural transmissions (for details see Segall *et al.*, 1990). Both socialisation and enculturation play a role in adjustment and once again it may be possible to use these for a group or culture. Cultures are said to develop in stages – lower, middle and upper status of savagery, lower, middle and upper status of barbarism, and then civilisation (Tylor, 1865; Morgan, 1877). There will be cultural differences in cognitive processes of members from any culture.

Values and beliefs but acculturation may change some or all of these. Cultural change and acculturation are universal (Segall *et al.*, 1990). These authors also note that acculturative pressures flow in an unbalanced way, reflecting power differential across cultures and among traditional (sociocentric) cultures. Some may be more susceptible to acculturative pressures than others. Internal cultural dynamics will bring about the cultural change when influenced by external cultural dynamics. Intercultural relationships will also be affected by in groups and out groups and their interactions with each other. Thus the sequelae of acculturation will lead to a number of changes, and different cultural groups will change at varying speed.

Acculturation: definitions

Migrants adjust to the influences of the new culture and its interaction with their own in various ways. Some tend to acquire characteristics of the host culture and reduce the dissonance between the two (assimilation). This is a complex process of redefining one's identity with retaining as well as giving up some characteristics of the culture of one's origin. Some, on the other hand, may struggle to do so and distance themselves (separation), while others are able to maintain their own cultural identities at the same time as becoming part of the host culture (biculturalism). People from minority cultural backgrounds can be accepted into the mainstream or feel alienated and marginalised by the dominant host culture, and these factors could be based on the level of difference between them in terms of race and culture.

Biculturalism is often seen in the children of those who have migrated and are brought up in the new culture. Some may find it easier navigating in both cultures, though some generational or cultural conflict may emerge. The intergenerational conflict between 'traditional' and 'less traditional' views can lead to tensions in the family and has been shown to be associated with psychiatric illness (Bhugra, 2004b). Awareness of one's own culture, cultural identity and differences with the other culture will influence one's cognitive and emotional responses. However, unless carefully nurtured, identity development may lead to a sense of confusion and changes in emotion, cognition, body and cultural values will all play a role in this. Migrants often describe personal sacrifices in order to help their families and others dependent upon them (see Ghuman 1994). Ghuman (1994, pp 32–32) notes that as the family (especially in sociocentric cultures) exerts a major influence on the identity development of adolescents, the differences across cultures become more intriguing to explore. It is obvious that the structure of the family and the family's own development both as individual members and a cohesive group will also play a role in the way children grow up to be. Stopes-Roe and Cochrane (1991) also point out the changes children of migrant parents are likely to go through. The behavioural changes in trying to conform with the larger society are more likely to occur sooner than attitudinal ones.

Cultural identity

Cultural identity includes various social characteristics that are shared within a certain group. Cultural identity helps define a person's uniqueness and is a composite of gender, ethnicity, race, religion, occupation, etc. It distinguishes a person from others by their social behaviour, clothes, food, lifestyle, religious beliefs, etc. Attempts at preservation of personal and cultural identity, especially in the face of an unwelcoming host environment, can lead to considerable conflict between the two as well as at a personal level. Discrimination (real and perceived) based on one's racial and cultural identities and mutual mistrust/misunderstanding can lead to social marginalisation of individuals and ethnic minority groups, contributing to behavioural problems, under-achievement and over-representation of these people in mental health and criminal justice systems.

Prevalence of mental disorders

Studies over the past century have repeatedly identified migration as an important factor in the development of mental disorders in migrant communities. With increasing globalisation this is gaining further importance from a preventative and aetiological point of view. The large number of studies that have found increased prevalence of psychoses, e.g. schizophrenia in migrants, have led to various social aetiological concepts. The high rates of schizophrenia amongst African and African-Caribbean migrants to western countries like the UK and the Netherlands (compared to natives and other racial groups) have been scrutinised (Bhugra, 2004b, c). Even after controlling for various confounding factors there are consistent findings of increased prevalence of psychotic disorders. Discrimination, social disadvantage, under-achievement and ethnic density have all been linked to this.

Greater globalisation leading to increased movement of people across cultures has highlighted the need for more epidemiological studies in this area. Services in host culture should also prepare for this and develop culturally sensitive mental health services to cope with growing demands and reduce illness burden. Preventative strategies can also go a long way if health and political systems have better understanding of factors leading to increased mental health morbidities in ethnic communities.

As seen in the chapters by Kirkbride and Jones (Chapter 2) and Liu and Cheng (Chapter 3) in this volume, epidemiological data provide only one side of the picture. There are issues related to epidemiological methods where denominators and numerators can both be confusing. Definitions of ethnicity and comparative data can provide additional problems. However, a combination of qualitative and quantitative data is the best way forward. As Kleinman (1980) has highlighted, if the assessment tools developed in one culture are used blindly without taking into account conceptual equivalence it is likely that a category fallacy will occur which will produce inaccurate figures. Using emic approaches in understanding and measuring culturally appropriate norms is more likely to give a true picture both of prevalence and burden and disease in a community. There is a limit to how many assessment tools can be developed and cross-cultural comparisons carried out, hence combining quantitative and qualitative approaches will benefit the researcher and the clinician alike.

Conclusions

Globalisation has both positive and negative aspects. Of these, positive factors include reduction in emotional distance, increasing interconnectedness; an awareness of other cultures' strengths and weaknesses will provide a way forward for cultures in transition. There are serious dangers that some cultures may feel taken over and feel decultured and may respond by reverting back to more religious or fundamentalist positions. Having started as a broadly economic perspective it is likely that economic factors will continue to influence these processes and cultures will respond and mould accordingly. The process of globalisation will also influence models of explaining distress and help-seeking. With economic perspectives shifting, the healthcare delivery systems will also change. The response of stakeholders and the need for adequate resources will also change. For the researchers and clinicians it is worth noting that cultures themselves and individuals will change at different paces. This may also be seen in the same family, where members may acculturate at different levels. Globalisation will not necessarily lead to total homogenisation across cultures but levels of cultural relativism may change. A better awareness of these factors will help policy-makers, planners and mental heath-care professionals.

References

Arnett, J. J. (2002). The psychology of globalization. *American Psychologist*, **57**, 774–83.

Becker, A. E. (2004). Television, disordered eating and young women in Fiji. *Culture Medicine and Psychiatry*, **28**, 533–59.

Berry, J. W. (1992). Acculturation and adaptation in a new society. *International Migration*, **30**, 69–85.

Berry, J. W. (1997). Immigration, acculturation and adaptation. *Applied Psychology: An International Review*, **46**, 5–68.

Berry, J. W. (2007). Acculturation and identity. In D. Bhugra and K. S. Bhui, eds. *Textbook of Cultural Psychiatry*. Cambridge: Cambridge University Press.

Bhugra, D. (2004a). Migration, distress and cultural identity. *British Medical Bulletin*, **69**(1), 129–41.

Bhugra, D. (2004b). *Culture and Self-harm: Attempted Suicide in South Asians in London*. Maudsley Monographs 46. London: Psychology Press.

Bhugra, D. (2004c). Migration and mental health. *Acta Psychiatrica Scandinavica*, **109**(4), 243–58.

Bhugra, D., Mallett, R., Leff, J. (1999). Schizophrenia and African-Caribbeans: a conceptual model of aetiology. *International Review of Psychiatry*, **11**(2), 145–52.

Charlesworth, S. J., Gilfillan, P., Wilkinson, R. (2004). Living inferiority. *British Medical Bulletin*, **69**, 49–60.

Ghodse, H. (2003). Commentary on globalization and psychiatry. *Advances in Psychiatric Treatment*, **9**, 470–3.

Ghuman, P. A. S. (1994). *Coping with Two Cultures*. Cleveden: Multilingual Matters.

Gupta, S., Bhugra, D. (2009). Globalization, economic factors and prevalence of psychiatric disorders. *International Journal of Mental Health*, **38**(3), 53–65.

Hertzman, C. *et al.* (2010). Tackling inequality: get them while they are young. *British Medical Journal*, **340**, 346–8.

Hofstede (1980/2001). *Culture's Consequences: International Differences in Work-Related Values*. Newbury Park, CA: Sage.

Hunter, D., Popay, J., Tanahill, C., Whitehead, M. (2010). Getting to grips with health inequalities at last. *British Medical Journal*, **340**, 323–4.

Jones, K., Woollard, J., Bhugra, D. (2010). Modern social networking and mental health. In C. Morgan and D. Bhugra, eds. *Principles of Social Psychiatry*. London: Wiley-Blackwell.

Kleinman, A. (1980). *Patients and their Healers in the Context of their Culture*. Berkeley, CA: University of California Press.

Layton-Henry, Z. (1992). *The Politics of Immigration*. Oxford: Blackwell.

Marmot, M. (2004). *Status Syndrome: How Your Social Standing Directly Affects Your Health and Life Expectancy*. London: Bloomsbury.

Marmot, M. (2010). *Strategic Review of Health Inequalities in England*. UCL: London, final report.

Morgan, L. H. (1877). *Ancient Society*. NY: Henry Holt.

Okasha, A. (2005). Editorial: globalization and mental health. *World Psychiatry*, **4**, 1–2.

Patel, V., Boardman, J., Prince, M., Bhugra, D. (2006). Returning the debt: how rich countries can invest in mental health capacity in developing countries. *World Psychiatry*, **5**(2), 67–70.

Pickett, K. E., James, O. W., Wilkinson, R. G. (2006). Income inequality and the prevalence of mental illness. *Journal of Epidemiology & Community Health*, **60**, 646–7.

Rex, J. (1987). *Race Relations in Sociological Theory*. London: Routledge and Kegan Paul.

Rose, N. (1996). *Inventing Ourselves: Psychology, Power and Personhood*. Cambridge: Cambridge University Press.

Sashidharan, S. (1993). Afro Caribbeans and schizophrenia. *International Review of Psychiatry*, **5**, 129–44.

Segall, M. H., Dasen, P. R., Berry, J. W., Poortinga, Y. H. (1990). *Human Behaviours in Global Perspective*. NY: Pergamon Press.

Stiglitz, J. (2002). *Globalization and its Discontents*. London: Allen Lane.

Stopes-Roe, M., Cochrane, R. (1991). *Citizens of this Country*. Cleveden: Multilingual Matters.

Tseng W-S. (2004). *Handbook of Cultural Psychiatry*. San Diego, CA: Academic Press.

Tylor, E. B. (1865). *Researches into the Early History of Mankind and Development of Civilization*. London: John Murray.

Wilkinson, R. G. (2005). *The Impact of Inequality: How to Make Sick Societies Healthier*. NY: New Press.

Pre-migration, personality and precipitating factors

Thomas Stompe, David Holzer, Alexander Friedmann[1] and Dinesh Bhugra

Editors' introduction

The period prior to the actual process of migration can be significant for individuals in terms of preparation for the sojourn and also in getting ready for the process of acculturation and adjustment. This preparation, however, is not always possible as it depends upon a number of other factors. The period of pre-migration will also depend upon the reasons for the migration. Biological, cultural or social and psychological factors will influence the response to the act of migration. In this chapter Stompe *et al.* illustrate that there are cultural differences in the prevalence of psychiatric disorders among these groups. In addition, differences in personality characteristics also affect the migration process, along with other factors such as education and socio-economic status. It is therefore likely that the pre-migration period may play a role in future adjustment and settlement. Stompe and colleagues conclude that high rates of schizophrenia in migrants may be related to the voluntary nature of migration. It is useful to understand individual experiences in the pre-migration phase to develop treatment strategies which may be acceptable to individuals.

Introduction

Migrants are not a homogeneous group and neither is migration a homogeneous phenomenon. Large numbers of migrants move for a number of a reasons and varying distances. It is the actual process of migration that will inevitably lead to a number of stressful life events in different spheres of life, depending upon the circumstances leading to migration, levels and degree of social support and the reasons for migration. The migration process will be affected by personality characteristics and other factors such as education, socio-economic status, previous experience of migration and the social capital which people bring with them when they migrate. As stated elsewhere in this volume, the actual process of migration is divisible into three stages: pre-migration, migration and post-migration. These three stages allow us to look at precipitating factors in different ways. The pre-migration period can be a few days or years in length, depending upon possible reasons for migration and the time available for preparation. In circumstances where reasons are for education, the potential migrant may have a longer period to prepare and get ready for the process. Where political reasons lead to migration, escape may have to be very quick. We know that under some circumstances

---

[1] Alexander Friedmann, head of the outpatient department for migrants, died in March 2008.

Migration and Mental Health, ed. Dinesh Bhugra & Susham Gupta. Published by Cambridge University Press. © Cambridge University Press 2011.

migration may be very short-term or temporary, whereas in others it may be permanent with no likelihood of return at all. Thus stresses faced by migrants will depend upon the underlying motives. Migration may be voluntary as by labour, students, diplomats, charity workers, etc. or involuntary, as in seeking asylum or refuge for political or religious reasons and persecution. There is no doubt that migration will offer new opportunities for personal, educational and financial growth, but high rates of several psychiatric disorders have been reported among migrants in different countries. These conditions include schizophrenia (Ödegaard, 1932; Cochrane and Bal, 1987; Harrison *et al.*, 1997; Hutchinson and Haasen, 2004; Cantor-Graae, and Selten, 2005; Fearon *et al.*, 2006; Cooper *et al.*, 2008), mood disorders (Bhugra, 2003; Fazel *et al.*, 2005; Swinnen and Selten, 2007) and, especially, post-traumatic stress disorder (Fazel *et al.*, 2005); also see chapters by Kirkbride and Jones and by Cheng in this volume. In this chapter, we focus on the impact of factors related to pre-migration in precipitating mental disorders and their link with pre-morbid personality.

Background

Several biological, psychological and social environmental and cultural factors interact and lead to the development of a bio-psycho-social model of aetiology and management. Thus the individual at the heart of this interaction is surrounded by environmental and cultural factors. Developing a response will be influenced by the interaction of these factors and the social response to the individual's distress. Personality factors and experiences of resilience in the past will affect how an individual deals with life events and how they adjust in the new environment. The processes of acculturation will depend upon various factors, including the previous experiences, social expectations and personality traits.

The gene patterns across cultures and ethnic groups vary in a complex manner. In the past quarter of a century, huge amount of data have been collected and studied. It is inevitable that human genome will allow individuals to deal with stress and stressors (de Jong, 2007). Dietary patterns, pre-natal care and infections in the ante-natal period are likely to influence personal, social and cognitive development (Mung'Ala-Odera *et al.*, 2004; Bangirana *et al.*, 2006). The core genetic patterns are carried across migratory borders and the response to stress as well as infections may vary, thereby creating another vulnerability factor. Biological and genetic factors are likely to carry on influencing individual development throughout one's life.

Cultural factors

Culture is defined as a distinct pattern of living and sharing values, attitudes, beliefs as they are embedded in art, folk tales, law and other features (Assman, 1988). Individuals are born into a culture and not with a culture. Cultures are dynamic and keep changing as a result of coming into contact with other cultures, through direct or indirect contact. In addition, the individuals carry multiple cultural identities, which may be related to culture, ethnicity, gender, training, education, etc. Culture has been defined in multiple ways (Kroeber and Kluckhohn, 1952). Cultures carry with them cultural memory, which is essential for child development and cognitive development. Moreover, cultural memory becomes extremely significant when individuals migrate. Memories of the past, culture, kinship and family ensure generational continuity. Loss of such memory may produce cultural bereavement (see later in this volume). Cultural memory allows individuals to identify themselves as one group as opposed to another group. This creation of memory may be romantic, rejecting or made up. This may be used in dealing with acculturation and how individuals settle down in other cultures, which will carry their own memory and sometimes these memories may clash. This creation or retention of memory is both historical and fresh for migrants as they come to deal with new contacts, new settings and tensions in the new place to which they have migrated. The communication of cultural memory within the same culture, or to members of other cultures, is important. However, this communication may cause conflict, especially if the memory is idealistic and is not matched by reality or by the other (new) culture's memory and perceptions. The communicated meaning embedded in the cultural memory will influence genuine or mixed interpretations of what's going on. This memory will shape self-image and self-esteem as well. The transmission of cultural memory is important in developing the cultural identity both of the individual belonging to a cultural group and of the cultural group itself. Cultural memory is vital in maintaining core cultural values such as symbols and beliefs.

Ethnic groups also carry collective memory related to shared beliefs and common features of life style, shared traditions and values (Weber, 1972). Ethnicity is self-ascribed and thus becomes a social category, whereas race is a biological concept. Race as a concept came into its own in Britain in the nineteenth century, relying on physical appearance – focusing on skin colour, shape of lips, colour of eyes, etc. Racism is thus a phenomenon where one group, by virtue of its race, takes on the privileges related to education, politics and health. This interaction between an individual's self-identity on the basis of culture, race or ethnicity will also play a role in preparation for migration and post-migration adjustment to the new culture.

Cultural factors directly influence the cognitive development of the child, which is indirectly affected by child rearing patterns. The child rearing and child development will influence personality development. As note above, the concepts of the self are influenced by culture (Markus and Kitayama, 1991). Personality development and personality types will be shaped by cultural values and norms (Triandis and Suh, 2002). For example, antisocial personality characteristics will be determined by the culture once what is social is defined and deemed acceptable. Cultural schema thus influence regulation of the self (Tweed and Lehman, 2002), and both internally and externally. Culture produces both internal and external regulations. The individual personality will respond to external regulations and also develop internal values. The concepts of the self will also ensure different strategies in coping with change and stress.

Cross (1995) reported that independent self-concept is positively related to coping strategies. Thus the way individuals see themselves and their esteem becomes important in dealing with adjustment. The relationship between what the migrant hopes to achieve after they migrate in terms of social, economic or financial status will be influenced by cultural and personal values. This discrepancy between aspiration and achievement has been suggested as a potential contributing factor in explaining the high rates of schizophrenia (Bhugra *et al.*, 1999; Mallett *et al.*, 2003). Illness beliefs will affect help-seeking and therapeutic adherence. As noted above, high rates of schizophrenia among African-Caribbeans in the UK have been confirmed in several studies (Harrison *et al.*, 1997; Bhugra *et al.*, 1997; Sharpley *et al.*, 2001; Kirkbride and Jones in this volume), with similar high rates among some migrants in the Netherlands (Selten *et al.*, 2001). In some of these studies, individuals from minority communities are not migrants, thus raising interesting questions about ethnicity and race in explaining the high rates. These differences are less likely to be genetic and more likely to be socially influenced. This is where the social defeat hypothesis (Selten and Cantor-Graae, 2005) or discrepancy between aspiration and achievement may play a role. However, both these hypotheses need to be tested in the pre-migration stage. It is inevitable that aspirations will be different and may indeed be higher if migration is planned and is for education or economic reasons. If the migration is sudden and the individual has not had time to plan, aspirations may be relatively lower. This needs to be investigated further. In the case of political migrants or refugees, aspirations may be basic in terms of physical survival.

Social factors

Social factors such as unemployment, poor housing, urbanisation, over-crowding and changes in family structure (as, for instance, moving from a joint family set-up to a nuclear family one) have been shown to be related to poor mental health. When people migrate, they may face one or more of these factors, even further if they have experienced these in the pre-migration phase. As rapid social change has also been linked with poor mental health (Rumble *et al.*, 1996), and it is possible that such pre-existing vulnerability to poor mental health may lead to mental illness after migration, especially if social support is poor.

The accumulation of social factors and the correlation between such an interaction and poor mental health can prove to be difficult to disentangle. Social factors such as poor housing, unemployment and poor education are also linked with poverty, which by itself is correlated with increased rates of certain types of mental illness. Furthermore, in periods of economic downturn and debt, it is inevitable that rates of mental disorders will increase. Poverty and malnutrition may further contribute to poor physical and mental health and lead to accidents (Patel and Kleinman, 2003). Pre-migration experiences thus may make the individuals more vulnerable to stresses of migration, especially if it is sudden and urgent.

Economic factors

Migrants who are rich and who may have frequent experiences of migrating will have very different experiences after migration. Film stars, pop stars, diplomats, military personnel and other groups who may move around regularly will have varying pre-migration expectations and post-migration experiences. In addition, taking money with them or access to financial resources will be very different. Poverty may also contribute to family disruption when its members move around in the same country or across boundaries, thereby providing limited social support. These experiences, especially if associated with poor childhood attachment, will be reflected in adult life and social isolation, which may be worse after migration. Economic factors will also influence settling down in the new country.

Education

Poor educational background will influence pre- and post-migration experiences. Those who have high educational achievements may find it difficult to adjust into the new culture if their qualifications are not recognised. For example, a lawyer in one country may find their experiences and education not relevant and may have to take on jobs inferior to their capability and achievements. This may be relevant when aspirations may not be achieved, thereby affecting self-esteem. Similarly, other professions, such as training in medicine, may not be approved in the new country. People with higher or poor education may find it difficult to adjust in the new settings.

Personality

The personality of individuals is a mixture of genetic and environmental factors, but cultures and societies define and dictate what is branded as normal and what is seen as deviant. At the core of an individual's personality is the notion of the self, which is very strongly influenced by culture (Morris, 1994). Cultural meanings of the self are related to social structures, thus the concept of the self has to be seen as both from within and from outside. Morris (1994) argues that cultural paradigms describe people's conceptions of the person as a cultural category. Therefore, notions of the self are culturally influenced and thus amenable to change. The self is a constant factor in the human personality structure and is also intrinsic to the operation of human society, according to Morris (1994) and consequently at the core of social interaction. Personal identity therefore gets defined by the structures of the culture, i.e. whether the culture is collectivist or individualistic. Thus personal identity may be bound in the type of culture an individual comes from: it is not possible that every member of a collectivist culture will have collectivist values. Of course, as a result of acculturation, these values may change. Our contention is that egocentric individuals from collectivist societies may have an easier time adjusting in egocentric societies, though this needs to be tested empirically (see Bhugra, 2005 for a detailed discussion).

It is inevitable that, in some cultures, both men and women will be expected to behave in culture-specific and culturally-normative ways. Castillo (1997) pointed out that men in Swat Valley and hailing from the Pushtun tribe own guns, 'trust no one' and are constantly vigilant (even hyper-vigilant) and protect their honour and personal interests at all costs, indicating a possessive and perhaps maladaptive behaviour according to Western standards, but not a personality disorder. These notions of honour killings in Western society, where women may be consorting with others from outside the tribe, arouse passion, which is clearly seen as pathological by Western standards. Similarly, Castillo (1997) uses the example of schizoid personality to illustrate the similarities in Hindu culture where being detached, and unmoved by good or bad news, is the epitome of good behaviour. Such behaviour will be seen as pathological in Western cultures. Another example highlighted by Castillo (1997) is that of machismo, in which a male Hispanic will demonstrate similar behaviours to a histrionic personality. Paniagua (2000) illustrates that symptoms of narcissistic personality may be seen in many cultures without these being pathological. Paniagua (1998) points out that counter to machismo in the Hispanic culture is marianisma, where the women are expected to be submissive, obedient, dependent, timid and docile, especially with men – many of these features appear in the dependent personality. These examples indicate two things: first, that some personality traits are common in some cultures and should not be pathologised; and second, that these traits will be carried into the new culture and may become exaggerated or diminished in response to migration, although this also remains a further avenue to be explored in research.

MacLachlan (1997) notes very cogently that culture has a strong influence on the construction of the self, and that by comparing ourselves with other people we are able to describe ourselves. As a consequence, social identity of the individual becomes absolutely crucial in relation to 'the other'. Culture inevitably will contain expectations of what is normal. Personality disorders therefore become a source of difficulty in that not only are they influenced by Western cultural norms and included in Western diagnostic classifications, but intriguingly the line between the abnormal and the normal is very thin and is sometimes based on legal concepts.

There are two issues which must be remembered: first, the normality of some traits in some cultures and their potential misuse in the new culture, which may lead to misdiagnosis;

second is the vulnerability of some personality traits to the process of migration and how it would predispose them to migrate.

Taking the presence of some personality traits in some cultures as the starting point, Alarcón and Foulks (1995a, 1995b) highlight some key issues. They argue very persuasively that personality disorder brings into play cultural and social factors in determining which behaviours are valued more and which behaviours are valued less.

Alarcón and Foulks (1995a) indicate that the debate regarding personality disorders is likely to escalate, possibly as a result of biological factors. Moreover, whether these disorders are distinct, lie on a spectrum or can be applied to individuals or cultures, raises interesting questions in exploring and understanding the relationship between culture, personality traits and personality disorders. Personality is typical of a person, thereby distinguishing them from others, and is the outcome of a life-long process of interaction between organism and environment (Berry et al., 1992). These authors (p. 69) challenge clinicians to think of differences in behaviour of individuals to be understood in terms of more permanent psychological dispositions or responses to specific situations. Thus psychodynamic theories, trait theories and social learning theories all play a role, and all of these are culturally influenced. Traits across cultures, according to Berry et al. (1992), will deal with issues to do with locus of control (where an individual explains their distress as being placed internally or externally), expressions of emotions and communication and styles of communication. National character or personality features related to a particular culture allow individuals to use shortcuts to identify individuals, their traits and personality types. The problem, of course, in taking shortcuts is ignoring the individual as well as relying on stereotypes. For example, Sow (1977, 1978) highlights concentric layers of African personality, the outermost being the body and the innermost being the spiritual principle. In this way, the notions of the self as explained by Morris (1994) start to make sense.

Alarcón and Foulks (1995a) also raise significant issues about the distinction between the separateness and the spectrum notions of personality. They point out that gradually a more cogent conceptualisation has emerged, which uses culture as an exploratory, pathogenic or diagnostic tool. Personality styles, they argue, contribute to delineating strategies of action for the handling of concrete situations. Normal development will carry many influences, from child rearing to peer pressures and interactions with the environment, whether that is within the family, the kinship or society as a whole. The process related to individuation will be influenced by a number of factors, including whether the culture is sociocentric or egocentric. The egocentric view considers the individual as a discrete identity and therefore the boundaries between the individual and the environment are likely to be more rigid. However, the social expectations and individual rebellion may turn the individual to become their own master and develop their traits at their own pace.

When individuals from one culture enter another culture as a result of migration, the changes in their behaviour as a result of acculturation are likely to be influenced at different levels. Some behaviours will change more rapidly than others and different members of the kinship, family or the group will be at different levels of changes, thereby making clinical interventions more difficult. Slow acculturation is likely to be criticised by the new culture and fast acculturation by members of their own group.

As noted above, gender roles and gender role expectations play an important role in the development of personality, as well as the expectations of an individual. Masculinity and femininity may carry different meanings in different cultures. Furthermore, as Hofstede (2000) has described, cultures themselves may be divided into masculine and feminine. As

Table 5.1 Some personality traits and DSM-IV categories (also see MacLachlan, 1997 and Alarcón and Foulks, 1995a)

	Behaviour	Common in cultures	DSM-IV categories
1.	Secretive/mistrustful	Arabs, Mediterranean	Paranoid
2.	Speaking in tongues Peculiar religious ideas	Evangelical religions	Schizotypal
3.	Indifference Not attached	Hindus	Schizoid
4.	Self-harm	Arabs, Native Americans	Borderline
5.	Emotionality Seductiveness Self-centred Dramatic	Mediterranean Hispanics	Histrionic
6.	Flamboyant Self-important	Latin Americans	Narcissistic
7.	Distrust Oversensitive Withdrawal	Oppressed groups	Avoidant
8.	Passive Deferential	Latin American women	Dependent

Alarcón and Foulks (1995a) recommend, it is crucial to apply the principles of cultural contextualisation of behaviour as well as personality.

The role of culture in leading to an explanation and an interpretation of psychopathology has been alluded to earlier. Research assessment using appropriate diagnostic tools and development must be culturally sensitive. Culture allows the interpretation of behaviour. However, what is conceivably 'normal' in the pre-migration phase may become abnormal, especially as the cultural context changes dramatically or even very slightly when normal behaviour is reclassified as abnormal or deviant. Emphasis on types of personality traits which are seen as a problem verging on personality disorders brings with it a further series of problems.

Table 5.1 illustrates some of the issues derived from the descriptions by Alarcón and Foulks and maps these on to DSM-IV diagnostic categories. Some of the examples have already been used earlier in the chapter.

DSM-IV remains an important system, but is very strongly influenced by the US culture. Personality is also an important aspect of response from the other in the new culture. For example, if an individual acts rigidly or is suspicious of the officialdom, particularly in these days of increased security awareness, the officials may respond inappropriately, thus escalating paranoid responses. Through family-based learning, the individual may develop defenses which may lead to borderline or antisocial behaviours (Alarcón and Foulks, 1995a).

Alarcón and Foulks (1995b) raise the important point that a major issue for the diagnostician working across cultures is the requirement to differentiate the ideal personality type, the typical personality and the atypical personality from the cultural perspective. In spite of the fact that personality disorders have rather poor diagnostic validity and reliability, for the clinician, underlying personality traits are significant in understanding the normative behaviour of people belonging to one culture. Humans have a genetic inheritance that is born into them and a cultural inheritance into which they are born

(Lidz, 1979). Culture is one of many factors that contribute to human development; therefore when working across cultures, the clinician must look around for a number of factors and the potential for complex interaction between these factors.

Clinicians may find it possible to accept research criteria and diagnostic tools (Loranger *et al.*, 1994) but these arguably are related to categories created in different cultures. Prevalence rates of various personality disorders vary across cultures (Compton *et al.*, 1991) – the challenge is whether these are true differences related to cultural differences or artificial differences as a result of different methods being used. As Tseng (2001) notes, there is no argument that in each society there will be people whose behaviours will deviate markedly from what the culture expects of them, but the threshold to identify such deviation will vary too.

Self-selection or drift hypothesis

Another key factor in the pre-migration phase is the process of social drift, which may occur from rural to urban areas or that movement may be preferred by these individuals. This process may also lead to forced migration, as has been seen in recent times in Romas being expelled from France. Thus both national policy and traumatic events may contribute to this. In this chapter, we do not propose to discuss post-traumatic stress disorder (PTSD), which may precipitate migration by itself or may be a sequel to the process of traumatic sudden migration.

Role expectations may be worth exploring further, both at pre-migration and post-migration levels. Role stress is said to be related to role conflict, ambiguity regarding role expectations and ambiguity regarding role evaluations (Naditch and Morrissey, 1976). Combined with personality traits, these may give a clue to coping strategies people may use while migrating and in the post-migration period of adjustment.

Therefore, the process of migration, heterogeneity in the group, expectations of the new country and aspirations, along with the response of the new country will determine how individuals settle down and adjust to new settings and get acculturated. Reasons for migration and time made available to prepare for the process will influence post-migration settling down, especially if there are cultural factors at play as well. Stompe *et al.* (2010) reported that voluntary migrants in their sample were more likely to develop schizophrenia, whereas forced migrants developed neuroses. Interestingly, migrants from Muslim countries had lower rates of substance abuse disorders. Those who had experienced traumatic stress in the pre-migration phase developed neurotic disorders and stress-related disorders after migration. This study illustrates in some depth experiences in the pre-migration period and their impact on post-migration adjustment. However, the data were collected from an outpatients' facility over a 12-year period in Vienna. The study illustrates the differences in outcome and also the role of religion and other factors in the pre-migration phase.

In the process of migration, the individual migrant's personality traits, along with cultural values or "personality of the culture", will interact and play a key role in settling down and enabling the migrants to acculturate.

Conclusions

Response to the process of migration will be influenced by previous experiences of coping with positive and negative life events. Childhood development and personality will contribute to coping strategies. After migration, the possibility of cultural bereavement, culture shock or cultural conflict will play a role in adjustment to the new culture. Not every migrant is likely to go through this process, but clinicians must be aware of this, especially if the migration is involuntary. Further work is necessary in understanding the role of personality and the period of pre-migration in adjustment of the migrants to the next stages of settlement, whether these are acculturation at an individual level or at a group level. The stressful pre-migration period may lead to neurotic disorders after arrival in the new country. However, these experiences do not fall into neat packages, and other factors – such as education, economic status and social capital, along with the nature of the new culture, acceptance and welcome by the new culture – will also play a role. Cultural identity of the migrant and personality factors, along with idioms of distress and explanatory models, as well as coping strategies, will also play a role in post-migration adjustment. Clinicians must take individual processes into account, keeping the individual at the centre of the assessment but ensuring that the individual migrant's culture and larger (new) culture are also part of the process in understanding individual distress.

References

Alarcón, R. D., Foulks, E. F. (1995a). Personality disorders and culture: contemporary clinical views (Part A). *Cult Diversity and Mental Health*, **1**, 3–17.

Alarcón, R. D., Foulks, E. F. (1995b). Personality disorders and culture: contemporary clinical views (Part B). *Cult Diversity and Mental Health*, **1**, 79–91.

Assmann, J. (1988). Kollektives Gedächtnis und kulturelle Identität. In J. Assmann and T. Hölscher, *Kultur und Gedächtnis*. Frankfurt am Main: Suhrkamp, 9–19.

Bangirana, P., Idro, R., John, C. C., Boivin, M. J. (2006). Rehabilitation for cognitive impairments after cerebral malaria in African children: strategies and limitations. *Tropical Medicine & International Health*, **11**, 1341–9.

Berry, J., Poortinga, Y. H., Segall, M. H., Dawson, P. R. (1992). *Cross-Cultural Psychology*. Cambridge: Cambridge University Press.

Bhugra, D. (2003). Migration and depression. *Acta Psychiatrica Scandinavica* Suppl., **418**, 67–72.

Bhugra, D. (2005). Cultural identities and cultural congruency: a new model for evaluating mental distress in immigrants. *Acta Psychiatrica Scandinavica*, **111** (2), 84–93.

Bhugra, D., Leff, J., Mallett, R., Der, G., Corridan, B., Rudge, S. (1997). Incidence and outcome of schizophrenia in Whites, African-Caribbeans and Asians in London. *Psychological Medicine*, **27** (4), 791–8.

Bhugra, D., Mallett, R., Leff, J. (1999). Schizophrenia and African-Caribbeans: a conceptual model of aetiology. *International Review of Psychiatry*, **11** (2), 145–52.

Cantor-Graae, E., Selten, J. (2005). Schizophrenia and migration: a meta-analysis and review. *American Journal of Psychiatry*, **162**, 12–24.

Castillo, R. J. C. (1997). *Culture and Mental Illness*. Pacific Grove, CA: Brooke/Cole.

Cochrane, R., Bal, S. (1987). Migration and schizophrenia: an examination of five hypotheses. *Social Psychiatry*, **22**, 181–91.

Compton, W., Helzer, J., Hwu, H. *et al.* (1991). New methods in cross cultural psychiatry: Psychiatric illness in Taiwan and the US. *American Journal of Psychiatry*, **148**, 1697–1704.

Cooper, C., Morgan, C., Byrne, M. *et al.* (2008). Perceptions of disadvantage, ethnicity and psychosis. *British Journal of Psychiatry*, **192**, 185–90.

Cross, S. E. (1995). Self-construals, coping, and stress in cross-cultural adaptation. *Journal of Cross-Cultural Psychology*, **26** (6), 673–97.

de Jong, J. T. (2007). Traumascape: an ecological – cultural – historical model for extreme stress. In D. Bhugra and K. Bhui, eds. *Textbook of Cultural Psychiatry*. Cambridge: Cambridge University Press, pp. 347–63.

Fazel, M., Wheeler, J., Danesh, J. (2005). Prevalence of serious mental disorder in 7000 refugees resettled in western countries: a systematic review. *Lancet*, **36**, 1309–14.

Fearon, P., Kirkbride, J. B., Morgan, C. *et al.* (2006). AESOP Study Group. Incidence of schizophrenia and other psychoses in ethnic minority groups: results from the MRC AESOP Study. *Psychological Medicine*, **36**, 1541–50.

Harrison, G., Glazebrook, C., Brewin, J. *et al.* (1997). Increased incidence of psychotic disorders in migrants from the Caribbean to the United Kingdom. *Psychological Medicine*, **27**, 799–806.

Hofstede, G. (2000). *Culture's Consequences: Comparing Values, Behaviors, Institutions, and Organizations across Nations* (2nd edn). Thousand Oaks, CA: Sage Publications.

Hutchinson, G., Haasen, C. (2004). Migration and schizophrenia. *Social Psychiatry and Psychiatric Epidemiology*, **39**, 350–7.

Kroeber, A. L., Kluckhohn, C. (1952). *Culture: A Critical Review of Concepts and Definitions*. New York: Vintage Books.

Lidz, T. (1979). Family studies and changing concepts of personality development. *Canadian Journal of Psychiatry*, **24**, 621–3.

Loranger, A. W., Sartorius, N., Andreoli, A. *et al.* (1994). The international personality disorder examination. *Archives of General Psychiatry*, **51**, 215–24.

MacLachlan, M. (1997). *Culture and Health.* Chichester: John Wiley & Sons.

Mallett, R., Leff, J., Bhugra, D., Takei, N., Corridan, B. (2003). Ethnicity, goal striving and schizophrenia: a case-control study of three ethnic groups in the United Kingdom. *International Journal of Social Psychiatry*, **50**, 331–4.

Markus, H. R., Kitayama, S. (1991). Culture and self: implications for cognition, emotion, and motivation. *Psychological Review*, **98**, 224–53.

Morris, B. (1994). *Anthropology of the Self.* London: Pluto Press.

Mung'Ala-Odera, V. Snow, R. W., Newton, C. R. (2004). The burden of the neurocognitive impairment associated with *Plasmodium falciparum* malaria in sub-saharan Africa. *American Journal of Tropical Medicine and Hygiene*, **71** (2 Suppl.), 64–70.

Naditch, M. P., Morrissey, R. F. (1976). Role stress, personality and psychopathology in a group of immigrant adolescents. *Journal of Abnormal Psychology*, **85**, 115–18.

Ödegaard, Ö. (1932). Emigration and insanity: a study of mental disease among the Norwegian-born population of Minnesota. *Acta Psychiatrica Neurologica Scandinavica*, **4**, 1–206.

Paniagua, F. A. (1998). *Assessing and Treating Culturally Diverse Clients: A Practical Guide.* Newbury Park, CA: Sage.

Paniagua, F. A. (2000). Culture bound syndromes. In I. Cuéllar and F. A. Paniagua, eds. *Handbook of Multicultural Mental Health.* San Diego: Academic Press, pp. 142–69.

Patel, V., Kleinman, A. (2003). Poverty and common mental disorders in developing countries. *Bulletin of the World Health Organization*, **81**, 609–15.

Rumble, S., Swartz, L., Parry, C., Zwarenstein, M. (1996). Prevalence of psychiatric morbidity in the adult population of a rural South African village. *Psychological Medicine*, **26**, 997–1007.

Selten, J. P. Cantor-Graae, E. (2005). Social defeat: risk factors for schizophrenia. *British Journal of Psychiatry*, **187**, 101–2.

Selten, J. P., Veen, N., Feller, W. *et al.* (2001). Incidence of psychotic disorders in immigrant groups to The Netherlands. *British Journal of Psychiatry*, **78**, 367–72.

Sharpley, M., Hutchinson, G., McKenzie, K., Murray, R. M. (2001). Understanding the excess of psychosis among the African-Caribbean population in England. Review of current hypotheses. *British Journal of Psychiatry*, Suppl. **40**, S60–8.

Sow I. (1977). *Psychiatrie Dynamique Africaine.* Paris: Payot.

Sow I. (1978). *Les Structures Anthropologiques de la Folie en Afrique Noire.* Paris: Payot.

Stompe, T., Holzer, D., Friedmann, A. (2010). Premigration and mental health of refugees. In D. Bhugra, T. Craig, and K. Bhui, eds. *Mental Health of Refugees and Asylum Seekers*. Oxford: Oxford University Press, pp. 23–38.

Swinnen, S. G., Selten, J. P. (2007). Mood disorders and migration: meta-analysis. *British Journal of Psychiatry*, **190**, 6–10.

Triandis, H. C., Suh, E. M. (2002). Cultural influences on personality. *Annual Review of Psychology*, **53**, 133–60.

Tseng, W-S, (2001). *Handbook of Cultural Psychiatry*. San Diego: Academic Press.

Tweed, R. G., Lehman, D. R. (2002). Learning considered within a cultural context: Confucian and Socratic approaches. *American Psychologist*, **57**, 89–99.

Weber, M. (1972). Ethnische Gemeinschaftsbeziehungen. In M. Weber ed. *Wirtschaft und Gesellschaft*. Tübingen: Mohr Siebeck, pp. 234–40.

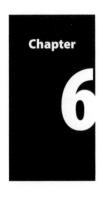

Ethnicity, migration and mental health: the role of social and economic inequalities

James Nazroo and Karen Iley

Editors' introduction

Migrants often end up doing unpopular jobs in the new country. As the aim is to settle down as soon as practically possible and financial imperatives dictate, migrants may take up work which locals may reject. From manual work to unpopular specialties in professions, it is likely that migrants may face a discrepancy between their aspirations and their achievements. After migration, further social and economic inequalities may contribute to a sense of low achievement and contribute to low self-esteem and chronic stress. Nazroo and Iley argue that economic inequalities may contribute to possible explanations of elevated rates of different illnesses in different ethnic groups. These inequalities are related to low income, poor housing, unemployment, social support, etc. Other factors, such as access to healthcare, will determine pathways into care, and attitudes of service providers will determine what is available, appropriate and used by patients. There is no doubt that treatment-based statistics have problems but conflation of ethnicity or race with culture also adds to problems of healthcare delivery. The challenge for policy-makers and clinicians is to look beyond simple epidemiological data.

Introduction

One of the most striking findings in the literature on inequalities in health in the UK is that black Caribbean people are three to five times more likely to be admitted to a psychiatric hospital with a diagnosis of first episode of psychosis than white people (Cochrane and Bal, 1989; Harrison *et al.*, 1988; McGovern and Cope, 1987; Van Os *et al.*, 1996), and some have reported even higher rates (Fearon *et al.*, 2006). This difference is larger than that for any other condition or ethnic group in the UK except diabetes, where differences between white and most ethnic minority groups are of a similar order of magnitude (Erens *et al.*, 2001; Nazroo, 2001; Sproston and Mindell, 2006). This greater risk of psychotic illness is apparent for black populations in other developed countries (for example, Breshnahan *et al.*, 2007; Cantor-Graae and Selton, 2005; Cantor-Graae *et al.*, 2005; Robins and Reiger, 1991; Selten *et al.*, 1997, 2001; Veling *et al.*, 2006). Although there is universal agreement that such findings are a matter of great concern, variations in how they are interpreted, and therefore the object of such concern, have led to great disagreement and controversy. This is, perhaps, not surprising, given that the topic has the potential to align mental disorder with ethnic/racial identity (Sashidharan, 1993), whereby the increased risk of such illnesses is considered to be driven by essential characteristics of the ethnic/racial group.

Migration and Mental Health, ed. Dinesh Bhugra & Susham Gupta. Published by Cambridge University Press. © Cambridge University Press 2011.

The variations in how such findings are interpreted range from the view that they reflect the character and circumstances of people in different ethnic/race groups to the claim that they reflect racism and racist research agendas. So, if the research evidence is accepted at face value, it can be seen as an opportunity for a further exploration of risk factors for mental illness, through an exploration of the characteristics of those ethnic minority groups with higher rates. And, insofar as such differences might be considered to be a consequence of the social and economic inequalities that ethnic minority groups face, such evidence can be used to press for policy development to address these inequalities. However, those who have regarded the data more critically have identified a range of methodological flaws in existing research, leading them to question the uncritical acceptance of the findings by the majority of the research and policy community, how this aligns with existing stereotypes about the lives and experiences of ethnic minority people, and how this leads to a reinforcing of racial stereotypes and the failure to identify racism as a key component of ethnic/racial minority people's interactions with both psychiatric services and the research community. These contrasting positions are reflected in the comments of Singh and Burns (2006) and Fernando (2003). Singh and Burns state:

> The excess of psychosis in the African-Caribbean community in the UK is real and well accepted by epidemiologists and researchers (page 649)

and

> Construing racism as the main explanation for the excess of detentions [under the Mental Health Act] among ethnic minorities adds little to the debate and prevents the search for the real causes of these differences (pages 649–50).

Their targets in making these comments are those who claim that psychiatric practice is institutionally racist. Fernando (2003) is an example of this. He writes:

> There is now an extensive body of theory and research documenting the ways in which race, ethnicity, gender and class . . . are causally linked to mental health problems, The problem is that none of this research seems to touch medical psychiatric research (page 203)

and

> The main and perhaps most serious problem is institutional racism that pervades all major systems affecting British people, including mental health services and the main disciplines that inform such services, namely psychology and psychiatry (page 25).

In this chapter we adopt a position that emphasises the role of social and economic inequalities in the production of both ethnic/racial differences in risk of mental illness, and in constructing the experience of ethnic/racial minorities in psychiatric care. We begin by outlining the key findings that have emerged on ethnic differences in mental illness in the UK, with a primary focus on psychotic illnesses. Following this we review potential explanations for the sometimes contradictory findings that have been reported. We will then critically review the sources of data that have produced these findings, particularly focusing on the validity of statistics based on treatment rates, with the intention of allowing the reader to more carefully judge the validity of the conclusions that have been drawn. This will be followed by a discussion of ethnic minority people's experiences of mental health services and the implications this has for healthcare provision and practice. We will finish with a discussion of the conclusions that can be drawn on ethnic inequalities in mental health, placing emphasis on how these are embedded in the social inequalities faced by ethnic minority people and how psychiatric institutions and practices are also embedded in these wider inequalities.

Ethnicity/race and mental illness: a summary of key findings

Ethnic differences in risk of psychotic illnesses have been the primary focus of research in the mental health field, and most of this work has been based on studies of treatment rates. This is not surprising: the low prevalence of these conditions (about one in 100 people), the difficulty of their measurement and the relatively small proportion of the population made up of ethnic minorities in the UK (only 7.9% of the population described themselves as non-white at the 2001 Census) makes the conduct of such studies in the community extremely difficult. Over the past three decades, studies of treatment rates in the UK have consistently shown elevated rates of schizophrenia among black Caribbean people compared with the white population. Black Caribbean people are typically reported to be three to five times more likely than whites to be admitted to hospital with a first diagnosis of schizophrenia (Bagley, 1971; Cochrane and Bal, 1989; Harrison *et al.*, 1988; Littlewood and Lipsedge, 1988; McGovern and Cope, 1987; Van Os *et al.*, 1996). These findings have been repeated in studies that have looked at first contact with all forms of treatment, rather than just hospital services (Fearon *et al.*, 2006; King *et al.*, 1994), although the rates in one such study were only twice those of the white population (Bhugra *et al.*, 1997). Some of the more recent of these studies have also looked at those of African ethnicity and have reported similarly raised rates of psychotic illness in this group (Fearon *et al.*, 2006; King *et al.*, 1994; Van Os *et al.*, 1996). Explorations of the demographic characteristics of black people admitted to hospital with a psychotic illness suggest that these illnesses are particularly common among young men (Cochrane and Bal, 1989), and some studies have suggested that the rates of schizophrenia for black Caribbean people born in Britain are even higher than for those who migrated – one widely cited study reported that young British-born black Caribbean men were 18 times more likely than average to experience an admission for a first episode of psychosis (Harrison *et al.*, 1988; see also McGovern and Cope, 1987).

Given the consistency of the evidence based on treatment statistics, it is somewhat surprising that they are not repeated in the two national community-based surveys of mental illness among ethnic minority groups in the UK, the Fourth National Survey of Ethnic Minorities (FNS) (Nazroo, 1997) and the EMPIRIC study (Sproston and Nazroo, 2002). Overall, these studies found that Caribbean people had rates of psychotic illness that were at most twice as high as those in the general population. For example, in the FNS (Nazroo, 1997) the annual prevalence of psychotic illness for black Caribbean people was 14 per 1000, in comparison with the rate of 8 per 1000 for the white group (that is 75% higher in the Caribbean group). When differences were considered across gender, age and migrant/non-migrant groups it was found that the prevalence of psychotic illness among men, young men and non-migrant men was no greater than that for equivalent white groups. For example, the annual prevalence of psychotic disorder among Caribbean men was estimated as 10 per 1000 while among white British men it was estimated as 8 per 1000 (Nazroo, 1997). This contrasts with treatment data, where the largest differences have been reported for young men; indeed, the higher rate found for Caribbean people in the community surveys was entirely driven by the higher rate found for Caribbean women.

Findings on rates of psychotic illness among other ethnic minority groups are more mixed. Studies of hospital-based treatment suggest that rates of admission for psychotic illness among South Asian people are similar to those among white people (Cochrane and Bal, 1989). A more comprehensive prospective study of first contact for schizophrenia with *all* treatment services in one area of London (whose South Asian population is predominantly of Indian origin) confirmed this (Bhugra *et al.*, 1997), but an earlier study using the same methods in another London district suggested that rates of psychotic illness among South Asian people (of Indian and Pakistani origin) were raised to similar levels to those found among black Caribbean people (King *et al.*, 1994). Indeed, King *et al.*'s study suggested that rates of psychotic illness among all ethnic minority groups studied were similarly raised in comparison with a white group, and that among the white people identified as having a first onset of psychotic illness the majority were not of British origin (King *et al.*, 1994). Elsewhere the authors state that: 'Most [patients] were from an ethnic minority background, including those people defined as White' (Cole *et al.*, 1995, page 771). This, of course, suggests that it is misleading to maintain an exclusive focus on those of black Caribbean origin when examining ethnic differences in psychotic illness.

In contrast to some of the findings for contact with treatment services, the community-based FNS and EMPIRIC prevalence studies suggested that rates of psychotic illness might not be raised for South Asian people generally, and may be lower for Bangladeshi people than for white British people (Nazroo, 1997; Sproston and Nazroo, 2002). In support of the conclusions drawn by King *et al.* (1994) and Cole *et al.* (1995), the FNS data also showed a high rate of psychosis among white people who were not of British origin, who had a 75% higher rate than the white British group (Nazroo, 1997), although this finding was not replicated in the oversample of Irish people in the EMPIRIC study (Sproston and Nazroo, 2002).

Returning to the situation of black Caribbean people, it is worth noting that treatment statistics suggest very low rates of depression compared with white people (Cochrane and Bal, 1989; Lloyd, 1993). This marked contrast with psychotic illness is a puzzle, because most (non-genetic) factors that might be implicated in the higher rates of psychotic disorders should also lead to a higher rate of other mental illnesses. Such statistics become more puzzling when considered alongside evidence from the FNS suggesting that the prevalence of depression among black Caribbean people in the community is, in fact, more than 50% higher than that among white people (Nazroo, 1997). Moreover, that study also suggested that, despite this higher prevalence, rates of treatment for depression among black Caribbean people were much lower than those for any other group and, unlike for other groups, were not related to level of depression symptoms – that is, treatment rates were low for black Caribbean people with and without a significant level of symptoms (Nazroo, 1997).

This review of evidence shows that the interpretation of statistics on the high rates of psychotic illness among black populations is problematic. Nevertheless, they have formed the basis for the discussion and research of possible underlying causes for the higher risk. So, before we go on to examine the methodological underpinnings of these statistics more critically, we discuss possible explanations for a higher risk, contrasting those that focus on the characteristics of ethnic/race groups and those that focus on the inequalities faced by minority groups.

Explaining ethnic inequalities in risk of mental illness

The kind of explanations suggested for the observed greater risk of psychotic illnesses among black Caribbean people are similar to those considered more generally in the epidemiological literature on ethnic inequalities in health (Nazroo, 2001, 2003), which in turn reflect those discussed as long ago as the Black Report on inequalities in health in the UK (Townsend and Davidson, 1982). Here we discuss non-health service-related factors (which are discussed fully in the next two sections of this chapter), under four broad headings. The first three, migration, genetics and culture, reflect identification of the characteristics of those at greater risk that are assumed to be relevant (the assumption being that ethnicity equates to genetic and cultural difference, and migration), while the final heading, social and economic inequalities, reflects the contexts of their lives.

Migration

Within the European context ethnic differences in health are often considered in relation to processes of migration, because the presence of significant non-white populations in Europe is a result of the relatively recent post-World War 2 migration. So, in this context different rates of psychotic illness across black Caribbean and white groups in the UK could be a consequence of factors related to the process of migration and post-migration life. Here most emphasis has been placed on two possibilities: that social selection into a migrant group could have favoured those with a higher (or, theoretically in this case, lower) risk of developing illness; and that the stresses associated with migration might have increased risks. There is evidence to both support and counter these suggestions. Investigations of the rates of schizophrenia in Jamaica and Trinidad suggest that they are much lower than those for black Caribbean people in the UK and, in fact, that they are similar to those of the white population of the UK (Bhugra *et al.*, 1996; Hickling, 1991; Hickling and Rodgers-Johnson, 1995). This would suggest that the higher rates for black Caribbean people in the UK are either a consequence of factors related to the migration process, and/or the greater stresses surrounding the lives of ethnic minority people in the UK.

However, if the higher rates were a consequence of stress around migration, we would also expect other migrant groups to have higher rates of mental illness. As described earlier, evidence here is contradictory. On the whole studies have suggested that other migrants to the UK, in particular South Asian people, do not have similarly raised rates (Cochrane and Bal, 1989), although King *et al.* (1994) strongly came to the conclusion that the risk of schizophrenia was markedly higher in all migrant groups (including white migrant groups). In addition, if the higher rates of psychotic illness among black Caribbean people were a consequence of selection into a migrant group or the stresses associated with migration, one would expect the rates for those born in the UK to begin to approximate those of the white population. However, also as described earlier, studies have suggested that rates of schizophrenia for second generation black Caribbean people are markedly higher than for the first generation (Harrison *et al.*, 1988; see also McGovern and Cope, 1987). This indicates that factors relating directly to the process of migration may not be involved, although these data (like most work in this area) are dependent on a very small number of identified cases.

Genetic differences

In much of the research on ethnicity and health, ethnicity is equated with genetically defined races, and genetic difference is mobilised as a potential explanation for observed differences in health. Not surprisingly, then, there has been some discussion of the possibility that differences in risk of psychotic illness between black and white people may be a consequence of genetic factors that correlate with ethnic/racial background, but little supporting evidence has been marshalled. In fact, what evidence there is suggests large differences in risk within ethnic/racial categories, implying that any genetic basis for such mental illness does not correlate closely with ethnic/racial background. For example, the evidence on schizophrenia cited in the previous section, which shows that there are important differences between black Caribbean people who stayed in Jamaica or Trinidad (who do not have raised rates) those who migrated to Britain (who appear to have raised rates) and those who were born in Britain (who appear to have markedly raised rates), suggests that the higher rates cannot be a straightforward consequence of ethnic differences in genetic risk.

Culture

As for claims to genetic differences, explanations based on claims of the significance of cultural difference are often mobilised by those attempting to interpret research showing ethnic difference in health. And, perhaps not surprisingly, such an approach to this explanation typically bases the cultural argument on speculative and stereotyped characterisations of the cultures of ethnic minority groups, which do not acknowledge the dynamic and contextual nature of culture (Ahmad, 1996). An examination of discussions in the UK around the higher risk of death from suicide among young female migrants from South Asia is illustrative of the inadequacy of explanations that resort to such an approach.

Research evidence has shown that South Asian people in general have a low or average risk of depression (Cochrane and Bal, 1989; Cochrane and Stopes-Roe, 1981; Gilliam et al., 1989; Nazroo, 1997; Sproston and Nazroo, 2002), but that migrant women from South Asia in the 15–24-year age group have a two to three times greater risk of death from suicide than the national average – a greater risk that is not found for older women or men (Karmi et al., 1994; Soni Raleigh and Balarajan, 1992; Soni Raleigh et al., 1990). To explain both these low and high rates of illness, the same stereotype is used in markedly different ways. So, in language that is reminiscent of the concept of social capital (though it predates its popularity in the health inequalities field), it has been suggested that the overall lower rates of mental illness among South Asian people could be a consequence of an Asian culture that provides extended and strong communities with protective social support networks (Cochrane and Bal, 1989). In contrast, in the attempt to explain the high mortality rates from suicide among young women born in South Asia, close and extended South Asian communities are portrayed as demanding of young people, constraining and conflictual, leading to the oppression of young women and contributing to the higher suicide rates (Soni Raleigh and Balarajan, 1992), rather than as supportive and cohesive.

Of course, a closer examination shows that such stereotypes may not hold. For example, despite the focus on patriarchal 'South Asian' families, there are, in fact, great similarities between the motives of white and South Asian patients for their suicidal actions. In one study of attempted suicide, Handy et al. (1991) report that arguments with parents were a common factor for both white and Asian children, and in another study of attempted suicide Merrill and Owens' (1986) examples of 'restrictive Asian customs (for example, not allowing them to go out at night, mix with boys, or take further education)' (page 709) are not greatly different from what one might find in a dispute between a young white woman and her parents. Indeed, a study of coroners' reports on actual suicides in London found that only one-third of the 12 South Asian women who had committed suicide had 'family conflict' cited among the reasons for the suicide, and only by stretching the imagination could these be considered as specific to South Asian cultures (Karmi et al., 1994).

It is also worth noting that the literature attempting to explain these high rates of death from suicide was largely generated in the early 1990s. In contemporary times it seems strange to be talking of 'South Asian' women in this way; rather the stereotype offered is one that is now typically, and routinely, applied to Muslim communities and Muslim women. It is, then, perhaps surprising to find that these high death rates do not apply to women born in the predominantly Muslim countries of Pakistan and Bangladesh. A more recent paper showed that rates for those women are, in fact, very low, with the high rates exclusively present for those born in India and East Africa (Soni Raleigh, 1996). This example illustrates both how the significance of a particular ethnic identity can change dramatically over a short period of time, with a shift from a discussion of 'South Asians' to one of 'Muslims', and also how this shift in significance has the potential to shape how we respond to research evidence.

Socio-economic inequalities and the impact of racism

Inequalities in economic position across ethnic groups are marked. For example, in the UK 90% of Bangladeshi people are in the bottom third of household incomes, compared with 69% of Pakistani, 48% of Caribbean, 45% of Indian and 41% of Chinese people (Nazroo and Williams, 2005). However, a focus on social causation is rare in the literature examining the aetiology of psychotic illness (Jarvis, 2007), in part because in much of this literature social inequalities are hypothesised to result from illness rather than the other way around. Nevertheless, it would not be surprising if the poor, run down, inner city environments and poor housing in which many ethnic minority people live, and their poorer employment prospects and standards of living, led to greater mental distress and increased risk of psychotic illness (King *et al.*, 1994). Although many have speculated that this may be the case, socio-economic inequalities have not been a primary area of empirical investigation in this field, perhaps because of data limitations (studies of contact with treatment services do not, on the whole, collect information on socio-economic position). In addition, where socio-economic inequalities have been studied, the methods have often been inappropriate (Nazroo, 1998). There has been considerable criticism of this failure, with commentators suggesting that ignoring the possibility that the relationship between ethnicity and mental health is a consequence of social disadvantage allows the theoretical alignment of psychiatric disorder with an essentialised ethnic difference and encourages a focus on genetic or cultural explanations (Sashidharan, 1993; Sashidharan and Francis, 1993). Perhaps not surprisingly, where the connection with socio-economic inequalities has been investigated small numbers of cases have given limited statistical power, but suggested that socio-economic inequalities might be important for risk of psychotic illness in the black Caribbean group (Nazroo, 1997; Sproston and Nazroo, 2002). This effect is illustrated in Table 6.1, which uses data from the

Table 6.1 Ethnic group and presence of symptoms suggestive of psychosis. Values are percentages

	White	Irish	Caribbean	Indian	Pakistani	Bangladeshi
Occupation						
Non-manual	4.0	7.4	8.0	7.6	11.7	3.7
Manual	6.3	6.9	13.2	8.2	7.7	4.7
Not working	22.0	16.7	19.0	14.6	13.3	6.1

EMPIRIC study to show the relationship between reporting symptoms suggestive of psychosis and an occupational measure of socio-economic position. If a broader spectrum of mental illnesses is considered, findings from the FNS show a marked socio-economic patterning within all of the ethnic groups covered, and that this patterning contributes to differences across groups (Nazroo, 1997).

This is consistent with the broader literature on ethnic/racial inequalities in health, which clearly demonstrates the significance of socio-economic inequalities, both within and across ethnic groups (Nazroo, 1998, 2001, 2003). So, within an ethnic/racial group greater socio-economic resources correlate with better health, and differences between ethnic/racial groups in the level of health are largely accounted for by socio-economic inequalities. This is the case for a wide range of health outcomes and in a range of national contexts (Nazroo and Williams, 2005).

However, the study of socio-economic inequalities in health across ethnic groups is not straightforward. While Table 6.1 shows a clear socio-economic gradient *within* ethnic groups, differences *across* ethnic groups in particular occupations remain – for example, in the non-manual group 4% of white people have symptoms suggestive of psychosis compared with 8% of Caribbean people, and the figures are 6.3% and 13.2% for the manual group. A straightforward interpretation of these data assumes that when standardising for socio-economic position all necessary factors are accounted for by the measures available (Kauffman *et al.*, 1997, 1998), but this assumption is wrong in most cases. An analysis of ethnic differences in income within class groups showed that within each class group ethnic minority people had a smaller income than white people (Nazroo, 1998, 2001). Indeed, for the poorest group – Pakistani and Bangladeshi people – differences were two-fold and equivalent in size to the difference between the richest and poorest class groups in the white population. Similar findings have been reported in the USA. For example, within occupational groups white people have higher incomes than black people. Once below the poverty line black people are more likely to remain in this situation than white people, and within income strata black people have considerably lower wealth levels than white people and are less likely to be home owners (Oliver and Shapiro, 1995). This reflects both the particular economic location of ethnic minority groups and the multidimensional nature of the economic and social inequalities they face, covering: economic activity; employment levels; educational outcomes; housing; geographical location; area deprivation; racism and discrimination; citizenship and claims to citizenship. Studies are often designed in a way that is inadequate for the study of socio-economic inequalities. For example, the low prevalence of psychotic illness favours a case-control design, where cases are sampled from treatment centres and controls from the local population. However, those in the control group will be of similar socio-economic location to those in treatment, so while they may allow the study of individual risk factors, they face the same socio-economic hazards as the treatment group. The implication of this is clear: using either single or crude indicators of socio-economic position does not 'control out' the impact of socio-economic position. Within any given level of a particular socio-economic measure the circumstances of minority groups are less favourable than those of white people. Nevertheless, research typically presents data that are 'standardised' for socio-economic position, allowing both the author and reader to mistakenly assume that all that is left is an 'ethnic/race' effect, often attributed to 'cultural' or 'genetic' difference.

Different rates in mental health disorders across different ethnic groups might also be a consequence of the experiences of discrimination and racism that ethnic minority people face in developed countries. The empirical investigation of the relationship between experiences of racial harassment and discrimination and mental health is far from straight-forward (Karlsen and Nazroo, 2006). Most important is the difficulty in measuring exposure to racism and discrimination accurately, given that these are a central, but often subtly expressed, feature of the lives of ethnic minority people and one that may be more likely to be reported by those experiencing mental distress. Nevertheless, experiences of racial harassment and discrimination appear to be related to mental health in the few, but growing number of, studies that have been conducted. Studies in the USA and New Zealand have shown a relationship between self-reported experiences of racial harassment and a range of health outcomes, including psychological distress (Harris *et al.*, 2006; Williams *et al.*, 2003). In the UK, findings from the Fourth National Survey of Ethnic Minorities suggested a relationship between experiences of racial harassment, perceptions of racial discrimination and a range of health outcomes across ethnic groups, including psychotic illness (Karlsen and Nazroo, 2002). This analysis showed that for ethnic minority people as a whole, reporting experiences of racial harassment and perceiving employers to discriminate were related to an increased likelihood of having a psychotic illness independently of each other, and that this relationship was also independent of socio-economic effects as indexed by occupational class. More recent analysis of the EMPIRIC study confirmed this, and was able to show that risk of psychotic illness for black Caribbean people was greatly increased by experiencing any of racial harassment/attack, discrimination in employment, or believing that British employers discriminate (Karlsen *et al.*, 2005).

Perhaps the most important conclusion to be drawn from these findings is that there is nothing inevitable, or inherent, in being a member of a particular ethnic/race category and risk of psychotic illness. It is misleading to consider black Caribbean people to be uniformly at higher risk; those who are in a higher occupational class, for example, have a lower risk. This points to the need to move beyond explanations that appeal to essentialised, or fixed, ethnic/race effects, and to consider context and socio-economic inequalities. It could be argued that the measures of socio-economic inequality that have been considered in empirical work represent three dimensions operating simultaneously: economic disadvantage (as measured by occupational class), a sense of being a member of a devalued, low status, group (for example, reporting the belief that British employers discriminate), and the personal insult and stress of being a victim of racial harassment or discrimination. Broadly, these inequalities can be considered to be a consequence of the ways in which ethnic minority groups are racialised in contemporary societies, which in turn reflects a historical legacy of racism. This relates to claims that both psychiatric practice and psychiatric research reflect a racist agenda, as demonstrated by the uncritical acceptance of findings based on evidence drawn from treatment settings. We now turn to a discussion of the use of treatment data.

Using treatment data to identify differences in risk of mental illness

One of the central problems with work on ethnicity and mental illness arises from the reliance of most work on data based on contact with treatment services. Contact with treatment services, even when access is universal as in the UK, reflects illness behaviour (that is, the way that symptoms are perceived, evaluated and acted upon), rather than illness per se (Blane *et al.*, 1996). This raises a number of linked problems when interpreting differences in treatment rates across ethnic groups, particularly as illness behaviour is likely to be affected by a number of factors that vary by ethnicity, such as socio-economic position, health beliefs, expectations of the sick role and lay referral systems. These problems become particularly important for work on rates of psychosis, where contact with services might be against the patient's wishes. So, despite the consistency of research findings showing that black Caribbean people have higher rates of treatment for psychosis, some commentators have not accepted the validity of the interpretation of these data and continue to suggest that a higher incidence (rather than a higher treatment rate) remains unproven, because of the serious methodological flaws with the research that has been carried out (Sashidharan, 1993; Sashidharan and Francis, 1993).

There are, as with all research, a number of technical problems facing studies using treatment data. For example, although these data can identify the number of patients, alternative data sources need to be used to identify the size of the population from which they are drawn. Typically this would be estimated from a population census, but the use of census data to provide a denominator requires: collection of appropriate data in the census; treatment data that are collected at the same time as the census and using census categories to classify patients; and accurate estimations of the geographical limit of the population that is covered by the treatment service. Here it is worth noting that a census typically under-estimates the numbers of certain groups in the population, including ethnic/racial minority groups (OPCS, 1994), that the 'catchment' areas covered by treatment centres are rarely tightly defined, and that both of these make it difficult to estimate the size of the population from which cases are drawn (although not to the extent that could explain the many times higher rates of admission that are reported for black Caribbean people and psychotic illnesses).

It is also possible that there are problems with the count of cases, with an overestimation of first onsets of psychosis, because of a variation across ethnic/race groups in the degree of under-identification of previous episodes. In the UK context it has been argued that this overestimation may occur for black Caribbean people because of high geographical mobility leading to records of previous admissions being missed and a reluctance to disclose previous diagnoses because of a concern about the impact of these on how they might be managed (Lipsedge, 1993). The count of those receiving treatment might also be biased by variations in the route of admission to treatment by ethnicity, with black people over-represented among patients compulsorily detained in psychiatric hospital, more likely to have been in contact with the police or forensic services prior to admission, and more likely to have been referred to these services by a stranger rather than by a relative or neighbour. And this is despite studies in the UK showing that black Caribbean patients are both less likely than whites to display evidence of self-harm and are no more likely to be aggressive to others prior to admission (Davies et al., 1996; Harrison et al., 1989; McKenzie et al., 1995; Rogers, 1990). Of course this might not be significant if all cases appeared in the treatment settings used for studies, but this is unlikely to be the case – a recent US study indicates that 39 of 183 (21%) people with possible psychosis had not received hospital treatment over a 16-year follow-up (Bresnahan et al., 2007), and within the UK those who are treated in the private healthcare sector (estimated to be 14% of patients) are not included in either treatment statistics or research studies (Raleigh and Deery, 2008).

It is also possible that differences in the attitudes of healthcare workers to different ethnic groups coupled with difficulties in the diagnosis of schizophrenia may be involved. For example, McKenzie et al. (1995) showed that black Caribbean people with psychosis were less likely than equivalent whites to have received psychotherapy or antidepressants; Harrison et al. (1989)

showed that although black Caribbean people were no more likely to have been aggressive at the time of admission, once admitted staff were more likely to perceive them as potentially dangerous both to themselves and to others; and Rogers (1990) showed that psychiatrists were *more* likely than police to consider black Caribbean patients detained in an emergency as dangerous to others. Coupled with difficulties in diagnosis, these pieces of evidence suggest that the stereotypes that inform the behaviour of heathcare workers may make them more likely to diagnose black Caribbean people as psychotic. Although studies based on case notes show that the validity of diagnosis does not relate to the ethnicity of the patient, such studies cannot account for the ways in which race is written into such case notes. In contrast, studies examining diagnostic practice (Neighbors *et al.*, 1989; 2003; Strakowski *et al.*, 1993) and robust studies using vignettes (Loring and Powell, 1988) suggest that black people are more likely than white people to be diagnosed as schizophrenic and more likely to be seen as dangerous.

Taken together, the comments above suggest that there are a variety of potential problems with studies based on treatment rates and, consequently, that their findings should not be taken at face value. There must remain some doubt about the claims of studies based on treatment rates regarding the higher rates of psychosis among black Caribbean people.

Of course other approaches to the study of mental illness also face methodological problems, including survey data, such as those provided by the FNS and EMPIRIC studies. First, many surveys of ethnic minority people are carried out in particular locations and consequently have restricted generalisability beyond that geographical context (for example, Bhugra *et al.*, 1997). Second, many studies that claim to be nationally representative often only cover areas with large ethnic minority populations, so ethnic minority people living in predominantly white areas are not included. Third, even survey data that address these sampling biases, such as the FNS and EMPIRIC studies, inevitably suffer from a non-response problem, where some of those who are identified for inclusion in the survey refuse to cooperate, and such non-response may be related to the condition under study. Fourth, the condition under study might be sufficiently rare in the community and be sufficiently hard to detect (as, for example, in the case of psychotic disorders) as to require both large samples and complicated procedures for estimating prevalence, making the estimate imprecise (so leaving large standard errors).

Mental health services

In addition to considering the impact of racism on health, either direct or through consequent adverse socio-economic circumstances, it is also important to explore and address how such social disadvantage influences ethnic minority patients' experiences of and uptake of mental health services, and the implications of this for practice.

Generally, regardless of their ethnic background, people with mental health problems are critical of the services they receive (Keating *et al.*, 2003; Sainsburys Centre for Mental Health (SCMH), 1998a, b). Common criticisms revolve around the fact that the mainstay of services are acute hospital units that are poorly staffed, leading to a lack of therapeutic intervention and a lack of information giving. These complaints have been echoed in recent comments from the President of the UK Royal College of Psychiatrists (Bhugra, 2008; Observer, 2008). Not surprisingly, this has led to suggestions that services could be improved by providing more support in the community and by engaging with service-user groups.

A number of more specific issues have been raised when the mental healthcare needs of ethnic minority people have been considered (King's Fund, 1998; SCMH, 1998a). Common criticisms have included a feeling that the contact they have with mental health services show staff to be culturally insensitive and that treatment is based on standard assessment tools that do not reflect their or their families' needs, of not being listened to, and families and carers feeling that they are not respected (Bowl, 2007a, b; SCMH, 2002). Such cultural insensitivity is likely to be reflected in the stereotypes used by healthcare workers when dealing with ethnic minority people (Audini and Lelliott, 2002; Keating et al., 2003). Stereotypes such as Caribbean people being considered as 'big, black and dangerous' (Keating, 2007; Webbe, 1998) or 'loud and difficult to manage' (Keating et al., 2003) continue to exist and it has been suggested that they contribute to the higher rates of detention experienced by such patients (SCMH, 2002). There is a clear possibility that such cultural stereotypes extend to other elements of psychiatric practice. For example, one study has shown that when South Asian patients consult with their GPs about mental health problems, their symptoms often go undiagnosed (Commander et al., 1997). The FNS found that Caribbean people who had scored on a depression inventory were far less likely than white people with equivalent scores to be receiving treatment, despite being as likely to have contacted their GP (Nazroo, 1997). This is further borne out by studies that show that black Caribbean people are less likely than white or South Asian people to be referred to specialist services (Bhui and Bhugra, 2002; Burnett et al., 1999; Commander et al., 1997).

Ethnic minority carers and users of mental health services have also indicated that they are suspicious of statutory mental health services, a suspicion that appears to be based on previous negative experiences. Some users have reported that they are fearful of dying in hospital as a result of the overuse of medication and the aggressive restraining techniques employed by staff (SCMH, 2002, 2006). This view fits with evidence that black patients are more likely to be compulsorily treated, despite not being more likely to be a danger to themselves or others (Audini and Lelliot, 2002; Davies et al., 1996; Harrison et al., 1989; McKenzie et al., 1995; Morgan et al., 2005; Rogers, 1990; SCMH, 2006). So they are more likely to be in psychiatric intensive care units and medium secure units, and more likely to be secluded or physically restrained (SCMH, 2006). They are also more likely to have contact with assertive outreach teams in the community, suggesting a lack of engagement with communities until crisis levels are reached (SCMH, 2006). Similarly, black Caribbean patients with a diagnosis of psychosis remain in acute hospital care longer than white patients and have more frequent outpatient follow-up contacts, despite having fewer negative symptoms (Commander et al., 2003; Takei et al., 1998). Yet, despite this over-representation in the acute sector, when discharged into the community it seems that black Caribbean patients receive variable and often inadequate support from community mental health teams and primary care services (Bhui and Bhugra, 2002; Bhui et al., 2003).

Such findings have led to a concern to address possible 'institutional racism' in the provision of services (Blofeld, 2003; DoH, 2005), defined as:

> The collective failure of an organisation to provide an appropriate and professional service to people because of their colour, culture or ethnic origin. It can be seen or detected in processes, attitudes and behaviour which amount to discrimination through unwitting prejudice, ignorance, thoughtlessness and racist stereotyping which disadvantages ethnic minority people. (Macpherson, 1999, page 28)

Not surprisingly, an acknowledgement of institutional racism has not sat easily with some psychiatrists, who are concerned that they and their services are being labelled as racist and that this will have a negative impact on patient care (Murray and Fearon, 2007; Patel and

Heginbotham, 2007; Singh, 2007). Nevertheless, several policy initiatives in the UK have been established to tackle ethnic inequalities in psychiatric care. For example, the National Service Framework for Mental Health (DoH, 1999) explicitly acknowledges the over-representation of black groups in secure services and their greater likelihood to receive physical rather than psychological treatments. More recently, the Delivering Race Equality in Mental Health Care document (DoH, 2005) provided a 5-year action plan to develop mental health services and improve the training of healthcare professionals. It has also led to the appointment of a National Director for mental health and ethnicity, who is supported by nine regional 'race equality leads' concerned with eliminating discrimination (Bhui and Bhugra, 2002; DoH, 2005). Such initiatives are clearly intended to tackle a range of connected problems; however, it remains uncertain whether they can be successful. For example, Fernando (2005) has pointed out that the 'race equality leads' have only an advisory role, so may have limited effectiveness.

A related and recurring theme in discussions of how to improve services is the need for healthcare professionals to receive training and education about cultural diversity. This need is seen across UK health services (DoH, 2005), where it is suggested that stereotypical images of ethnic minority people continue to persist, in part because of the lack of cultural diversity and cultural competence training (Gerrish et al., 1996; Webbe, 1998). In the mental health field, it has been noted that many healthcare professionals are uncomfortable about discussing race, culture and racism (Keating, 2007; SCMH, 2002). To address such concerns, cultural competency training and the promotion of anti-discriminatory practice has now been incorporated into healthcare education; for example, there has been a focus on this both in the pre-registration education programmes for mental health nurses and as a component of their continuing education post-qualification (DoH, 2006). However, effective cultural competency training is neither easy, nor straightforward, to achieve. Certainly, many attempts to address cultural diversity in educational materials have failed or, worse still, been based on stereotypical images of ethnic minority groups. It has been suggested that, in this new culturally aware climate, service users experience a new form of stereotyping, where practitioners make assumptions about their culture and identity as a result of simple generalisations (Challal and Iqbal, 2004; Keating, 2007; SCMH, 2002). Fernando (2003) argues that this is exactly why an approach that focuses on cultural difference can reinforce a racist environment. So, although these recent policy shifts have produced some optimism, it is by no means straightforward to tackle the institutional racism that lies at the root of these problems (Burr and Chapman, 1998). It is possible that legislation and policies to overcome discrimination will not have a great impact on practice.

Concluding comments

The account presented here suggests that many basic questions concerning the relationship between ethnicity/race and mental health remain unanswered. Treatment-based statistics have a number of problems, both for the estimation of incidence and prevalence, and for an investigation of factors that might lead to differences in risk. In addition, they reflect more than the health experiences of the populations from which those in treatment are drawn, they also reflect the operation of public institutions in an environment where social identities remain racialised. Population studies (surveys) also have to deal with issues of representa-tiveness and generalisation, and with the difficulty of accurate measurement of illness. The investigation of these issues is far from straightforward, not least because such phenomena are deeply embedded in specific contexts. Complex social phenomena are not easily reduced to gross empirical observations.

This is very apparent when we reflect on how ethnicity/race becomes reduced to simple observed categories, including within our own research. Within the wider theoretical literature many writers emphasise a notion of ethnicity as a social identity that reflects self-identification with cultural traditions that provide meaning, but also boundaries (fluid) between groups. Although such a conceptualisation of ethnicity reflects identification with sets of shared values, beliefs, customs and lifestyles, it has to be understood dynamically, as an active social process (Smaje, 1996). In particular, the influence of a cultural affiliation on individuals and groups, and on their health, has to be properly contextualised to take account of different periods and different elements of an identity, such as class, gender and caste (Ahmad, 1996). What it means, for example, to be black Caribbean might vary greatly in the different contexts of the USA and the UK (Nazroo et al., 2007). So, ethnicity is also a hybrid identity (Hall, 1992; Modood, 1998) that is not just given, but which is also the target of social action, changing across contexts and over time, fused with elements from other cultures, and which exists alongside other competing and complementary identities (such as gender and class).

Nevertheless, and as any discussion of racism or socio-economic inequality implies, it is important to consider the structural determinants of ethnicity/race. Here Miles' (1989) portrayal of racism as central to an understanding of ethnic/race relations is of great use. When discussing the emergence of ethnic or 'race' categories within a society (the 'ethnic moment'), Miles emphasises how ethnic difference can be essentialised as a product of 'nature' and how this becomes a justification for exclusionary and discriminatory treatment (Miles, 1996). In addition to the implicit critique of health research that adopts essentialist notions of ethnicity as culture or biology, this also reminds us that a core component of ethnic relations involves the categorisation of the 'other' and the exclusion of the 'other'. This is a reminder that ethnic identity – and the meaning of particular ethnic identities – are assigned as well as adopted (and assigned on the basis of power relations), and brings us back to the importance of the social and economic inequalities that flow from this.

Such complexity indicates that explaining ethnic/race differences in mental illness, or the role of psychiatric institutions, is not a straightforward task. Perhaps, as others have pointed out (Sashidharan and Francis, 1993), the most important conclusion to draw is that it is vital to avoid essentialising ethnic differences in mental health (that is, reducing them to stereotyped notions of cultural or biological difference), and there is a need to explore the factors associated with ethnicity that may explain any relationship between ethnicity and mental health, such as the various forms of social disadvantage that ethnic minority people face. It also remains important to explore how racism and the social disadvantages that this leads to structure the experiences of ethnic minority people when they come into contact with mental health services. Despite this, the focus on biological explanations for mental illness and neglect of social explanations continues in both the USA and the UK (Jarvis, 2007; Munro, 1999), and media-fuelled public concerns about the dangers associated with mental illness appear to continue to influence policy (Munro, 1999). This has implications for the success of attempts to reform mental health services, with a risk of a return to more coercive services in a context where young men are racialised as 'big, black and dangerous' (Keating, 2007; Webbe, 1998).

References

Ahmad, W. I. U. (1996). The trouble with culture. In D. Kelleher and S. Hillier, eds. *Researching Cultural Differences in Health*. London: Routledge.

Audini, B., Lelliott, P. (2002). Age, gender and ethnicity of those detained under Part ll of the Mental Health Act 1983. *British Journal of Psychiatry*, **280**, 222–6.

Bagley, C. (1971). The social aetiology of schizophrenia in immigrant groups. *International Journal of Social Psychiatry*, **17**, 292–304.

Bhugra, D. (2008). Renewing psychiatry's contract with society. *Psychiatric Bulletin*, **32**, 281–3.

Bhugra, D., Hilwig, M., Hossein, B. *et al.* (1996). First-contact incidence rates of schizophrenia in Trinidad and one-year follow-up. *British Journal of Psychiatry*, **169**, 587–92.

Bhugra, D., Leff, J., Mallett, R. *et al.* (1997). Incidence and outcome of schizophrenia in whites, African-Caribbeans and Asians in London. *Psychological Medicine*, **27**, 791–8.

Bhui, K., Bhugra, D. (2002). Mental illness in black and Asian ethnic minorities: pathways to care and outcomes. *Advances in Psychiatric Treatment*, **8**, 26–33.

Bhui, K., Stansfield, S., Hull, S. *et al.* (2003). Ethnic variations in pathways to and use of specialist mental health services. *British Journal of Psychiatry*, **182**, 105–16.

Blane, D., Power, C., Bartley, M. (1996). Illness behaviour and the measurement of class differentials in morbidity. *Journal of the Royal Statistical Society*, **156**(1), 77–92.

Blofeld, J. (2003). *Independent Inquiry into the Death of David Bennett*. Norwich: Norfolk, Suffolk and Cambridgeshire Strategic Health Authority.

Bowl, R. (2007a). The need for change in UK Mental Health Services: South Asian service user's views. *Ethnicity and Health*, **12**, 1–19.

Bowl, R. (2007b). Responding to ethnic diversity: black service users' views of mental health services in the UK. *Diversity in Health and Social care*, **4**, 201–10.

Bresnahan. M., Begg, M. D., Brown, A. *et al.* (2007). Race and risk of schizophrenia in a US birth cohort: another example of health disparity? *International Journal of Epidemiology*, **36**, 751–8.

Burnett, R., Mallet, R., Bugra, D. *et al.* (1999). The first contact of patients with schizophrenia with psychiatric services: social factors and pathways to care in a multi-ethnic population. *Psychological Medicine*, **29**, 475–83.

Burr, J. A., Chapman, T. (1998). Some reflections on cultural and social considerations in mental health nursing. *Journal of Psychiatric and Mental Health Nursing*, **5**, 431–7.

Cantor-Graae, E., Selten, J. P. (2005). Schizophrenia and migration: a meta-analysis and review. *American Journal of Psychiatry*, **162**, 12–24.

Cantor-Graae, E., Zolkowska, K., McNeil, T. F. (2005). Increased risk of psychotic disorder among immigrants in Malmo: a 3-year first-contact study. *Psychological Medicine*, **35**, 1155–63.

Challal, K., Iqbal, A. (2004). *Foundations Experiencing Ethnicity: Discrimination and Service Provision*. York: Joseph Rowntree Foundation.

Cochrane, R., Bal, S. S. (1989). Mental hospital admission rates of immigrants to England: a comparison of 1971 and 1981. *Social Psychiatry and Psychiatric Epidemiology*, **24**, 2–11.

Cochrane, R., Stopes-Roe, M. (1981). Psychological symptom levels in Indian immigrants to England – a comparison with native English. *Psychological Medicine*, **11**, 319–27.

Cole, E., Leavey, G., King, M., Johnson-Sabine, E., Hoar, A. (1995). Pathways to care for patients with a first episode of psychosis: a comparison of ethnic Groups. *British Journal of Psychiatry* **167**, 770–6.

Commander, M. J., Dharan, S. P., Odell, S. M., Surtees, P. G. (1997). Access to mental health care in an inner city health district. II: Association with demographic factors. *British Journal of Psychiatry*, **170**, 317–20.

Commander, M., Odell, S., Surtees, P., Sashidharan, S. (2003). Characteristics of patients and patterns of psychiatric service user in ethnic minorities. *International Journal of Social Psychiatry*, **49**, 216–24.

Davies, S., Thornicroft, G., Leese, M. *et al.* (1996). Ethnic differences in risk of compulsory psychiatric admission among representative cases of psychosis in London. *British Medical Journal*, **312**, 533–7.

DoH (Department of Health). (1999). *The National Health Framework for Mental Health*. London: Department of Health.

DoH (Department of Health). (2005). *Delivering Race Equality in Mental Health Care: an Action Plan for Reform Inside and Outside Services: and the Government's Response to the Independent Inquiry into the Death of David Bennett*. London: Department of Health.

Department of Health. (2006). *From Values to Action: The Chief Nursing Officer's Review of Mental Health Nursing*. London: Department of Health.

Erens, B., Primatesta, P., Prior, G. (2001). *Health Survey for England 1999: The Health of Minority Ethnic Groups*. London: The Stationery Office.

Fearon, P., Kirkbiride, J. B., Morgan, C. *et al.* (2006). Incidence of schizophrenia and other psychoses in ethnic minority groups: results from the MRC AESOP Study. *Psychological Medicine*, **36**, 1541–50.

Fernando, S. (2003). *Cultural Diversity, Mental Health and Psychiatry. The Struggle Against Racism*. Hove and New York: Brunner-Routledge.

Fernando, S. (2005). Multicultural mental health services: projects for ethnic minority communities in England. *Transcultural Psychiatry*, **42**, 420–36.

Gerrish., K., Husband, C., Mackenzie, J. (1996). Ethnicity, the minority ethnic community and health care delivery. In W. I. U. Ahmad and C. Husband, eds. *'Race', Health and Social Care*. Birmingham, Open University Press.

Gilliam, S. J., Jarman, B., White, P., Law, R. (1989). Ethnic differences in consultation rates in urban general practice. *British Medical Journal*, **299**, 953–7.

Hall, S. (1992). The question of cultural identity. In S. Hall, D. Held and T. McGrew, eds. *Modernity and its Futures*. Cambridge: Polity.

Handy, S., Chithiramohan, R. N., Ballard, C. G., Silveira, W. R. (1991). Ethnic differences in adolescent self-poisoning: a comparison of Asian and Caucasian groups. *Journal of Adolescence*, **14**, 157–62.

Harris, R., Tobias, M., Jeffreys, M. *et al.* (2006). Racism and health: the relationship between experience of racial discrimination and health in New Zealand. *Social Science and Medicine*, **63**(6), 1428–41.

Harrison, G., Owens, D., Holton, A., Neilson, D., Boot, D. (1988). A prospective study of severe mental disorder in Afro-Caribbean patients. *Psychological Medicine*, **18**, 643–57.

Harrison, G., Holton, A., Neilson, D. *et al.* (1989). Severe mental disorder in Afro-Caribbean patients: some social, demographic and service factors. *Psychological Medicine*, **19**, 683–96.

Hickling, F. W. (1991). Psychiatric hospital admission rates in Jamaica. *British Journal of Psychiatry*, **159**, 817–21.

Hickling, F. W., Rodgers-Johnson, P. (1995). The incidence of first contact schizophrenia in Jamaica. *British Journal of Psychiatry*, **167**, 193–6.

Jarvis, G. E. (2007). The social causes of psychosis in North American psychiatry: a review of a disappearing literature. *The Canadian Journal of Psychiatry*, **52**, 287–94.

Karlsen, S., Nazroo, J. Y. (2002). The relationship between racial discrimination, social class and health among ethnic minority groups. *American Journal of Public Health*, **92**(4), 624–31.

Karlsen, S., Nazroo, J. (2006). Measuring and analyzing 'race', racism and racial discrimination. In J. Oakes, and J. Kaufman, eds. *Methods in Social Epidemiology*. Francisco: Jossey-Bass, pp. 86–111.

Karlsen, S., Nazroo, J. Y., McKenzie, K., Bhui, K., Weich, S. (2005). Racism, psychosis and common mental disorder among ethnic minority groups in England. *Psychological Medicine*, **35**(12), 1795–1803.

Karmi, G., Abdulrahim, D., Pierpoint, T., McKeigue, P. (1994). *Suicide Among Ethnic Minorities and Refugees in the UK*. London: NE and NW Thames RHA.

Kauffman, J. S., Cooper, R. S., McGee, D. L. (1997). Socioeconomic status and health in blacks and whites: the problem of residual confounding and the resiliency of race. *Epidemiology*, **8**(6), 621–8.

Kauffman, J. S., Long, A. E., Liao, Y., Cooper R. S., McGee D. L. (1998). The relation between income and mortality in U.S. blacks and whites. *Epidemiology*, **9**(2), 147–55.

Keating, F. (2007). *African and Caribbean Men and Mental Health*. Better Health Briefing 5. London: Race Equality Foundation.

Keating, F., Robertson, D., Kotecha, N. (2003). *Ethnic Diversity and Mental Health in London: Recent Developments*. Working Paper, Kings Fund.

King, M., Coker, E., Leavey, G., Hoare, A., Johnson-Sabine, E. (1994). Incidence of psychotic illness in London: comparison of ethnic groups. *British Medical Journal*, **309**, 1115–19.

King's Fund. (1998). *London's Mental Health. The Report to the King's Fund London Commission*. London: King's Fund Publishing.

Lipsedge, M. (1993). Mental health: access to care for black and ethnic minority people. In A. Hopkins and V. Bahl, eds. *Access to Health Care for People from Black and Ethnic Minorities*. London: Royal College of Physicians.

Littlewood, R., Lipsedge, M. (1988). Psychiatric illness among British Afro-Caribbeans. *British Medical Journal*, **296**, 950–1.

Lloyd, K. (1993). Depression and anxiety among Afro-Caribbean general practice attenders in Britain. *International Journal of Social Psychiatry*, **39**, 1–9.

Loring, M., Powell, B. (1988). Gender, race and DSM-III: a study of the objectivity of psychiatric diagnostic behavior. *Journal of Health and Social behavior*, **29**, 1–22.

McGovern, D., Cope, R. (1987). First psychiatric admission rates of first and second generation Afro-Caribbeans. *Social Psychiatry*, **22**, 139–49.

McKenzie, K., van Os, J., Fahy, T. *et al.* (1995). Psychosis with good prognosis in Afro-Caribbean people now living in the United Kingdom. *British Medical Journal*, **311**, 1325–8.

Macpherson, W. (1999). *The Stephen Lawrence Inquiry: Report of an inquiry by Sir William Macpherson of Cluny*, Cm 4261–1. London: The Stationery Office.

Merrill, J., Owens, J. (1986). Ethnic differences in self-poisoning: a comparison of Asian and white groups. *British Journal of Psychiatry*, **148**, 708–12.

Miles, R. (1989). *Racism*. London: Routledge.

Miles, R. (1996). Racism and nationalism in the United Kingdom: a view from the periphery. In R. Barot, ed. *The Racism Problematic: Contemporary Sociological Debates on Race and Ethnicity*. Lewiston: The Edwin Mellen Press.

Modood, T. (1998). Anti-essentialism, multiculturalism and the 'recognition' of religious groups. *The Journal of Political Philosophy*, **6**(4), 378–99.

Morgan, C., Mallet, R., Hutchinson, G. *et al.* (2005). Pathways to care and ethnicity. 1: Sample characteristics and compulsory admission. *British Journal of Psychiatry*, **186**, 281–9.

Munro, R. (1999). There's sin in them there genes. *Nursing Times*, **95**(33), 28–9.

Murray, R., Fearon, P. (2007). Searching for racists under the psychiatric bed: commentary on . . . institutional racism in psychiatry. *Psychiatric Bulletin*, **31**, 365–6.

Nazroo, J. Y. (1997). *Ethnicity and Mental Health: Findings from a National Community Survey*. London: Policy Studies Institute.

Nazroo, J. Y. (1998). Genetic, cultural or socio-economic vulnerability? Explaining ethnic inequalities in health. *Sociology of Health and Illness*, **20**(5), 710–30.

Nazroo, J. Y. (2001). *Ethnicity, Class and Health*. London: Policy Studies Institute.

Nazroo, J. (2003). The structuring of ethnic inequalities in health: economic position, racial discrimination and racism. *American Journal of Public Health*, **93**(2), 277–84.

Nazroo, J. Y., Williams, D. R. (2005). The social determination of ethnic/racial inequalities in health. In M. Marmot and R. G. Wilkinson, eds. *Social Determinants of Health*, 2nd edn. Oxford: Oxford University Press, pp. 238–66.

Nazroo, J., Jackson, J., Karlsen, S., Torres, M. (2007). The black diaspora and health inequalities in the US and England: does where you go and how you get there make a difference? *Sociology of Health and Illness*, **26**, 811–30.

Neighbors, H. W., Jackson, J. S., Campbell, L., Williams, D. (1989). The influence of racial factors on psychiatric diagnosis. *Community Mental Health*, **44**, 237–56.

Neighbors, H. W., Trierweiler, S. J., Ford, B. C., Murof, J. R. (2003). Racial differences in DSM diagnosis using a semi-structured instrument: the importance of clinical judgement in the diagnosis of blacks. *Journal of Health and Social Behaviour*, **44**, 237–56.

Nursing Midwifery Council. (2004). *Standards of Proficiency for Pre-registration Nurse Education*. London: Nursing Midwifery Council.

Observer. (2008). Psychiatric patients 'feel lost and unsafe.' 29 June, http://www.guardian.co.uk/society/2008/jun/29/mentalhealth.health3 (last accessed 24 October 2008).

OPCS (Office of Population Censuses and Surveys). (1994). *Undercoverage in Great Britain (Census User Guide no. 58)*. London: HMSO.

Oliver, M. L., Shapiro, T. M. (1995). *Black Wealth/White Wealth: A New Perspective on Racial Inequality*. New York: Routledge.

Patel, K., Heginbotham, C. (2007). Institutional racism in mental health services does not imply racism in individual psychiatrists: commentary on institutional racism in psychiatry. *Psychiatric Bulletin*, **31**, 367–8.

Raleigh, V., Deery, A. (2008). Care quality data on mental health is too hard to pin down. *Health Service Journal*, 10 April 2008.

Robins, L. N., Reiger, D. A. (1991). *Psychiatric Disorders in America: The Epidemiologic Catchment Area Study*. New York: Free Press.

Rogers, A. (1990). Policing mental disorder: controversies, myths and realities. *Social Policy and Administration*, **24**(3), 226–36.

SCMH (Sainsburys Centre for Mental Health). (1998a). *Keys to Engagement: Review of Care for People with Severe Mental Illness who are Hard to Engage with Services*. London: Sainsburys Centre for Mental Health.

SCMH (Sainsburys Centre for Mental Health). (1998b). *Acute Problems: A Survey of the Quality of Care in Acute Psychiatric Wards*. London: Sainsburys Centre for Mental Health.

SCMH (Sainsburys Centre for Mental Health). (2002). *Breaking the Circles of Fear*. London: Sainsburys Centre for Mental Health.

SCMH (Sainsburys Centre for Mental Health). (2006). *Policy Paper 6. The Costs of Race Inequality*. London: Sainsburys Centre for Mental Health.

Sashidharan, S. P. (1993). Afro-Caribbeans and schizophrenia: the ethnic vulnerability hypothesis re-examined. *International Review of Psychiatry*, **5**, 129–44.

Sashidharan, S., Francis, E. (1993). Epidemiology, ethnicity and schizophrenia. In W. I. U. Ahmad, ed. *'Race' and Health in Contemporary Britain*. Buckingham: Open University Press.

Selten, J. P., Slaets, J. P. J., Kahn, R. S. (1997). Schizophrenia in Surinamese and Dutch Antillean immigrants to The Netherlands: evidence of an increased incidence. *Psychological Medicine*, **27**, 807–11.

Selten, J. P., Veen, N. N., Feller, W. *et al.* (2001). Incidence of psychotic disorders in immigrant groups to The Netherlands. *British Journal of Psychiatry*, **178**, 367–72.

Singh, S. (2007). Institutional racism in psychiatry. *Psychiatric Bulletin*, **31**, 363–5.

Singh, S. P., Burns, T. (2006). Race and mental health: there is more to race than racism. *British Medical Journal*, **333**, 648–51.

Smaje, C. (1996). The ethnic patterning of health: new directions for theory and research. *Sociology of Health and Illness*, **18**(2), 139–71.

Soni Raleigh, V. (1996). Suicide patterns and trends in people of Indian subcontinent and Caribbean origin in England and Wales. *Ethnicity and Health*, **1**(1), 55–63.

Soni Raleigh, V., Balarajan, R. (1992). Suicide and self-burning among Indians and West Indians in England and Wales. *British Journal of Psychiatry*, **161**, 365–8.

Soni Raleigh, V., Bulusu, L., Balarajan, R. (1990). Suicides among immigrants from the Indian subcontinent. *British Journal of Psychiatry*, **156**, 46–50.

Sproston, K., Mindell, J. (2006). *Health Survey for England 2004: The Health of Minority Ethnic Groups*. London: National Centre for Social Research.

Sproston, K., Nazroo, J. (eds.) (2002). *Ethnic Minority Psychiatric Illness Rates in the Community (EMPIRIC)*. London: The Stationery Office.

Strakowski, S. M., Shelton, R. C., Kolbrener, M. L. (1993). The effects of race and comorbidity on clinical diagnosis in patients with psychosis. *Journal of Clinical Psychiatry*, **54**, 96–102.

Takei, N., Persaud, R., Woodruff, P., Brockington, I., Murray, R. M. (1998). First episodes of psychosis in Afro-Caribbean and white people. *British Journal of Psychiatry*, **172**, 147–53.

Townsend, P., Davidson, N. (1982). *Inequalities in Health (the Black Report)*. Middlesex: Penguin.

Van Os, J., Castle, D. J., Takei, N., Der, G., Murray, R. M. (1996). Psychotic illness in ethnic minorities: clarification from the 1991 Census. *Psychological Medicine*, **26**, 203–8.

Veling, W., Selten, J. P., Veen, N. *et al.* (2006). Incidence of schizophrenia among ethnic minorities in the Netherlands: a four-year first-contact study. *Schizophrenia Research*, **86**, 189–93.

Webbe, A. (1998). Ethnicity and mental health. *Psychiatric Care*, **5**(1), 12–16.

Williams, D. R., Neighbors, H. W., Jackson, J. S. (2003). Racial/ethnic discrimination and health: findings from community studies. *American Journal of Public Health*, **93**, 200–8.

Risk and protective factors in mental health among migrants

Driss Moussaoui and Mohamed Agoub

Editors' introduction

Individuals who migrate bring with them to the new society a number of factors relating to adjustment and resilience. However, their personality traits and characteristics, which may not be vulnerability factors in their own culture, may become so in the new culture. Personal experiences, histories and vulnerabilities will vary from individual to individual. Migrant individuals adapt and change in response to the process of migration according to a number of reasons and factors and coping strategies. Personal and social circles related to migration and post-migration experiences influence adjustment towards the new society. In this chapter, Moussaoui and Agoub point out that risk factors for deteriorating mental health among migrants are not only multiple but also multidimensional and interactive. Gender, traumatic events, past history of psychiatric disorders and substance abuse, unemployment and poverty have all been noted to be risk factors which may cause further mental health problems after migration. After migration, individual characteristics, such as unemployment, language proficiency and substance use, and cultural characteristics, such as discrimination and attitudes of the new society, may play a role. Social support and protective factors – including coping skills, better self-esteem and better adaptation skills – will also act as buffers from developing psychiatric disorders.

Introduction

Migration is a universal phenomenon and is inherent to the human condition. Reasons for migration are diverse, usually seeking a better life through economic and material improvement, but also for psychological reasons (Moussaoui and Ferrey, 1985). Migration has been legally controlled since the nineteenth century, and this trend has been accentuated in the twentieth and twenty-first centuries. The economic and security gaps between developed and middle-income countries will increase illegal transnational migration. The biggest rate of migration happens inside each country, especially in low to middle-income countries, from rural to urban areas. According to the United Nations (UN), one out of every three human beings lives and works in a different geographical site than birth place.

Over the past two decades, there has been an increasing interest in the impact of migration on mental health. It has been identified as a stressful process, which can generate a risk for the psychological and physical health of migrants (Bhugra and Jones, 2001). The process of migration may be associated not only with great hope for a better life, but also with distressing experiences that can lead to psychological distress.

Migration and Mental Health, ed. Dinesh Bhugra & Susham Gupta. Published by Cambridge University Press. © Cambridge University Press 2011.

The migratory process can be divided into three stages:

- The first is the pre-migration stage, when the individuals decide to migrate and plan to move from one zone to another, from one country to another or from one continent to another.
- The second stage involves the process of migration itself and the physical transition from one place to another, involving all the necessary psychological and social steps. It is best described metaphorically by the concept of transplant.
- The third stage in the process is the post-migration stage, when the individuals deal with the social and cultural environments of the new society, learn new roles and become interested in transforming their group (Bhugra and Jones, 2001).

As personal history is diverse among migrants, both before, during and after migration, the process of migration will hence differ from one migrant to another. This complex process is not always linear, and what helps the adaptation of a migrant at the beginning may hamper it some years later, and the opposite is true. Migrants develop their capacities to confront the difficult task to settle and be integrated in the host society. On a personal level, migration necessitates stages of adaptation from loss of previous life experiences and values to the acceptance of the benefits and difficulties of the new society and culture. On a professional level, it requires the acquisition of a new culture of work, with integration of previous knowledge and experience on multiple levels. Integration means recognition, understanding and acceptance within the new society, despite continuing differences. The personal and professional experiences of migration are interconnected and can interfere with each other (Goldner-Vukov, 2004).

Once difficulties arise, cultural factors can play an important role in the expression of the psychological distress. In western developed countries, individuals tend to localise pathological processes in the body and view illness primarily as the malfunctioning or failure of an affected organ, including the brain. In southern developing countries, like Mediterranean societies, illness is frequently viewed as something that comes from the outside; explanations and actions based on the supernatural are hence frequent (Schouler-Ocak and Reiske, 2008).

Mental disorders among migrants

The prevalence of mental disorders among migrants is one of the aspects of the impact of migration on mental health. The epidemiology of the association between migration and mental disorders shows inconsistent results (Kinzie, 2006). The results are conflicting because of the methods used or because of differences between populations, making the comparability of results limited. The prevalence of mental disorders varies depending on the type of assessed mental disorder and the stage of migration. The majority of studies investigating the effects of migration on the mental health of migrants show a higher prevalence of mental disorders, but some empirical studies have revealed that at least some migrant groups may experience better mental health when compared with the local populations (Bhugra, 2003; Levecque et al., 2009; Takeuchi et al., 2007a; Wong and Leung, 2008).

For example, in the meta-analaysis performed by Cantor-Graae and Selten (2005), the mean weighted relative risk for developing schizophrenia among first generation migrants was 2.7. However, the risk is low when sending and receiving countries are similar (western to western country) and higher when sending and receiving countries are dissimilar, for example Surinam to the Netherlands or African and Caribbean migrants to the UK (Kinzie, 2006).

The incidence of psychotic disorders varies depending on the origin of migrants in the Netherlands. The risks for Turkish immigrants, first or second generation, and for immigrants from western countries were not significantly increased, but the risks were increased for subjects born in Morocco, Surinam, the Netherlands Antilles and other non-western countries. This risk was also increased for Moroccans and Surinamese of the second generation (Selten *et al.*, 2001).

In a study investigating psychiatric admission in Switzerland, findings suggested significantly lower admission rates among immigrants from southern, western and northern European countries, and former Yugoslavia, with relative risks ranging from 0.70 to 0.54 compared to Swiss people of the same gender; there were high admission rates for male immigrants originating from Turkey, eastern European and 'other' countries (rates >6 per 1000 population/year versus 4.3 per 1000 for the Swiss) (Lay *et al.*, 2007). Using data from the Danish Civil Registration System, the relative risk of developing schizophrenia was 2.45 and 1.92 among first and second generation immigrants, respectively (Cantor-Graae *et al.*, 2003).

For mood disorders, Swinnen and Selten (2007), using a meta-analysis, examined whether migration is a risk factor. The mean relative risk of developing bipolar disorder among migrants was 2.47. However, after excluding people of African-Caribbean origin in the UK, this risk was no longer significantly increased.

Levecque *et al.* (2007) retrieved a higher prevalence of depressive symptoms among persons of Turkish and Moroccan origin as compared to Belgians or people from other European Union member states.

Another aspect of the impact on mental health and psychosocial wellbeing is the use of mental health services by migrants. Many studies have documented low rates of utilisation of mental health services by immigrants (Kinzie, 2006; Lay *et al.*, 2006). This cannot be attributed to lower rates of distress or to the use of alternative sources of help, but most probably reflects cultural and linguistic barriers to care (Kirmayer *et al.*, 2007).

Risk factors for migrants

Since migration is not just one phenomenon, but a whole process involving a series of events, it will be influenced by a number of factors at social and individual levels. Risk factors for a deteriorating mental health of the migrant are multiple, multidimensional and interactive. Sometimes, risk factors may trigger resilience in some migrants and reinforce them. Their impact on the migrant can occur during one of the phases of the migratory process.

Risk factors during pre-migration stage

During this stage, risk factors can be divided into two categories: factors depending on personal characteristics of migrants and those linked to environmental factors.

Gender is a significant personal factor. Female gender is a predictor of minor mental disorders among recent Chinese migrants to New Zealand (Abbott *et al.*, 1999*)*. Women from low-income countries who migrate for economic reasons represent a more vulnerable population (Anbesse *et al.*, 2009).

Subjects with a history of mental disorders and alcohol and substance abuse are among the most vulnerable. Ryan *et al.* (2006) found that a history of depression in Ireland and childhood emotional abuse among Irish migrants living in London were potential pre-migration predictors of current depression.

Region of origin may be considered as a risk factor for some mental disorders, especially when the migrants come from remote and poor environments, such as the Rif region in Morocco. Migrants moving from a low-income country to a developed country are exposed to more psychological distress. In a Belgian community-based sample, Turkish and Moroccan immigrants are found to have higher rates of depression and severe anxiety symptoms compared to Belgians and immigrants coming from the European Union (Levecque *et al.*, 2007).

Pre-migration traumatic events (violence, sexual abuse during childhood, civil war, ethnic cleansing and being close to death or suffering serious injury) are all risk factors for developing mental disorders, particularly depression and anxiety (Bhui *et al.*, 2003; Yearwood *et al.*, 2007).

Economic conditions are also a predictor of psychological distress. Poverty and unemployment lead to migration and to vulnerability among migrants (Bhui *et al.*, 2003). We can mention here perinatal consequences of poverty when it leads to malnutrition and its impact on the development of the fetal brain.

Motivations to migration play a great role in migrant mental health. In the case of forced migration, subjects are not prepared and are traumatised by the decision to move and leave their home, their country and family.

Risk factors during migration stage

Age at migration plays an important role in the adaptation and adjustment to the new society and may represent a risk factor for psychological distress. Immigrants who reach the host country as adults will have more difficulties learning the new language and will have fewer opportunities to develop social relationships outside of their families and members of their community (Takeuchi *et al.*, 2007b). In a study of psychiatric morbidity of recent Chinese immigrants in New Zealand, being aged 26–35 years or over 45 was a predictor of mental disturbance (Abbott *et al.*, 1999). Stevens and Vollebergh (2008) reviewed the literature regarding mental health of migrant children to explain differences in mental health problems between migrants and native children. They did not confirm that migrant youths are at higher risk of developing mental health problems.

The association between poorly planned migration and current depression was stronger for younger than for older migrants, although the results were only significant in men (Ryan *et al.*, 2006).

Illegal immigration also increases the difficulties, dangers and traumas significantly, and leads to more psychological distress (Segal *et al.*, 2010).

Risk factors during post-migration stage

The post-migration factors that are associated with psychological distress and mental disorders can be divided into two categories: the first is related to the individual's characteristics, including unemployment, language proficiency and substance use, while the second category has to do with the new environment of the migrant, such as rejection by the new society, discrimination and racism.

The economic situation of the migrant plays a crucial role in the integration and adjustment of the individual. Many studies reported this factor as a predictor of mental disorder (Ryan *et al.*, 2006; Zunzunegui *et al.*, 2006). Disadvantageous economic conditions reduce the chances of having adequate socialisation, and may reinforce isolation, discrimination, low self-esteem and the occurrence of mood disorders and anxiety, as well as substance and alcohol abuse.

Absence of or inadequate social support is another factor that can cause psychological distress (Ryan et al., 2006). Poor social support has been identified as significantly related to the onset, course and outcome of many psychological disorders (Pantelidou and Craig, 2006). Ethnic density, defined by the concentration of the same ethnic group around an individual, does not always represent an adequate social support. It may play a significant role in genesis and maintenance of some types of psychological distress (Bhugra and Jones, 2001).

One question must be raised concerning the results of studies showing that the incidence rate of psychotic disorders seems to be higher among migrants scattered in neighbourhoods inhabited by local people, as compared to high ethnic density neighbourhoods (Veling et al., 2008): is it a cause or a consequence of schizophrenia? Is schizophrenia secondary to the social and cultural isolation/deprivation, or is the latter a behavioural consequence of the illness?

Post-migration detention is another traumatic experience and is associated with poor mental health. Sometimes, mental disturbance continues several years after release (Ichikawa et al., 2006; Phillips, 2010). Difficulties in interpersonal relationships are also common risk factors in migrants, particularly those who have more marital and work conflicts (Wong and Leung, 2008). On the other hand, occurrence of physical illness, particularly chronic diseases like cardiovascular and respiratory diseases, negatively affects the mental health of migrants (Lai, 2005; Ortega et al., 2006; Silveira and Ebrahim, 1998). This kind of comorbidity weakens the status of the migrant both economically, socially and psychologically by reducing his or her 'health capital'.

Self-esteem is highly linked to the sense of achieving the aspirations and goals planned before migration. If an individual migrates and is unable to obtain an appropriate job to his status and his aspirations, it is likely that this will increase stress and psychological distress (Bhugra, 2004).

On the second category of risk factors related to the new environment, 'culture shock' has been suggested to be a major predictor of psychological distress. The concept of 'culture shock' comprises six distinct aspects, including the strain of adapting to the new culture, a sense of loss of culture and values of society of origin, confusion in role expectations and self-identity, a feeling of being rejected by members of the new culture, and anxiety and feelings of impotence owing to not being able to cope with the new environment (Pantelidou and Craig, 2006). Reasons for the 'culture shock' may be of economic, cultural (way of life), political, religious and educational nature. When the process is started and maintained, it leads to psychological distress and to mental disorders.

Migration involves the loss of a familiar environment, including the mother tongue, attitudes, values, social structure and support networks. Grieving for this loss can be viewed as a healthy reaction. However, if the symptoms cause significant distress or persist, this can be considered as pathological (Bhugra and Becker, 2005).

Contact between the migrant and the host community may lead to assimilation (a person entering a new culture is absorbed into the dominant culture), rejection, integration or deculturation (act of causing a person or group to abandon its culture) (Bhugra and Becker, 2005). A good example is the necessity of abandoning the sheep sacrifice during Eid El Adha by Muslims in their homes when they migrate to European countries.

Another concept is acculturation. It means that a person must become a competent participant in the majority culture, but will always be identified as a member of the minority culture.

Cultural changes in identity can be stressful and may result in problems with self-esteem and mental health. Jasinskaja-Lahti and Liebkind (2007) mentioned the existence of various acculturative stressors such as: (1) perceiving oneself as having been treated unfairly, or being a victim of discrimination; (2) lacking social support; (3) inadequate language proficiency; (4) low socio-economic status; and (5) length of stay in the host country.

Discrimination may be an important predictor of poor mental health and occurrence of psychological disturbance (Gee *et al.*, 2006); it is also a decisive factor regarding access to healthcare services (Agudelo-Suàrez *et al.*, 2009). The migrants in Spain reported examples of discrimination in their community and working life, characterised by experiences of racism, mistreatment and precarious working conditions in comparison to the Spanish-born population (Agudelo-Suàrez *et al.*, 2009). Perceived discrimination is positively correlated with acculturative stress (Tartakovsky, 2007).

Protective factors for migrants

Protective factors prevent psychological distress and mental illness among migrants. It covers, like risk factors, pre-migration, migration and post-migration stages.

Protective factors during pre-migration stage

Having good physical and mental health helps the prevention of the migrant from other vulnerabilities. Good academic background and professional skills may help the migrant in the integration into the host country.

Psychological resources in the pre-migration phase are a key element in preventing psychological distress during the migration process. These resources include normal personality traits, adequate coping skills, the ability to solve problems and no mental disorder.

Protective factors during migration

Migration during childhood does not in itself represent a risk factor. Takeuchi *et al.* (2007b) found that subjects who arrived when they were children (12 years and younger) had a lifetime rate of any disorder similar to that in US-born subjects. Perhaps, immigrants arriving as children learn English more easily and schools serve as the primary socialisation institution outside of the family (Takeuchi *et al.*, 2007b). The same results were reported by Vollebergh *et al.* (2005); children from immigrant families do not appear to experience more problems than their non-immigrant peers in the Netherlands. Young age might, to a certain extent, be considered as a protective factor.

On the contrary, for those with substance use disorders, coming to the USA as an adult, after age 25, might protect against exposure to risky social networks linked to drug use and subsequently substance and alcohol abuse and dependence (Alegria *et al.*, 2007).

If the country of immigration is the country of choice, the departure from homeland is planned and arrival in the host country is unequivocally welcoming, the experience of immigration is positive. The availability of economic resources increases the probability of rapid independence and adjustment in new countries (Segal *et al.*, 2010).

Protective factors during post-migration stage

Migration may have positive outcomes such as personal growth, self-affirmation and learning new social and adaptation skills (Walsh *et al.*, 2008). In this case, mental health may be satisfactory and even excellent.

Social support plays an essential role in the maintenance of a good mental health. An adequate social support, a coethnic presence and a low expressed emotion are protective factors against alcohol use behaviours and mental disorders. It is predictive of greater happiness and less depression (Bhugra and Jones, 2001; Shin *et al.*, 2007). Social network should include not only migrants from the same country of origin, but should be broader, especially subjects from the host society, in order to integrate and be accepted better in the new country.

Low perceived discrimination and high perceived social support in the host country are the keys of a successful integration and a good mental health.

Conclusion

The process of migration and subsequent cultural and social adjustments play a key role in the mental health of migrants. Mental health professionals must be aware of the problems of migrants. More specific training should be available at training centres for caregivers (e.g. medical school, teaching hospitals, training centres for nurses and social workers). They must take into account risk and protective factors both at the time of the assessment of difficulties and mental health problems and at the time of therapeutic interventions and in planning of preventive actions.

There is a need for more research in the field of migration by integrating different variables using the biopsychosocial model. Finally, and in order to treat and manage care for migrants, specialised services for education, training and third referral must be established in hosting countries.

References

Abbott, M. W., Wong, S., Williams, M., Au, M., Young, W. (1999). Chinese migrants' mental health and adjustment to life in New Zealand. *Australian and New Zealand Journal of Psychiatry*, **33**, 13–21.

Agudelo-Suàrez, A., Gil-Gonzàlez, D., Ronda-Pérez, E. *et al.* (2009). Discrimination, work and health in immigrant populations in Spain. *Social Science & Medicine*, **68**, 1866–74.

Alegria, M., Shrout, P. E., Woo, M. *et al.* (2007). Understanding differences in past year psychiatric disorders for Latinos living in the U.S. *Social Science & Medicine*, **65**, 214–30.

Anbesse, B., Hanlon, C., Alem, A., Packer, S., Whitley, R. (2009). Migration and mental health: a study of low-income. *International Journal of Social Psychiatry*, **55**, 557–68.

Bhugra, D. (2003). Migration and depression. *Acta Psychiatrica Scandinavica*, **418**(Suppl.), 67–72.

Bhugra, D. (2004). Migration and mental health. *Acta Psychiatrica Scandinavica*, **109**, 243–58.

Bhugra, D., Becker, M. A. (2005). Migration, cultural bereavement and cultural identity. *World Psychiatry*, **4**, 18–24.

Bhugra, D., Jones, P. (2001). Migration and mental illness. *Advances in Psychiatric Treatment*, **7**, 216–23.

Bhui, K., Abdi, A., Abdi, M. *et al.* (2003). Traumatic events, migration characteristics and psychiatric symptoms among Somali refugees. *Social Psychiatry and Psychiatric Epidemiology*, **38**, 35–43.

Cantor-Graae, E., Selten, J. P. (2005). Schizophrenia and migration: a meta-analysis and review. *American Journal of Psychiatry*, **162**, 12–24.

Cantor-Graae, E., Pedersen, C. B., McNeil, T. F., Mortensen, P. B. (2003). Migration as a risk factor for schizophrenia: a Danish population-based cohort study. *British Journal of Psychiatry*, **182**, 117–22.

Gee, G. C., Ryan, A., Laflamme, D. J., Holt, J. (2006). Self-reported discrimination and mental health status among African descendants, Mexican-Americans, and other Latinos in the New Hampshire REACH 2010 Initiative: the added dimension of immigration. *American Journal of Public Health*, **96**, 1821–8.

Goldner-Vukov, M. (2004). A psychiatrist in cultural transition: personal and professional dilemmas. *Transcultural Psychiatry*, **41**, 386–405.

Ichikawa, M., Nakahara, S., Wakai, S. (2006). Effect of post-migration detention on mental health among Afghan asylum seekers in Japan. *Australian and New Zealand Journal of Psychiatry*, **40**, 341–6.

Jasinskaja-Lahti, I., Liebkind, K. (2007). A structural model of acculturation and well-being among immigrants from the former USSR in Finland. *European Psychologist*, **12**, 80–92.

Kinzie, J. D. (2006). Immigrants and refugees: the psychiatric perspective. *Transcultural Psychiatry*, **43**, 577–91.

Kirmayer, L. J., Weinfeld, M., Burgos, G. *et al.* (2007). Use of health care services for psychological distress by immigrants in an urban multicultural milieu. *The Canadian Journal of Psychiatry*, **52**, 295–304.

Lai, D. W. L. (2005). Prevalence and correlates of depressive symptoms in older Taiwanese immigrants in Canada. *Journal of the Chinese Medical Association*, **68**(3), 118–25.

Lay, B., Lauber, C., Nordt, C., Rössler, W. (2006). Patterns of inpatient care for immigrants in Switzerland: a case control study. *Social Psychiatry and Psychiatric Epidemiology*, **41**, 199–207.

Lay, B., Nordt, C., Rössler, W. (2007). Mental hospital admission rates of immigrants in Switzerland. *Social Psychiatry and Psychiatric Epidemiology*, **42**, 229–36.

Levecque, K., Lodewyckx, I., Vranken, J. (2007). Depression and generalised anxiety in the general population in Belgium: a comparison between native and immigrant groups. *Journal of Affective Disorders*, **97**, 229–39.

Levecque, K., Lodewyckx, I., Bracke, P. (2009). Psychological distress, depression and generalized anxiety in Turkish and Moroccan immigrants in Belgium. *Social Psychiatry and Psychiatric Epidemiology*, **44**, 188–97.

Moussaoui, D., Ferrey, G. (1985). *Psychopathologie des Migrants*. Paris: Presses Universitaires de France, 96 pp.

Ortega, A. N., Feldman, J. M., Canino, G., Steinman, K., Alegria, M. (2006). Co-occurrence of mental and physical illness in US Latinos. *Social Psychiatry and Psychiatric Epidemiology*, **41**, 927–34.

Pantelidou, S., Craig, T. K. J. (2006). Culture shock and social support: a survey in Greek migrant students. *Social Psychiatry and Psychiatric Epidemiology*, **41**, 777–81.

Phillips, C. B. (2010). Immigration detention and health. *Medical Journal of Australia*, **192**, 61–2.

Ryan, L., Leavey, G., Golden, A., Blizard, R., King, M. (2006). Depression in Irish migrants living in London: case-control study. *British Journal of Psychiatry*, **188**, 560–6.

Schouler-Ocak, M., Reiske, S. L. (2008). Cultural factors in the diagnosis and treatment of traumatised migrant patients from Turkey. *Transcultural Psychiatry*, **45**, 652–71.

Segal, U. A., Mayadas, N. S., Elliott, D. (2010). The migration process. In U. A. Segal, D. Elliott, N. S. Mayadas, eds. *Immigration Worldwide: Policies, Practices and Trends*. New York: Oxford University Press, pp. 3–16.

Selten, J. P., Veen, N., Feller, W. *et al.* (2001). Incidence of psychotic disorders in immigrant groups to The Netherlands. *British Journal of Psychiatry*, **178**, 367–72.

Shin, H. S., Han, H. R., Kim, M. T. (2007). Predictors of psychological well-being amongst Korean immigrants to the United

States: a structured interview survey. *International Journal of Nursing Studies*, **44**, 415–26.

Silveira, E. R. T., Ebrahim, S. (1998). Social determinants of psychiatric morbidity and well-being in immigrant elders and whites in East London. *International Journal of Geriatric Psychiatry*, **13**, 801–12.

Stevens, G. W. J. M., Vollebergh, W. A. M. (2008). Mental health in migrant children. *Journal of Child Psychology and Psychiatry*, **49**, 276–94.

Swinnen, S. H. A., Selten, J. P. (2007). Mood disorders and migration: meta-analysis. *British Journal of Psychiatry*, **190**, 6–10.

Takeuchi, D. T., Alegría, M., Jackson, J. S., Williams, D. R. (2007a). Immigration and mental health: diverse findings in Asian, Black, and Latino populations. *American Journal of Public Health*, **97**, 11–12.

Takeuchi, D. T., Zane, N., Hong, S. *et al.* (2007b). Immigration-related factors and mental disorders among Asian-Americans. *American Journal of Public Health*, **97**, 84–90.

Tartakovsky, E. (2007). A longitudinal study of acculturative stress and homesickness: high-school adolescents immigrating from Russia and Ukraine to Israel without parents. *Social Psychiatry and Psychiatric Epidemiology*, **42**, 485–94.

Veling, W., Susser, E., van Os, J. *et al.* (2008). Ethnic density of neighbourhoods and incidence of psychotic disorders among immigrants. *American Journal of Psychiatry*, **165**, 66–73.

Vollebergh, W. A. M., Have, M. T., Dekovic, M. *et al.* (2005). Mental health in immigrant children in the Netherlands. *Social Psychiatry and Psychiatric Epidemiology*, **40**, 489–96.

Walsh, S., Shulman, S., Murer, O. (2008). Immigration distress, mental health status and coping among young immigrants: a one-year follow-up study. *International Journal of Intercultural Relations*, **32**, 371–84.

Wong, D. F. K., Leung, G. (2008). The functions of social support in the mental health of male and female migrant workers in China. *Health & Social Work*, **33**, 275–85.

Yearwood, E. L., Crawford, S., Kelly, M., Moreno, N. (2007). Immigrant youth at risk for disorders of mood: recognizing complex dynamics. *Archives of Psychiatric Nursing*, **21**, 162–71.

Zunzunegui, M. V., Forster, M., Gauvin, L., Raynault, M. F., Willms, J. D. (2006). Community unemployment and immigrants' health in Montreal. *Social Science & Medicine*, **63**, 485–500.

Psychosis, migration and ethnic minority status: a story of inequality, rejection and discrimination

Tom K. J. Craig

Editors' introduction

Social inequalities have been associated with prevalence of mental disorders for a considerable period of time. It is interesting to see whether people with mental illness drift down to a lower socio-economic status or whether low socio-economic status contributes to aetiology of mental illness. Low socio-economic status, related to unemployment and poor housing, will certainly contribute to stress being experienced by individuals. For migrants and ethnic minority groups such an experience may add to a sense of alienation and isolation. Obviously, the response to these factors will depend upon the resilience of the migrants and personality factors, but also on the reasons for migration and educational and economic factors. In this chapter, Craig highlights some of the recent research evidence. In conjunction with other chapters, Craig is able to demonstrate that the aetiology of schizophrenia and other psychoses may well be related to ethnicity, discrimination and low social status, as well as to the discrepancy between achievement and expectations. A sense of alienation and experiences of rejection will also add to the stress the individuals are dealing with. Childhood sexual and physical abuse may further add to this sense of distress. Migration as an act needs to be disentangled from the status as a migrant.

Introduction

There is a growing consensus that the incidence of schizophrenia is increased among migrant populations. Studies carried out over the past 30 years into African and African-Caribbean migrants and their offspring in England report rates between 2 and 14 times higher than that seen in the native-born white population (Fearon *et al.*, 2006) and similarly elevated rates have been observed among migrants to other countries (Cantor-Grae and Selten, 2005; also see Chapters 2 and 3 for detailed discussions). Although many of the studies can be individually criticised for problems in the classification of ethnicity, inaccuracy of estimates of the numbers of ethnic minorities in the general population or for errors of measurement of mental disorder in minority groups, taken as a whole the consistency of the findings leads to the near inevitable conclusion that this is a real effect and not one easily dismissed as an artefact of bias or poor measurement. Cantor-Graae and Selten (2005), in summarising the findings of these studies to date, point out that the

Migration and Mental Health, ed. Dinesh Bhugra & Susham Gupta. Published by Cambridge University Press. © Cambridge University Press 2011.

findings are most robust for migrants from developing versus developed countries, and for those from areas where the majority population is black. Second and third generation offspring of these migrants remain at higher risk.

Recent findings

One of the more recent confirmations of this elevated risk comes from the aetiology and ethnicity in schizophrenia and other psychoses (AESOP) study. This comprised the identification of all first contact cases of psychosis in three English city areas (South London, Nottingham and Bristol) with nested case-control studies to explore hypotheses concerning social and biological factors that might account for the increased incidence of psychosis in ethnic minority populations. All people presenting for the first time to secondary mental health services with psychotic symptoms and aged 16–64 years were screened and a diagnosis established using the Schedules for Clinical Assessment in Neuropsychiatry (WHO, 1992). There was a leakage study at the end to determine any cases that might have been missed. A total of 308 cases was identified over 2 years in South London, 203 in Nottingham and 57 in Bristol (the latter in 1 year only). Standardised incidence rates for all diagnoses of psychotic conditions were calculated. Compared with the native white British population, all other ethnic groups had elevated incidence rates of psychosis. This was particularly marked for those of African-Caribbean and African ethnicity and was observed for both schizophrenia (African IRR 5.8, African-Caribbean 9.1) and mania (African 6.2, African-Caribbean 8.0). Rates were elevated for both men and women, and across the age span (Fearon *et al.*, 2006).

Urbanicity

The AESOP study was carried out in cities where migrants, their children and grandchildren have lived for many years. Many live in the poorer parts of town, in dense inner city relatively deprived environments that have also long been known to be associated with high rates of psychosis. As long ago as 1939, Faris and Dunham published the results of a detailed study of the distribution of mental illness in Chicago, showing very convincingly that schizophrenia was not evenly distributed across the population but occurred in clumps that broadly mapped on to the more deprived and downtrodden parts of the city (Faris and Dunham, 1939). More recent replications and extensions of these findings have included some impressive epidemiology. For example, one Swedish study (Sundquist *et al.*, 2004) screened the national health records of some 4.4 million men and women aged 24–64 between 1997 and 1999 for any admission to hospital for treatment of psychosis or depression. The residential address of each was mapped to a database that allowed each residential location to be assigned to one of five levels of population density. The hazard ratio for psychosis and depression for each of the four increasingly urbanised areas was compared with the most rural/least urbanised area. There was a near linear increase from low to highly dense urban dwelling for both men and women. In addition, the authors examined marital status as a crude index of social support, educational attainment as an indicator of social economic status and immigrant status (whether economic migrants from southern Europe or refugees from eastern Europe). All three measures were also related to incidence – people living alone had higher incidence rates, as did people with lower educational attainment and those categorised as refugees or economic migrants. However, the urban differences remained even after these effects were taken into account (Sundquist *et al.*, 2004).

Of course, this study reported residency at admission to treatment and not necessarily at the time of onset of psychosis so that the association may be inflated by people moving into the more downtrodden urban areas after the onset of their illness or during its prodrome but before their first contact with mental health services. However, other studies suggest this is an insufficient explanation of the findings. For example, Pedersen and Mortensen (2001) used data from the Danish Civil Registration system to obtain a large, representative population sample of 1.9 million people with an address in Denmark or Greenland and emigrations/ immigrations to and from other countries. The addresses of each person could be located in one of 276 municipalities in Denmark that in turn were classified according to the degree of urbanisation. Finally, the residential location of each resident could be tracked from birth to their fifteenth birthday, thus allowing the investigators to see whether any increased rate of schizophrenia in highly urbanised areas was determined by the age at which the person first lived in the area and the length of time or exposure involved. As in the Swedish study, there was a strong association between urban density and the incidence of psychosis . Furthermore, those living in areas of higher urban density on their fifth birthday than they were at birth had a significantly greater relative risk of schizophrenia compared to those whose living circum- stances were unchanged. This was even more marked at the tenth birthday – so that for a fixed urbanicity at birth, risk increased with increasing degree of urbanisation at successive years. It was also possible to examine this association more directly for a subsample whose accom- modation was known across their upbringing – thus they were able to add up the number of years lived consecutively in each level of urban density. When this was done, it appears that the more years lived in the higher degree of urbanicity, the greater the risk of schizophrenia.

It appears also that the effect of urban living is not confined to help-seeking populations. Several studies have shown that psychosis-like experiences such as brief auditory hallucina- tions, overvalued ideas and even delusions are prevalent in the general population and show longitudinal, epidemiological and neuropsychological continuities with schizophrenia (King et al., 2005; Morgan et al., 2008a; Vanheusden et al., 2008). They also show an association with urban density. For example, in one Dutch study the lifetime prevalence of both clinical disorder and psychotic symptoms in the general population increased as the level of population density increased, and this remained even after adjusting for age, sex, level of education, country of birth of subject and parents. The prevalence of symptoms in the most dense areas of the city was twice that seen in the least dense area. Importantly, the association remained even when subjects with a psychosis diagnosis were excluded and there was no interaction with lifetime mental health treatment (van Os et al., 2001).

So, to summarise, we have two well established and likely related macro-social observa- tions: that the incidence of schizophrenia and other psychoses is increased by prolonged living in dense inner city locations and among migrants – most of whom, in the studies reported to date, live in these inner city settings.

In the AESOP study, the rates of schizophrenia and mania were elevated in South London compared to those in Nottingham and Bristol, and this difference persisted even when adjusting for differences in age and sex. Although some of the variation could be explained by differences in the proportions of ethnic minority populations in each centre, there was still a significant excess morbidity in South London (Kirkbride et al., 2006). There are several possible explanations for this excess. These include greater economic deprivation, lower social cohesion, the relative inaccessibility of key social supports and resources, or the prolonged exposure to a poor quality environment characterised by delinquency, vandalism and criminality. For example, Allardyce et al., (2005) showed that economic deprivation and social fragmentation (defined as high residential mobility, single person households and numbers of single people) were both strongly associated with psychosis. In the AESOP data, compared with a general population sample, cases were more deprived on measures of educational attainment, employment, housing, living alone and being without long-term relationships. Similar patterns were observed across ethnic subgroups, but deprivation and social isolation were consistently more common among black African-Caribbean participants than their white British counterparts, with black African-Caribbean patients being the most disadvantaged of all. These findings held even when making adjustments for pre-morbid IQ, and the duration of untreated psychosis (DUP). Furthermore, these findings held when only cases with a clear recent onset were examined (Morgan *et al.*, 2008b).

It seems, therefore, that social deprivation and social isolation might explain at least part of the observed increase in incidence of psychosis among migrant minorities. In turn, deprivation and social isolation may have subtly different underlying sources in minority populations, including some that are a consequence of racial discrimination. In one intriguing hint of the impact of hidden discrimination at work, Boydell *et al.*, (2001) compared incidence rates for schizophrenia across 15 electoral wards in South London and found the incidence of schizophrenia in non-white ethnic minorities was significantly increased among those living in predominantly white areas. Most strikingly, the incidence rate ratios varied in a dose–response fashion from 2.28% in the electoral wards where the non-white population formed the largest proportion of the total to 4.4% in the wards where they formed the smallest proportion (Boydell *et al.*, 2001).

Whether racial discrimination can explain the difference in incidence, black participants in the AESOP study certainly thought they were unfairly discriminated against. The proportion of those who reported being disadvantaged due to culture, religion or skin colour was considerably greater in black than in white respondents. In a logistic regression of factors predicting case status, being younger, black unemployed and the perception of disadvantage all increased the risk of psychosis (Cooper *et al.*, 2008).

Restricted access

One consequence of living in a deprived environment may be restricted access to resources – be these directly because of personal hardship, poverty or because of the lack of opportunity to access resources in the community. The idea of 'social capital' encompasses a broad range of social involvement from civic participation, through involvement in social networks and through these to access of resources and, eventually, a sense of coherence and 'trust' in the society in which one is embedded. Links between poor social capital and incident schizophrenia have been reported in some studies (Boydell *et al.*, 2002) but not others (Drukker *et al.*, 2006). The AESOP data suggested that as much as 25% of the variance in the incidence of schizophrenia could be attributed to neighbourhood level factors, including ethnic density, fragmentation and voter turnout (Kirkbride *et al.*, 2007). In an attempt to take these observations further, Kirkbride *et al.*, (2008) carried out a cross-sectional survey of 5% of the general population in the south-east London area of the AESOP study to collect detailed social capital data at the neighbourhood level. Individual questionnaires concerning measures of social cohesion and trust (SC&T) and of social disorganisation (e.g. graffiti, vandalism, theft of/from vehicles etc.) were obtained from 4231 respondents (around 26% of those approached but lower for some key groups such as black Caribbeans). Analyses were conducted using both SC&T scores as well as a categorical approach assigning each neighbourhood as high, medium or low. A very similar percentage (25%) of the variation in incidence rates could be attributed to neighbourhood level effects. Lower ethnic fragmentation was associated with lower incidence and higher socio-economic deprivation, with higher incidence reflecting findings from other studies, but surprisingly, incidence rates were not linearly related to the measure of SC&T. Instead, compared to areas with medial levels of SC&T, incidence rates were higher in both those with lower as well as higher levels of SC&T. This rather counterintuitive observation might well be a consequence of problems in the data – a very low response rate particularly from the most socially disorganised areas or the over-representation of white, older females in responses – but it could also be that some of the people living in the high social capital environments are none the less excluded from accessing this social capital in the way hinted at by the earlier Boydell *et al.* (2001) study.

Childhood factors

In their seminal work, Faris and Dunham (1939) suggested that a high proportion of people living alone was indicative of 'social isolation.' They in turn suggested that this had a causal influence on the development of psychotic symptoms. Social isolation has long been noted to be a common antecedent in the history of people who develop a psychosis (e.g. Hare, 1956; Jablensky, 1997). In a case register study in the Netherlands, van Os and colleagues showed a 'neighbourhood' effect of higher rates of schizophrenia from neighbourhoods with a high proportion of people living alone. In addition, in areas where the proportion of persons living alone was below the Maastricht mean, the effect of single marital status was more than twice as large as the effect in neighbourhoods with values above the mean (van Os *et al.*, 2000).

So, as we saw for ethnicity, being the odd one out seems to be important. Perhaps this is because such relative isolation reflects alienation from the social milieu and experiences of rejection. This exposure may well be over many years as there is increasing evidence for the importance of experiences earlier in life and how these can shape lives in such a way as to make exposure to adversity in adulthood both more likely as well as more toxic. The most comprehensive examples of these longitudinal effects can be found in the literature of depression and common mental disorder but is now being unravelled for psychosis as well. In the AESOP study, Morgan *et al.* (2007) ascertained histories of separation from one or other parent for a year or more prior to age 16. These separations were further characterised on the basis of whether they were part of a planned stage in the migration experience, whether because of employment or schooling or whether they were for more 'aberrant' and rejecting reasons such as parental divorce, death or being abandoned. Compared with a general population sample, such aberrant separations were some two to three times more commonly reported by people who had experienced a psychotic illness. The strength of the associations were similar for both the white British and black African-Caribbean participants although separation from a parent was more common among the African-Caribbean participants. That it is aberrant separations that distinguished cases and controls is lent further support by the observation of increased rates of psychosis among those living in institutional care (Bebbington *et al.*, 2004), and both observations hint at some unpleasant quality in the family environment such as family conflict or abuse. Of the latter, Morgan and Fisher (2007), in a comprehensive review of the literature, concur that despite methodological limitations of many studies, the rates of childhood sexual and physical abuse do appear elevated compared to those reported for the general population. Several large general population studies have found childhood maltreatment to be associated with psychotic symptoms (Bebbington *et al.*, 2004; Janssen *et al.*, 2004). In the AESOP sample, detailed retrospective ratings of childhood experience were available for 181 patients and

246 healthy comparison subjects. Severe physical abuse was defined as repeated episodes involving at least two occurrences of being hit by a stick, punched or kicked resulting in significant injury including broken bones and a description suggesting that the perpetrator was 'out of control' during the assault. Similarly, severe sexual abuse was defined as unwanted sexual contact carried out by a relative or household member, involving genital contact, including intercourse. At this threshold of severity, psychosis cases were three times more likely than their healthy counterparts to have experienced severe physical abuse at the hands of their mother before the age of 12 years and twice as likely to report sexual abuse in childhood although the latter difference fell just short of significance (Fisher *et al.*, 2010). In a separate analysis, it appeared that the impact of physical abuse was particularly marked among female patients (Fisher *et al.*, 2009).

Of course it is a long leap between showing association between psychosis and adverse childhood experiences to a causal interpretation. Parental maltreatment may for example reflect parental mental illness and although a history of this was controlled for in the analyses, it seems likely that only the most conspicuous disorders will have been identified and other possibly untreated and unrecognised common mental disorders went unrecorded. Similarly, there are limitations of reliance on retrospective reports of parenting, although in this regard some comfort can be taken from the use of a detailed measure with clearly defined inclusion criteria, good test–retest reliability with high specificity over time (i.e. low false positive rate) and also in the fact that the rates of abuse reported by the control group in this study closely reflect those reported by published data from other UK surveys.

One impressive longitudinal study of the impact of parenting on later psychosis is that of Tienari and colleagues in Finland (Tienari *et al.*, 2004). The medical records of 19 447 women in Finnish psychiatric hospitals between 1960 and 1997 were examined to identify those with a diagnosis of schizophrenia and who had at least one child who had been adopted away. These adopted offspring ('high genetic risk') and their adoptive families were then matched with control families where the adoptee had come from a family where there was no diagnosis of schizophrenia spectrum disorder ('low genetic risk'). Both sets of offspring and their adoptive families were assessed using interviews with all the family members and with the parental couples. A rating was made of the family relationships across a range of scales that covered such areas as empathy, criticism and communication that were collapsed into a smaller number of overarching dimensions reflecting levels of criticism/conflict; communication and boundary/ enmeshment. These could be further subcategorised into broad indices of family function, distinguishing 'healthy' from 'dysfunctional' family environments. The adoptee children were then assessed after a median interval of 12 years by clinicians blind to the initial evaluations using clinical research diagnostic interviews and, finally, the diagnostic status of all adoptees checked at the end of a case register follow-up 21 years after initial assessment

The results were striking and showed a clear genetic versus environmental interaction (GxE). Low genetic risk children reared in healthy families had 0% morbid risk for schizophrenia spectrum disorders at follow-up, high genetic risk children reared in healthy families had a risk of just 1.49% while the morbid risk for schizophrenia for low risk adoptees in dysfunctional families was 4.48% and those high genetic risk adoptees in dysfunctional families was 13.04%. The findings suggest that adoptees with genetic risk were more sensitive then other adoptees to the adverse environments throughout their childhood. Further analyses were carried out of each of the separate family relationship scales although it appears that adoptees at high genetic risk were more sensitive to problems ascertained as scores on the individual domains as well as a total score across domains and no specific form of family problem, at least as conceptualised in these measures was more strongly associated in the model than any other (Tienari *et al.*, 2004).

Interactional mechanisms

There is, of course, a considerable gap between observing the association between childhood experiences, adult social behaviour and the mechanisms through which these are associated with psychosis. It has been known for many years from animal models that severely aberrant parenting can produce pathological social behaviours, including social avoidance (Harlow and Suomi, 1971), and this is also a consequence of childhood maltreatment in humans. Abused children are reported to be less well liked than their peers and to experience higher rates of rejection even by those they consider to be their friends (Salzinger *et al.*, 1993). They also appear to attend to and remember negative stimuli more than do non-abused children (Dodge *et al.*, 1995). There are also well established links between childhood maltreatment and downstream mood disorders. For example, the work of George Brown and colleagues has mapped out a causal pathway to depression in women that, in a nutshell, links early maternal maltreatment to the development of persisting low self-esteem, shame and withdrawal that in turn are associated with adult depression through environmental pathways involving early premarital pregnancy and unstable adult relationships (see, for example, Brown *et al.*, 2007, 2008). It is not a huge leap to speculate that something similar might be observed for schizophrenia with common social antecedents operating on a different biological vulnerability. One such speculation, put forward by Selten and Cantor-Graae (2005), suggests that it is the 'social defeat' of being in a subordinate or 'outsider' social position and which is reflected in repeated experiences of discrimination, frustrated ambition and rejection that lies behind the increased risk of psychosis in migrant groups. They suggest that defeat may be more common in migrants as their ambitions for upward mobility are thwarted by the lack of opportunities open to them in the host country. This hypothesis can be taken further by considering it in the light of processes of acculturation. Acculturation involves a process of retaining or relinquishing characteristics of one's own ethnic origin, resulting in higher or lower levels of ethnic identification (Szapocznik and Kurtines, 1980). The association between ethnic identification and distress are, however, mixed and complicated by contextual factors such as the host nation's reaction to ethnic minorities (Bhui *et al.*, 2005). To disentangle the disparate findings, it may be helpful to consider the nature of the social stress that is at play in the tensions of acculturation. It has long been established that inequality in social status (be this financial, educational or employment achievement) heightens social evaluation anxiety. This is anxiety linked to situations in which performance in personally important social tasks is open to being judged negatively by others – where one can be seen to do less well than others, to be ridiculed or devalued. It is most toxic when the failure and the devaluing involve a loss of social status and esteem. A migrant seeking to improve his prospects is faced with something of a dilemma. Achievement in the host country largely depends on how successful the migrant is at acculturation – 'fitting in' and adopting the cultural norms (behaviours and expressed beliefs/attitudes) of the host country. But the more the move in this direction, the greater the distance from his original culture and the greater the risk of alienation from his peers, at best diminishing the opportunity for their support should things go wrong and at worst raising the risk of their ridicule and rejection. The adaptive response to this tension is probably the capacity to alternate between the two cultures depending on context while less flexible responses such as the defensive assertion of the minority culture may be associated with greater risk of psychiatric disorder with the more flexible adaptive response being associated with lower risk. Just as the defensive assertion of minority culture might be one response to frustrated ambitions, another way of coping might well be a denial of weakness or personal responsibility for failure and an exaggerated expression of what has been and can still be achieved. Although only indirectly, this hypothesis is supported by another finding from AESOP that examined the 'achievement–expectation gap' for employment achievement among white British and African-Caribbean patients and healthy controls. A mismatch between high expectations and actual achievement was a risk factor for psychosis and applied equally to both ethnic groups, but the gap was most marked for the African-Caribbean cases who reported the highest expectations but the lowest objective achievement compared with either their counterparts in the general population or white British cases and controls (Reininghaus *et al.*, 2009).

To conclude, we are now at a point where the importance of the social environment for the aetiology of psychosis is beyond doubt, but we are only just beginning to unravel the more detailed social, psychological and biological mechanisms underlying schizophrenia and other psychoses. Further work is needed, for example, to disentangle aspects of process (migration) with that of status (the migrant, ethnicity) and how both work through experiences of discrimination, acculturation and adversity across the lifespan.

References

Allardyce, J., Gilmour, H., Atkinson, J. *et al.* (2005). Social fragmentation, deprivation and urbanicity. *British Journal of Psychiatry*, **187**, 401–6.

Bebbington, P., Bhugra, D., Singleton, N. *et al.* (2004). Psychosis, victimisation and childhood disadvantage: evidence from the second British National Survey of Psychiatric Morbidity. *British Journal of Psychiatry*, **185**, 220–6.

Bhui, K., Stansfeld, S., Head, J. *et al.* (2005). Cultural identity, acculturation and mental health among adolescents in east London's multiethnic community. *Journal of Epidemiology and Community Health*, **59**, 296–302.

Boydell, J., Van Os, J., Mckenzie, K. *et al.* (2001). Incidence of schizophrenia in ethnic minorities in London: ecological study into interactions with environment. *British Medical Journal*, **323**, 1336–8.

Boydell, J., McKenzie, K., Van Os, J. *et al.* (2002). The social causes of schizophrenia: an investigation into the influence of social cohesion and social hostility – report of a pilot study. *Schizophrenia Research*, **53**, 264–5.

Brown, G. W., Craig, T., Harris, T. O. *et al.* (2007). Child-specific and family-wide risk factors using the Childhood Experience of Care and Abuse (CECA) instrument: a life course study of adult chronic depression – 3. *Journal of Affective Disorders*, **103**, 225–36.

Brown, G. W., Craig, T. K., Harris, T. O. (2008). Parental maltreatment and proximal risk factors using the Childhood Experience of Care and Abuse (CECA) instrument: a life-course study of adult chronic depression – 5. *Journal of Affective Disorders*, **110**, 222–33.

Cantor-Graae, E., Selten, J. P. (2005). Schizophrenia and migration: a meta-analysis and review. *American Journal of Psychiatry*, **162**, 12–24.

Cooper, C., Morgan, C., Byrne, M. *et al.* (2008). Perceptions of disadvantage, ethnicity and psychosis. *British Journal of Psychiatry*, **192**, 185–90.

Dodge, K. A., Pettit, G. S., Bates, J. E. *et al.* (1995). Social information processing patterns partially mediate the effects of early physical abuse on later conduct problems. *Journal of Abnormal Psychology*, **104**, 623–43.

Drukker, M., Krabbendam, L., Driessen, G. *et al.* (2006). Social disadvantage and schizophrenia: a combined neighbourhood- and individual-level analysis. *Social Psychiatry and Psychiatric Epidemiology*, **41**, 595–604.

Faris, R. E., Dunham, H. W. (1939). *Mental Disorders in Urban Areas. An Ecological Study of Schizophrenia and Other Psychoses*, 2nd edn, 1960 edn. New York: Hafner.

Fearon, P., Kirkbride, J. K., Morgan, C. *et al.* (2006). Incidence of schizophrenia and other psychoses in ethnic minority groups: results from the MRC AESOP study. *Psychological Medicine*, **36**, 1541–50.

Fisher, H., Morgan, C., Dazzan, P. *et al.* (2009). Gender differences in the association between childhood abuse and psychosis. *British Journal of Psychiatry*, **194**, 319–25.

Fisher, H., Jones, P. B., Fearon, P. *et al.* (2010). The varying impact of type, timing and frequency of exposure to childhood adversity on its association with adult psychotic disorder. *Psychological Medicine*, doi:10.1017/S0033291710000231.

Hare, E. (1956). Mental illness and social conditions in Bristol. *Journal of Mental Science*, **102**, 349–57.

Harlow, H. F., Suomi, S. J. (1971). Production of depressive behaviors in young monkeys. *Journal of Autism and Childhood Schizophrenia*, **13**, 246–55.

Jablensky, A. (1997). The 100-year epidemiology of schizophrenia. *Schizophrenia Research*, **28**, 111–25.

Janssen, I., Krabbendam, L., Bak, M. *et al.* (2004). Childhood abuse as a risk factor for psychosis. *Acta Psychiatrica Scandinavica*, **109**, 38–45.

King, M., Nazroo, J., Weich, S. *et al.* (2005). Psychotic symptoms in the general population of England: a comparison of ethnic groups (the EMPIRIC study). *Social Psychiatry and Psychiatric Epidemiology*, **40**, 375–81.

Kirkbride, J., Fearon, P., Morgan, C. *et al.* (2006). Heterogeneity in incidence rates of schizophrenia and other psychotic syndromes: findings from the 3 centre AESOP study. *Archives of General Psychiatry*, **63**, 250–8.

Kirkbride, J., Morgan, C., Fearon, P. *et al.* (2007). Neighbourhood-level effects on psychoses: re-examining the role of context. *Psychological Medicine*, **37**, 1413–25.

Kirkbride, J. B., Boydell, J., Ploubidis, G. B. *et al.* (2008). Testing the association between the incidence of schizophrenia and social capital in an urban area. *Psychological Medicine*, **38**, 1083–94.

Morgan, C., Fisher, H. (2007). Environmental factors in schizophrenia: childhood trauma – a critical review. *Schizophrenia Bulletin*, **33**, 3–10.

Morgan, C., Kirkbride, J., Leff, J. *et al.* (2007). Parental separation, loss and psychosis in different ethnic groups: a case-control study. *Psychological Medicine*, **37**, 495–503.

Morgan, C., Fisher, H., Hutchinson, G. *et al.* (2008a). Ethnicity, social disadvantage and psychotic-like experiences in a healthy population based sample. *Acta Psychiatrica Scandinavica*, **119**, 226–35.

Morgan, C., Kirkbride, J., Hutchinson, G. *et al.* (2008b). Cumulative social disadvantage, ethnicity and first-episode psychosis: a case-control study. *Psychological Medicine*, **38**, 1701–15.

Pedersen, C. B., Mortensen, P. B. (2001). Urbanization and schizophrenia: evidence of a cumulative negative effect of urban residence during upbringing. *Archives of General Psychiatry*, **58**, 1039–46.

Reininghaus, U., Morgan, C., Simpson, J. *et al.* (2009). Unemployment, social isolation, achievement-expectation mismatch and psychosis: findings from the AESOP study. *Social Psychiatry and Psychiatric Epidemiology*, **43**, 743–51.

Salzinger, S., Feldman, R. S., Hammer, M. *et al.* (1993). The effects of physical abuse on children's social relationships. *Child Development*, **64**, 169–87.

Selten, J.-P., Cantor-Graae, E. (2005). Social defeat: risk factor for schizophrenia? *British Journal of Psychiatry*, **187**, 101–2.

Sundquist, K., Frank, G., Sundquist, J. (2004). Urbanisation and incidence of psychosis and depression: follow-up study of 4.4 million women and men in

Sweden. *British Journal of Psychiatry*, **184**, 293–8.

Szapocznik, J., Kurtines, W. (1980). Acculturation, biculturalism, and adjustment. In A. Padilla, ed. *Recent Advances in Acculturation Research*. New York: Westview Press.

Tienari, P., Wynne, L. C., Sorri, A. *et al.* (2004). Genotype–environment interaction in schizophrenia-spectrum disorder: long term follow-up study of Finnish adoptees. *British Journal of Psychiatry*, **184**, 216–22.

van Os, J., Driessen, G., Gunther, N. *et al.* (2000). Neighbourhood variation in incidence of schizophrenia. Evidence for person–environment interaction. *British Journal of Psychiatry*, **176**, 243–8.

van Os, J., Hanssen, M., Bijl, R. V. *et al.* (2001). Prevalence of psychotic disorder and commmunity level of psychotic symptoms: an urban–rural comparison. *Archives of General Psychiatry*, **58**, 663–8.

Vanheusden, K., Mulder, C. L., van der Ende, J. *et al.* (2008). Associations between ethnicity and self-reported hallucinations in a population sample of young adults in the Netherlands. *Psychological Medicine*, **38**, 1095–1102.

WHO (World Health Organization). (1992). *Schedules for Assessment in Clinical Neuropsychiatry*. Geneva, Switzerland: World Health Organization.

Migration and its impact on the psychopathology of psychoses

Thomas Stompe and David Holzer

Editors' introduction

As shown in several studies and chapters in this volume, rates of psychoses vary and are raised in some migrant groups. We already know that cultures influence the way symptoms are presented and mould the content of these symptoms. To understand the abnormal nature of symptoms and their contents, clinicians must remain aware of their patients' cultural norms and how these cultures define abnormality and deviance from the norm. In this chapter, Stompe and Holzer use comparative data across Austria, Georgia, Ghana, Lithuania, Nigeria, Pakistan and Poland and point out that paranoid schizophrenia was commoner in post-modern societies and migration status by itself had no impact on changing symptoms. Catatonic schizophrenia was less frequent in migrants in comparison with natives from traditional countries. Contents of delusions varied according to cultures as did the type of hallucinations. The subtypes of schizophrenia are not influenced by the process of migration. Clinicians must therefore be open to exploring cultural values and norms in understanding the patient's symptoms. Psychopathology and its contents will also change with adjustments and acculturation.

Schizophrenia and migration

The impact of migration on the incidence and prevalence of schizophrenia and related psychoses has been studied extensively since the 1930s (Ødegaard, 1932).

Studies in migrants provide compelling support for the notion that social factors contribute to the development of schizophrenia. Most analyses found an increased risk for schizophrenia among first generation but also among second generation migrants (Brugha et al., 2004; Cantor-Graae and Selten, 2005; Cantor-Graae et al., 2005; Hutchinson and Haasen, 2004; Selten et al., 2007). The mean weighted risk (RR) among first generation migrants was 2.7 (95% CI 2.3–3.2), and among second generation migrants it was even higher; however, with a broader range (RR 4.5; 95% CI 1.5–13.1). The meta-analysis of subgroups yielded a RR of 3.3 (95% CI 2.8–3.9) for migrants from developing countries compared to a RR of 2.3 (95% CI 1.7–3.1) for those from developed countries (Cantor-Graae and Selten, 2005). The greatest effect size was found in migrants from areas with a black majority (RR 4.8; 95% CI 3.7–6.2). This result was confirmed by a 3-year Swedish incidence study (Cantor-Graae et al., 2005). Here too, the highest risk of developing a psychotic disorder was found in the first generation of black immigrants (RR 5.8; 95% CI 2.8–13.4).

Migration and Mental Health, ed. Dinesh Bhugra & Susham Gupta. Published by Cambridge University Press. © Cambridge University Press 2011.

In a prevalence study among 10 000 people in the UK, Brugha *et al.* (2004) found an increased risk of developing a psychotic disorder in immigrant groups of African-Caribbean and Africans (odds ratio (OR) 4.5), but not in the South Asian ethnic groups. Important for the interpretation of these data is the fact that epidemiological studies performed in the countries of origin found incidence rates in the Caribbean population, similar to those for white Europeans in Europe (Bhugra *et al.*, 1997; Hickling and Rodgers-Johnson, 1995; Mahy *et al.*, 1999). Hutchinson *et al.* (1996) found an increased rate of schizophrenia in the siblings of second generation African-Caribbean index cases, as compared to the incidence of schizophrenia in the siblings of white index cases with schizophrenia, a result suggesting a lower threshold for the expression of the disorder in carriers of susceptibility alleles that might be induced by environmental stress. This environmental stress might comprise a lack of supportive community structure, acculturation stress, demoralisation resulting from racial discrimination and blocked opportunity for upward social mobility (Bhugra *et al.*, 1999). Migrants are exposed to higher levels of competition. Those migrant groups which are under social pressure in their host society (e.g. the Moroccan males in the Netherlands or the African-Caribbean in Great Britain) have the highest risk of developing schizophrenia (Fearon *et al.*, 2006; Haasen *et al.*, 2001; Kirkbride *et al.*, 2006, 2008; Morgan *et al.*, 2006, 2007; Norris and Inglehart, 2004; Veling *et al.*, 2006, 2007b, 2008). Therefore, several authors have suggested that the chronic experience of social defeat or discrimination might lead to sensitisation of the mesolimbic dopamine system (Hutchinson and Haasen, 2004; Selten and Cantor-Graae, 2005).

The phenomenology of schizophrenia in migrants

Compared to the amount of literature concerning the high risk of certain migrant groups developing schizophrenia or bipolar disorder, little is known about the impact of migration on the psychopathology of psychoses. In a comparative study on symptom differences in schizophrenia between white and Caribbean patients, Hutchinson *et al.* (1999) were able to identify six symptom dimensions by means of factor analysis: mania, depression, first-rank delusions, other delusions, hallucinations and a dimension which comprised both manic and catatonic symptoms. The only difference between the two ethnic groups was seen in the mixed mania–catatonia dimension with the Afro-Caribbean group being over-represented. Discriminant analysis, however, revealed no significant differences between the groups in any dimension. These results seem to indicate that the core symptoms of schizophrenia are very similar in white and African-Caribbean patients. Comparing 74 patients of Turkish and 48 of German origin, Haasen *et al.* (2001) found higher scores of depression and hostile excitement, but no differences in positive, negative or cognitive symptoms in Turkish patients. These results are in line with a study by Veling *et al.* (2007a). The authors compared the symptoms at first treatment contact for psychotic disorders between 117 native Dutch and 165 ethnic minority patients from Morocco, Surinam, Turkey, other non-western countries and western countries. They found a higher total psychopathology and higher total score for the assessment of negative symptoms (SANS) scores for Moroccans compared to the native Dutch. Particularly, delusions of persecution were more frequent in the Moroccan sample. One crucial limitation of these studies is the fact that it remained unclear whether the differences between the native populations and the migrant groups are because of the circumstances of migration and to problems of acculturation or, rather, to what degree they are caused by the cultural pattern in their countries of origin. In 2002, Suhail and Cochrane addressed this problem for the first time. The authors compared Pakistani groups living in Britain or in Pakistan with white British groups. The comparison of these three groups yielded greater differences in the phenomenology of delusions and hallucinations between both Pakistani groups compared with the white British. These findings suggested a strong influence of the immediate environment on the pathogenesis of delusions and hallucinations. The limitation of this study was the small database, the retrospective design and the fact that the authors investigated only one ethnic minority group.

To throw further light on this topic, we combined the data of two Austrian studies, as detailed below.

The international study on psychotic symptoms

This study was conducted between 1995 and 2004 in Austria, Poland, Lithuania, Georgia, Pakistan, Nigeria and Ghana. The inclusion criterion was a clinical diagnosis of schizophrenia in patients between 18 and 60 years of age. Subjects with a migration background were excluded. DSM-IV diagnoses were achieved by use of the structured clinical interview for DSM-IV – SCID1. Contents of delusions, hallucinations and first-rank symptoms were classified by means of the questionnaire for psychotic symptoms – a semi-structured instrument developed by our research group – which was translated into the languages of the countries included in the study. Meanwhile the psychometric properties of the questionnaire have been published (Stompe and Friedmann, 2007; Stompe et al., 1999, 2004, 2006). The final sample under study consisted of 1080 subjects from Austria ($n = 350$), Poland ($n = 80$), Lithuania ($n = 73$), Georgia ($n = 74$), Pakistan ($n = 103$), Nigeria ($n = 324$) and Ghana ($n = 76$).

The Austrian migration and mental health survey

The data of 1770 migrants (958 male and 913 female; age 35.6 ± 10.5 years; age of migration 24.8 ± 10.8 years) from 93 countries were consecutively collected between 1995 and 2007 at the outpatient facility for migrants at the Department of Psychiatry and Psychotherapy of the Medical University of Vienna. All patients were classified according to ICD-10 and DSM-IV. SCID1 and CroCuDoc, an instrument for the acquisition of sociocultural data and of data related to traumatic experiences and migration, were administered, if necessary with the support of professional interpreters. All patients suffering from schizophrenia were additionally examined by means of the questionnaire for psychotic symptoms. Most patients came from Turkey ($n = 488$), followed by migrants from the former Yugoslavia and the states of the former USSR (GUS), most from civil war regions like Chechenia. There were 245 patients from Asia, 86 from sub-Saharan Africa, 137 from the EU, 29 from one of the EU-15 states and only 19 from America or Australia. Of these, 9.5% ($n = 169$) suffered from schizophrenia.

Comparison of natives and migrants suffering from schizophrenia

To compare the two samples, we subsumed the single countries into two groups, namely postmodern/modern countries and traditional countries. The classification followed the results of the world value survey (Inglehart, 1997; Norris and Inglehart, 2004). Traditional countries and postmodern/modern countries respectively share certain important cultural patterns independent of their localisation. In traditional countries, for example, family values are more important than individual self-actualisation. Religion and kinship systems are usually the central social subsystems, dominating other subsystems like economy, art, science or law. Personal relationships are more important than individual abilities; the individual has his or her place in a stable hierarchy. The central aim in modern countries is personal development and welfare with materialistic values dominating. The individual is more or less self-determined. In postmodern cultures other values like self-actualisation, emancipation or ecological thinking become more important than materialistic values. According to the world value survey, Austria, Poland and Lithuania belong to the (post)modern countries, while Georgia, Nigeria, Ghana and Pakistan belong to the group of traditional countries. The same classification was performed for the different ethnic groups living in Austria. The final sample consisted of 66 migrants from traditional and 103 migrants from (post)modern countries. Both groups were compared with the native sample of the international study on psychotic symptoms, divided into 564 inhabitants living in traditional countries and 516 natives in (post)modern countries.

We compared schizophrenia subtypes, contents of delusions, hallucinations and first-rank symptoms, calculating Chi squared for five pairs:

1. Migrants from traditional countries (A) versus migrants from (post)modern countries (B)
2. Natives from traditional countries (C) versus natives from (post)modern countries (D)
3. Migrants from traditional countries (A) versus natives from traditional countries (C)
4. Migrants from (post)modern countries (B) versus natives from (post)modern countries (D)
5. Migrants from traditional countries (A) versus natives from (post)modern countries (D).

Schizophrenia subtypes

Schizophrenia subtypes are complex phenotypes with more or less typical symptoms which often differ not only in the cross-sectional psychopathology but also in prevalence, age at onset, course and outcome of disease (Stompe *et al.*, 2005). Schizophrenia subtypes are distributed unequally over time and regions. Studies have shown that hebephrenia is most prevalent in South Asian countries (Inoue, 1993; Kraepelin, 1904a, 1904b; Stompe *et al.*, 2005), catatonic schizophrenia in sub-Saharan Africa and paranoid schizophrenia in Europe and North America (Pfeiffer, 1994). No current data on the distribution of schizophrenia subtypes in migrant samples are published. Our comparison of the four groups of our sample revealed substantial differences (Table 9.1).

In line with the literature, paranoid schizophrenia was more prevalent in (post)modern countries, in migrants as well as in natives. In contrast, catatonic and disorganised (hebephrenic) subtypes were more frequent in traditional countries. Schizoaffective disorders were more prevalent in traditional than in (post)modern countries. The difference was more explicit in natives than in migrants. The migration status had nearly no impact. Only catatonic schizophrenia and residual states were less frequent in migrants than in natives from traditional countries. Within the migrants from traditional countries and the inhabitants of the (post)modern countries, the distribution of most schizophrenia subtypes differed significantly.

Contents of delusions

The most distinct differences concerning contents of delusions were found between the two native groups. Natives in (post)modern countries more often showed delusions of grandeur, guilt and apocalypse; in contrast, inhabitants of traditional countries more often expressed hypochondriac delusions and delusions of poisoning. The process of migration is leading to a levelling of these differences. Migrants with different cultural background only differed concerning the frequency of delusions of grandeur, with lower rates in migrants from

Table 9.1 Prevalence of schizophrenia subtypes according to DSM-IV in migrants from traditional and postmodern/modern societies and inhabitants of traditional and postmodern/modern countries

Subtype	Migrants from		Natives in		Significance (P)				
	Traditional countries (n = 66) A	(Post) modern countries (n = 103) B	Traditional countries (n = 564) C	(Post) modern countries (n = 516) D	A versus B	C versus D	A versus C	B versus D	A versus D
Paranoid	23 (34.9)	61 (59.2)	239 (42.4)	349 (67.6)	**	***	n.s.	n.s.	***
Catatonic	11 (16.7)	7 (6.8)	69 (12.2)	28 (5.4)	n.s.	*	*	n.s.	**
Disorganised	13 (19.7)	9 (8.7)	60 (10.6)	36 (7.0)	***	***	n.s.	n.s.	***
Indifferent	2 (3.0)	7 (6.8)	34 (6.0)	19 (3.7)	n.s.	n.s.	n.s.	n.s.	n.s.
Residual	2 (3.0)	9 (8.7)	64 (11.3)	56 (10.9)	n.s.	n.s.	*	n.s.	*
Schizoaffective	15 (22.7)	10 (9.7)	98 (17.4)	28 (5.4)	*	***	n.s.	s.s.	***

Chi² test; * P < 0.05; ** P < 0.01; *** P < 0.001. n.s., Not significant. Values in parentheses are percentages.

Table 9.2 Lifetime prevalence of contents of delusions in schizophrenia in migrants from traditional and postmodern/modern societies and inhabitants of traditional and postmodern/modern countries

Delusions of:	Migrants from		Natives in		Significance (P)				
	Traditional countries ($n=66$) A	(Post) modern countries ($n=103$) B	Traditional countries ($n=564$) C	(Post) modern countries ($n=516$) D	A versus B	C versus D	A versus C	B versus D	A versus D
Persecution	61 (92.8)	93 (90.3)	478 (84.7)	442 (85.7)	n.s.	n.s.	n.s.	n.s.	n.s.
Grandeur	12 (18.7)	37 (36.3)	202 (35.9)	235 (43.0)	*	**	**	*	***
Religion	11 (16.7)	29 (28.2)	191 (33.8)	152 (29.5)	n.s.	n.s.	**	n.s.	*
Hypochondria	12 (18.2)	13 (12.6)	52 (9.2)	193 (20.0)	n.s.	**	n.s.	n.s.	n.s.
Guilt	2 (3.0)	7 (6.8)	32 (5.7)	83 (16.1)	n.s.	***	n.s.	*	**
Poisoning	10 (15.2)	11 (10.7)	162 (28.7)	88 (17.1)	n.s.	***	n.s.	s.s.	n.s.
Apocalypse	6 (9.1)	9 (8.7)	36 (6.4)	64 (12.4)	n.s.	**	n.s.	n.s.	n.s.
Being loved	4 (6.1)	4 (3.9)	36 (6.4)	32 (6.2)	n.s.	n.s.	n.s.	n.s.	n.s.
Jealousy	3 (4.4)	3 (2.9)	23 (4.1)	15 (2.9)	n.s.	n.s.	n.s.	n.s.	n.s.

Chi^2 test; * $P < 0.05$; ** $P < 0.01$; *** $P < 0.001$. n.s., Not significant. Values in parentheses are percentages.

Table 9.3 Lifetime prevalence of hallucinations in schizophrenia in migrants from traditional and postmodern/modern societies and inhabitants of traditional and postmodern/modern countries

Hallucinations	Migrants from		Natives in		Significance (P)				
	Traditional countries (n = 66) A	(Post)modern countries (n = 103) B	Traditional countries (n = 564) C	(Post)modern countries (n = 516) D	A versus B	C versus D	A versus C	B versus D	A versus D
Audible	61 (92.4)	78 (75.7)	446 (79.1)	362 (70.2)	**	**	n.s.	n.s.	***
Visual	20 (30.3)	16 (15.5)	220 (39.0)	128 (24.8)	*	***	n.s.	*	n.s.
Olfactory	4 (6.1)	5 (4.9)	32 (5.7)	30 (5.8)	n.s.	n.s.	n.s.	n.s.	n.s.
Gustatory	3 (4.5)	4 (3.9)	19 (3.4)	27 (5.2)	n.s.	n.s.	n.s.	n.s.	n.s.
Tactile	5 (7.6)	9 (8.7)	39 (6.9)	32 (6.2)	n.s.	n.s.	n.s.	n.s.	n.s.
Coenstethic	32 (33.3)	33 (32.0)	182 (32.2)	173 (33.5)	n.s.	n.s.	n.s.	s.s.	n.s.

Chi² test; * P < 0.05; ** P < 0.01; *** P < 0.001. n.s., Not significant. Values in parentheses are percentages.

Table 9.4 Lifetime prevalence of Schneiders' first-rank symptoms in schizophrenia in migrants from traditional and postmodern/modern societies and inhabitants of traditional and postmodern/modern countries

First-rank symptoms	Migrants from		Natives in		Significance (P)				
	Traditional countries (n = 66) A	(Post) modern countries (n = 103) B	Traditional countries (n = 564) C	(Post) modern countries (n = 516) D	A versus B	C versus D	A versus C	B versus D	A versus D
Delusional perception	52 (78.8)	83 (80.6)	386 (68.4)	419 (81.2)	n.s.	***	n.s.	n.s.	n.s.
Audible thoughts	8 (12.1)	17 (16.5)	90 (16.0)	85 (16.5)	n.s.	n.s.	n.s.	n.s.	n.s.
Thought broadcast	12 (18.2)	13 (12.6)	107 (19.0)	72 (14.0)	n.s.	*	n.s.	n.s.	n.s.
Thought insertion	27 (40.9)	37 (35.9)	176 (31.2)	182 (35.3)	n.s.	n.s.	n.s.	n.s.	n.s.
Thought withdrawal	9 (13.6)	9 (7.7)	47 (8.3)	60 (11.6)	n.s.	n.s.	n.s.	n.s.	n.s.
Commenting voices	29 (43.9)	47 (45.6)	279 (49.5)	200 (38.8)	n.s.	***	n.s.	s.s.	n.s
Dialogue voices	25 (37.9)	35 (34.0)	227 (40.2)	134 (26.0)	n.s.	***	n.s.	n.s.	n.s.
Made volition	8 (12.1)	9 (9.7)	65 (11.5)	109 (21.1)	n.s.	***	n.s.	**	n.s.
Somatic passivity	13 (19.7)	15 (14.6)	98 (17.4)	107 (20.7)	n.s.	n.s.	n.s.	n.s.	n.s.

Chi² test; * $P < 0.05$; ** $P < 0.01$; *** $P < 0.001$. n.s., Not significant. Values in parentheses are percentages.

traditional countries. In general, migration is leading to a decrease in delusions of grandeur in ethnic minorities. Religious delusions are more prevalent in natives than in migrants with a traditional background. In contrast, delusional guilt is reported more frequently in inhabitants of (post)modern countries than in migrants. The migrants from traditional countries showed fewer delusions of grandeur and guilt and also fewer religious delusions compared with the natives in (post)modern countries (Table 9.2).

Hallucinations

Differences were only seen in audible and visual hallucinations, in the so-called higher sensory perceptions. Independent of their migration status, subjects with a traditional cultural background show a higher prevalence for both types of hallucinations. The hallucinations of the so-called lower sensory perceptions were equally distributed in all four groups. Visual hallucinations were less prevalent in migrants than in natives with a (post)modern background. Migrants from traditional countries differed from native patients in (post) modern countries only in their higher rate of audible hallucinations (Table 9.3).

First-rank symptoms

The group comparisons mainly revealed differences between the two native populations. Natives living in traditional countries showed higher rates of thought broadcast and of audible first-rank hallucinations, while natives with a (post)modern background more often reported delusional perceptions and made volitions.

The distribution of these schizophrenia-typical symptoms did not vary statistically significantly between both migrant groups. The lower rates of made volition in migrants from (post)modern countries compared to the native population with the same background was the only difference between migrants and natives (Table 9.4).

Conclusion

The data presented here highlight the impact of migration on central symptoms of schizophrenia. We compared migrants from traditional and (post)modern countries with natives from the same cultural background. It became obvious that schizophrenia subtypes and hallucinations and their believed biological aetiology were not influenced by the process of migration. In contrast, comparable life circumstances in the post-migration period seem to cause a levelling of contents of delusions and first-rank symptoms in the migrant groups of different origin. The immediate environment might have a stronger impact on these psychotic phenomena than the cultural background.

References

Bhugra, D., Hilwig, M., Hossein, B. *et al.* (1997). First-contact incidence rates of schizophrenia in Trinidad and one-year follow-up. *British Journal of Psychiatry*, **169**, 587–92.

Bhugra, D., Mallett, R., Leff, J. (1999). Schizophrenia and the African-Caribbeans: a conceptual model of aetiology. *International Reviews of Psychiatry*, **11**, 145–52.

Brugha, T., Jenkins, R., Bebbington, P. *et al.* (2004). Risk factors and the prevalence of neurosis and psychosis in ethnic groups in Great Britain. *Social Psychiatry and Psychiatric Epidemiology*, **39**, 939–46.

Cantor-Graae, E., Selten, J. P. (2005). Schizophrenia and migration: a meta-analysis and review. *American Journal of Psychiatry*, **162**, 12–24.

Cantor-Graae, E., Zolkowska, K., McNeil, T. F. (2005). Increased risk of psychotic disorder among immigrants in Malmö: a 3-years first-contact study. *Psychological Medicine*, **35**, 1155–63.

Fearon, P., Kirkbride, J. B., Morgan, C. *et al.* (2006). Incidence of schizophrenia and other psychoses in ethnic minority groups: results from the MRC AESOP Study. *Psychological Medicine*, **36**, 1541–50.

Haasen, C., Yagdiran, O., Mass, R. *et al.* (2001). Schizophrenic disorders among Turkish migrants in Germany. A controlled clinical study. *Psychopathology*, **34**, 203–8.

Hickling, F., Rodgers-Johnson, P. (1995). The incidence of first contact schizophrenia in Jamaica. *British Journal of Psychiatry*, **167**, 193–6.

Hutchinson, G., Haasen, C. (2004). Migration and schizophrenia: the challenges for European psychiatry and implications for the future. *Social Psychiatry and Psychiatric Epidemiology*, **3**, 350–7.

Hutchinson, G., Takei, N., Bhugra, D. (1996). Morbid risk of schizophrenia in first-degree relatives of white and African-Caribbean patients with psychosis. *British Journal of Psychiatry*, **171**, 776–80.

Hutchinson, G., Takei, N., Sham, P. *et al.* (1999). Factor analysis of symptoms in schizophrenia: differences between white and Caribbean patients in Camberwell. *Psychological Medicine*, **29**, 607–12.

Inglehart, R. (1997). *Modernization and Postmodernization: Cultural, Economic, and Political Change in 43 Societies*. Princeton: Princeton University Press.

Inoue, S. (1993). Hebephrenia as the most prevalent subtype of schizophrenia in Japan. *Japanese Journal of Psychiatry & Neurology*, **47**, 505–14.

Kirkbride, J. B., Fearon, P., Morgan, C. *et al.* (2006). Heterogeneity in incidence rates of schizophrenia and other psychotic syndromes: findings from the 3-center AeSOP study. *Archives of General Psychiatry*, **63**, 250–8.

Kirkbride, J. B., Boydell, J., Ploubidis, G. B. *et al.* (2008). Testing the association between the incidence of schizophrenia and social

capital in an urban area. *Psychological Medicine*, **38**, 1083–94.

Kraepelin, E. (1904a). Vergleichende Psychiatrie. *Zentralblatt für Nervenheilkunde und Psychiatrie*, **27**, 433–7.

Kraepelin, E. (1904b). Psychiatrisches aus Java. *Zentralblatt für Nervenheilkunde und Psychiatrie*, **27**, 468–9.

Mahy, G. E., Mallet, R., Leff, J. *et al.* (1999). First-contact incidence rates of schizophrenia on Barbados. *British Journal of Psychiatry*, **175**, 28–33.

Morgan, C., Dazzan, P., Morgan, K. *et al.* (2006). First episode psychosis and ethnicity: initial findings from the AESOP study. *World Psychiatry*, **5**, 40–6.

Morgan, C., Kirkbride, J., Leff, J. *et al.* (2007). Parental separation, loss and psychosis in different ethnic groups: a case-control study. *Psychological Medicine*, **37**, 495–503.

Norris, P., Inglehart, R. (2004). *Sacred and Secular: Religion and Politics Worldwide*. Cambridge: Cambridge University Press.

Ødegaard, Ø. (1932). Emigration and insanity: a study of mental disease among Norwegian born population in Minnesota. *Acta Psychiatrica Neurologica Scandinavica*, **7**(Suppl. 4), 1–206.

Pfeiffer, W. (1994). *Transkulturelle Psychiatrie*. Stuttgart, New York: Thieme.

Selten, J. P., Cantor-Graae, E. (2005). Social defeat: risk factor for schizophrenia? *British Journal of Psychiatry*, **187**, 101–2.

Selten, J. P., Cantor-Graae, E., Kahn, R. S. (2007). Migration and schizophrenia. *Current Opinion in Psychiatry*, **20**, 111–15.

Stompe, T., Friedmann, A. (2007). Culture and schizophrenia. In D. Bhugra and K. Bhui, eds. *Textbook of Cultural Psychiatry*. Cambridge: Cambridge University Press, 314–22.

Stompe, T., Friedmann, A., Ortwein, G. *et al.* (1999). Comparison of delusions among schizophrenics in Austria and in Pakistan. *Psychopathology*, **32**, 225–34.

Stompe, T., Ortwein-Swoboda, G., Schanda, H. (2004). Schizophrenia, delusional symptoms and violence: the threat/control-override-concept re-examined. *Schizophrenia Bulletin*, **30**, 31–44.

Stompe, T., Ortwein-Swoboda, G., Ritter, K. *et al.* (2005). The impact of diagnostic criteria on the prevalence of schizophrenic subtypes. *Comprehensive Psychiatry*, **46**, 433–9.

Stompe, T., Bauer, S., Ortwein-Swoboda, G. *et al.* (2006). Delusions of guilt: The attitude of Christian and Islamic confessions towards good and evil and the responsibility of men. *Journal of Muslim Mental Health*, **1**, 43–56.

Suhail, L. K., Cochrane, R. (2002). Effect of culture and environment on the phenomenology of delusions and hallucinations. *International Journal of Social Psychiatry*, **48**, 126–38.

Veling, W., Selten, J. P., Veen, N. *et al.* (2006). Incidence of schizophrenia among ethnic minorities in the Netherlands: a four-year first-contact study. *Schizophrenia Research*, **86**, 189–93.

Veling, W., Selten, J. P., Mackenbach, J. P. *et al.* (2007a). Symptoms at first contact for psychotic disorder: comparison between native Dutch and ethnic minorities. *Schizophrenia Research*, **95**, 30–8.

Veling, W., Selten, J. P., Susser, E. *et al.* (2007b). Discrimination and the incidence of psychotic disorders among ethnic minorities in the Netherlands. *International Journal of Epidemiology*, **36**, 761–8.

Veling, W., Susser, E., van Os, J. *et al.* (2008). Ethnic density of neighborhoods and incidence of psychotic disorders among immigrants. *American Journal of Psychiatry*, **165**, 66–73.

Chapter 10

Identity, idioms and inequalities: providing psychotherapies for South Asian women

Kamaldeep Bhui and Tamsin Black

Editors' introduction

Identity is a multilayered and multifaceted concept. Every individual has several identities, but at any given time one identity takes precedence over the others. Of these, cultural identity, especially among migrants, presents great challenges and a strong aspect of personality is needed to cope with changes related to settling down in the new culture. The processes of acculturation will influence cultural identity. Expressions of distress are key to seeking help and these may or may not change even if an individual's cultural identity has begun to shift. In this chapter, Bhui and Black describe the link between culture and expression of symptoms and distress, and how culture influences help-seeking and affects recovery and health inequalities. Using clinical examples from South Asian women, they illustrate clinical management issues and what clinicians may find useful in dealing with the problems with which patients present. Changing notions of self and the importance of some symptoms in help-seeking will influence the presentation styles.

Introduction

In this chapter, South Asian refers to people with origins in or immigrant from India, Pakistan or Bangladesh. Migrants from these countries arrived in the UK in the 1950s and 1960s from India and Pakistan and Bangladesh, with a slower flow later; South Asian migrants arrived in the UK to improve their quality of life and to fill employment demands in the UK, and to avoid harsh treatment in the 1970s in Uganda. The societies from which South Asians migrated are an important context as they uphold particular forms of gender relations, hardship and experiences of poverty, and specific processes for coping with misfortune; health is seen not in a purely biomedical, physiological or western psychological form but as part of a harmonious existence in relation to family, community, supernatural forces and the Gods. It is known that ethnic minorities are on the whole more religious than white British subjects, and that they more often use religious and spiritual ways of coping with misfortune and distress (Bhui *et al.*, 2008a).

The literature on the role of culture in the development of mental illness and the promotion of mental health makes use of numerous terms to denote specific cultural, religious, ethnic and

---

Migration and Mental Health, ed. Dinesh Bhugra & Susham Gupta. Published by Cambridge University Press. © Cambridge University Press 2011.

racial groups. These are often talked about as if representing homogenous categories of people with similar characteristics and problems, and for whom similar solutions can be applied. A specific and useful definition of culture that captures this complexity is:

> a set of guidelines which individuals inherit as members of a particular society, and which tells them how to view the world, how to experience it emotionally, and how to behave in relation to other people, supernatural forces, or gods and to the environment. It is transmitted by symbols, language, art and ritual.   (Helman, 1991a, b)

While it is accepted that individuals within any category, including South Asian, can vary markedly (as set out in this chapter), it is also true that culture is a group and shared experience and some similarities between individuals within an ethnic group or any cultural group arise owing to their shared histories, religious practices, and shared homeland, shared traditions and ways of perceiving and relating to the world and people within it. The geographic origins are important as these provide a shared geopolitical location with particular local economies and social fabric and numerous closely related and connected subcultures. It is from these that South Asian women have migrated to the new economies and social fabric in the UK, mainly in urban environments where migrants are most likely to take up residence. These new environments, as well as those created and carried in tradition, will all influence the way mental distress is experienced and expressed, and managed. The new environments, for example, offer new forms of gender relations, new forms of social activities, including leisure and consumer goods, and new connections with other communities, perhaps with differing or even opposing world views; the ensuing accommodations or entrenchments can be understood and experienced as strains, and constraints, opportunities for growth and escape.

Families migrating together, single men or women coming to settle in the UK by marriage and the elderly joining the children in the UK – all have different profiles of 'push' and 'pull' factors for migration; and diaspora from South Asia reside in all parts of the world and remain connected through family ties, business relations, religious affiliations and shared interests in the plight of their own cultural heritage. However, the identification with the country of origin can vary, and shifts in lifestyle and beliefs are seen toward that of the host nation. However, this process is not linear, so more intensified and radical and traditional cultural and religious practices may be found in second and third generation migrants, where they are in search of positive identities. New cultures are therefore developed which are blended varieties of homeland and new world cultures, products of youth culture, globalisation, and are often borne out of a search for identity to combat social exclusion, isolation and discrimination.

Literature on South Asian women and mental health

The early literature on South Asian women refers to a higher suicide rate among young women of Indian origin, and greater levels of self-harm amongst South Asian women in general; the implication is that women of South Asian origin experience particular forms of strain, and gender roles and gender disadvantage are important (Bhui and McKenzie, 2008; Bhui et al., 2007; McKenzie et al., 2008; Raleigh, 1998, 2000), and there are significant strains on women with children and women of childbearing age (Woollett and Marshall, 1996; Woollett et al., 1994, 1995). Among South Asian migrants, depression was not originally asserted to be common (Gillam, 1990; Gillam et al., 1989), but somatic complaints were common among those seeking help from doctors in general, and women in particular. This finding is common to many immigrant groups, yet it is also reported that somatic complaints are common in all presenting patients, but appear to be more prominent in the therapeutic discourse with South Asians, especially women. These symptoms of physical bodily complaints have been understood in many ways:

- An idiom of distress found in the original language with no physical complaints
- A physical complaint associated with a change in perceived function of the self
- A physical complaint existing alongside emotional ones
- A physical complaint in the presence of a physical illness with confirmed diagnosis, yet the level of disability far exceeds what would be expected
- Pain syndromes.

Case study 1

A is a 44-year-old mother of four children (they are aged 4, 8, 11 and 12) living in a two-bedroom flat, with a husband who has diabetes. She has lived in the UK for 35 years, having grown up in Bangladesh. She speaks some English. No one in the house is working and her husband receives benefits. She is referred as her GP thinks she is depressed, as she has been neglecting the children and her husband for a year and no longer goes out shopping. Her main complaint is of heat emanating from the top of her head and aches in her limbs. She is self-caring and manages the house on her own. One son (aged 4) has been diagnosed as autistic and requires a great deal of individual attention. She attends a psychotherapy assessment, and spends 40 minutes talking about her physical complaints and lethargy. She does not seem to understand what psychotherapy means, and assumed she was coming to another department in the hospital for medical treatment.

Questions

Is this patient suitable for psychotherapy? What else needs to be assessed and what work might be done to assess her further before deciding she is not suitable?

One should not conclude that she is not suitable. Although physical complaints are prominent, some psychoeducational work may help her realise why she is being seen in psychotherapy. Information about the service, and emotional issues, and how physical symptoms can reflect these might be shared. A cognitive behavioural approach at testing her views about her symptoms may be helpful to establish the degree to which she might be able to take up alternative explanations for her illness. This will permit her to test her ability to take up the proposed solutions while accepting the gravity of her symptoms. She has numerous social stressors which are not easily relieved; however, these may be helped by social support and befriending, carer allowances and childcare; these may even be required before she can focus on her mind and before she can engage in a therapy that gives her the best chance of recovery.

Case study 2

S is a 17-year-old single woman who lives with her brother and mother. She has overdosed several times and fears her brother wants her to marry this year, before she is able to go to university. She was born in the UK as was her brother; her parents were from Pakistan. Her father died 3 years ago from a heart attack. When she goes home late after spending time with her friend (female in a neighbouring flat), her brother is offended and has threatened violence. She wishes to exercise her freedoms but also follows traditional religious practices with the family. She has suffered injury from her brother in the past, but accepts that he is her brother and she does not wish to seek help from the police or leave home. S feels she has a poor relationship with her brother, and that is her problem. She complains of weakness and depressive symptoms, but otherwise is highly functioning and continues to joke and smile with her friends, and to associate with them.

Questions

Why does she not leave home? What is her explanatory model? Why does her brother, despite being brought up here, still expect her to behave as though they live in Pakistan.

She may be suitable for psychotherapy, but this suitability cannot be assessed so quickly and in a linear fashion without some psychoeducation and then a trial of therapy. Although physical complaints are prominent, some psychoeducational work may help her realise why she is being seen in psychotherapy. Information about the service, emotional issues and how physical symptoms can reflect these might be shared.

Why does she put up with her situation and the way she is treated?

A more diffuse rather than individual sense of self, 'we-self' rather than 'I-self', loyalty to the family and an existence that is defined by the other makes it difficult for her to leave, despite risk to her. She thinks she has a relationship problem rather than a mental health problem, and sees overdoses as a rational attempt to remove the problem for her brother while ablating thoughts about how she can remove herself from this situation without changing her own identity and desires and without ridding herself of her family or showing disloyalty. She is clearly stuck and unable to consider taking action to remedy the relationship or help her safety, and any attempt to do so results in her breaking off treatment. Her brother has inherited a particular set of beliefs about gender relations and expectations of marriage, and as the elder male in the family, in the absence of their father, he considers it his duty to ensure that her and the family dignity is preserved. This seems like an over-intensified identification with the culture of origin, which differs from her own acculturation status, that tolerates and embraces aspects of the host and own culture (called bicultural or integrated).

The self

Tseng has reviewed the role of culture in different psychotherapies, emphasising that adaptations were needed to all forms of therapy; he proposed technical, philosophical and theoretical modifications to any intervention (Tseng, 2001). Most clinicians work on the technical and read around theoretical limitations, but do not address the philosophical challenges when encountering patients with diverse forms of self and identity, perhaps with varying degrees of individualisation and varying concepts of the person (Kirmayer, 2007). In a more sociocentric society, reflected in a more sociocentric experience of the self, mental distress and depression are experienced as an interpersonal problem; that is where remedy is sought, rather in embodied individual problems (Beliappa, 1991; Kirmayer, 2007; Tseng, 2001). Social support and resources for recovery are then also located in the family and in the social group to which the person belongs. If the self is identified strongly with supernatural or religious forces as part of the social and supernatural worlds, then these also form part of how the person copes with misfortune. Alternatively, some models of distress and healing require sitting in the presence of a holy or revered individual, a Guru, and perhaps even being blessed by the gaze and presence, rather than on introspection or active treatment (Neki, 1973). A patient with these notions of self and explanatory models may not seek active treatment but the presence and influence of a more powerful and authoritative other; our qualifications as therapists or health professionals may not be sufficient for us to be seen as influential among powerful supernatural or spiritual forces; our age, if young, may also work against us if the culture of the patient expresses particular emphases on age as the basis of wisdom, or age as needing to be compatible for certain intimate discussions.

Some studies suggest that more authoritative therapeutic relationships with didactic prescriptions of behaviour change are preferred by South Asians, including the prescription of injections and somatic bodily treatments rather than talking treatments; however, there is marked variation with background educational factors, literacy and exposure to psychoeducation, be it formally through primary care and public health campaigns or through watching soap operas, films and talk shows.

Patients presenting with alternative explanations for their illness, patients who seek miraculous cures, patients who seek your presence to recover rather than any specific treatment or patients who seek physical treatments including pharmacological interventions may also be misjudged to reflect non-psychological mindedness or even passivity and a lack of commitment. Many patients need to be encouraged and educated into psychotherapy, the rules explained and the processes experienced, while their own models of recovery are understood and streamlined with our interventions.

Idioms of distress and gender

Somatic idioms of distress are common. Classically Krause, (1989) described sinking heart among Punjabi women, but other somatic complaints include chest pain, shortness of breath, weakness in the limbs and heat coming out of the head. The presence of somatic complaints was initially seen as a form of masked depression or, in Freudian terms, a bodily container for emotional problems, expressed through conversion or hysterical mechanisms; such a view is now outdated and largely discredited although it is well established that physical symptoms can arise from emotional problems. This is often alongside emotional problems and the majority of patients can express them if encouraged. A small proportion do continue to deny any emotional component, to a point where physical investigations are necessary; however, these should be undertaken with caution and only if clearly indicated given the potential to reinforce illness behaviour positively. A good starting point is for the therapist to review with the patient what, if any, physical assessments are required, and more biological lines of enquiry have been followed and what conclusions were drawn by the health professional and by the patient. This can be rich ground for gaining a greater understanding of the patient's belief system and points of conviction and also engender a sense of trust and collaboration between therapist and patient. It also helps to establish areas on which there is disagreement, and issues that the patient feels are unresolved. In a small proportion, persistent physical complaints will ultimately be explained by later physical illness or points of inconsistency or misinformation discovered that might be maintaining health anxiety through uncertainty. So this possibility needs to be kept in mind and a delicate balance achieved between pursuing psychological explanations and interventions and ensuring physical health. The separate structures of services providing each of these interventions also impairs the ability of therapists to proceed without hesitation or concern if physical illness is suspected. However, it is well established that immigrants and minorities, although experiencing somatic complaints as much as other non-immigrant groups, tend to present to doctors more often with these.

One explanation is that somatic symptoms serve as a ticket to enter systems of care in a less stigmatising manner. Similarly, this way of expressing distress or inability to cope may have been reinforced within the patient's family or community. Once given permission by the therapist to talk about their struggle in a different way, many patients may be surprisingly eloquent and aware of the nature of their social, interpersonal or intrapsychic struggle. Also, somatic symptoms have been described as a form of social protest and social strain, communicated through physiology and idiom (Kirmayer *et al.*, 2004). Thus, adverse life events, financial strain, interpersonal difficulties and gender disadvantage, including through violence (Kumari, 2004), can all be expected to contribute to the development of somatic symptoms. It is possible if their existence is accepted for somatic experiences not to dominate the therapeutic discourse. The construction of an individualised symptom monitoring measure that incorporates affective, behavioural and somatic phenomena can be all it takes to broaden the range of material that is felt to be appropriate or acceptable for the patient to bring to therapy. Personality variables, including negative affectivity, repressive coping styles and somatic attributional style all need further investigation (Kirmayer *et al.*, 1994; 2004; Kumari, 2004).

Women may experience special strains where gender roles in specific cultures restrict their freedoms to travel alone, work in specific jobs or marry whom they choose (Gupta *et al.*, 2007). No single set of cultural expectations is found within any one ethnic or religious group and, as case study 2 shows, individuals living in similar environments may develop different patterns of acculturation and show different degrees of integration and marginalisation, or assimilation and/or traditionalism. The strain in identity only occurs if there is a mismatch between the predominant identity of the woman and that of her peers, or husband, family or society. A particular point of strain may be at the point of marriage.

Table 10.1 Somatic items and their association with morbidity in each cultural group (P, Punjabi; E, English)

Somatic symptom	Culture	Cases versus non-cases (%; on CIS-R; weighted)	OR	95% CI	P value
Pain and tension in shoulders and neck	P	53.2 vs 16.8	5.64	2.19–14.52	$P < 0.001$
	E	40.1 vs 15.2	3.83	1.37–10.72	$P < 0.01$
Severe headaches	P	55.3 vs 11.2	9.83	4.44–28.10	$P < 0.001$
	E	44.8 vs 16.4	4.13	1.42–12.0	$P < 0.01$
Fluttering in stomach as if something is moving	P	21.3 vs 1.9	14.23	1.71–118.25	$P < 0.01$
	E	20.5 vs 12.2	1.85	0.52–6.61	$P = 0.35$
Pain in chest or heart	P	42.6 vs 13.1	4.94	1.8–13.53	$P < 0.01$
	E	18.4 vs 13.0	1.52	0.45–5.15	$P = 0.5$
Mouth or throat felt dry	P	46.8 vs 15.6	4.76	1.67–13.57	$P < 0.01$
	E	32.5 vs 20.4	1.88	0.64–5.48	$P = 0.25$
Been sweating a lot	P	34.0 vs 20.5	2.0	0.79–5.06	$P = 0.14$
	E	42.7 vs 16.4	3.8	1.3–11.09	$P = 0.01$
Choking sensation in throat	P	34.0 vs 14.9	2.95	1.09–7.93	$P = 0.03$
	E	20.2 vs 8.2	2.85	0.67–12.08	$P = 0.16$
Aches and pains all over body	P	51.1 vs 22.4	3.62	1.48–8.9	$P < 0.001$

Table 10.1 (cont.)

Somatic symptom	Culture	Cases versus non-cases (%; on CIS-R; weighted)	OR	95% CI	P value
	E	24.6 vs 16.4	1.66	0.55–5.0	P = 0.37
Aware of palpitations or heart pounding	P	44.7 vs 9.3	7.86	2.59–23.8	P < 0.001
	E	30.7 vs 6.8	6.1	1.37–26.7	P = 0.02
Trembling or shaking	P	29.8 vs 5.6	7.16	1.87–27.41	P < 0.01
	E	24.6 vs 4.1	7.66	0.93–63.16	P = 0.06
Passing urine more frequently	P	48.9 vs 18.6	4.18	1.66–10.55	P < 0.01
	E	28.6 vs 13.6	2.55	0.79–8.24	P = 0.12
Feeling of pressure inside head as if going to burst	P	34.0 vs 18.6	2.25	0.88–5.79	P = 0.09
	E	4.3 vs 6.8	2.29	0.48–10.99	P = 0.30
Troubled by constipation	P	31.9 vs 5.6	7.91	2.08–30.12	P < 0.01
	E	22.5 vs 8.20	3.25	0.83–12.73	P = 0.09
Heart felt weak or shrinking	P	23.4 vs 7.5	3.79	1.09–13.15	P = 0.04
	E	0 vs 4.02	—	—	—
Suffered from excessive wind (gas or belching)	P	36.2 vs 15.6	3.06	1.06–8.85	P = 0.04
	E	20.5 vs 9.6	2.42	0.67–8.72	P = 0.18
Hands and feet felt cold	P	27.7 vs 3.7	9.9	2.06–47.45	P < 0.01
	E	20.5 vs 21.8	0.92	0.32–2.7	P = 0.88

So, in a geographical area in which a specific migrant community retains traditional practices, say Bangladeshi residents in East London, an individual deviating from cultural group norms (a body of rules and regulations which are implicit and influenced by the more powerful in society, men on the whole, rather than being available in a specific doctrine which might be scrutinised) may find themselves isolated and under internal and external pressures to conform. Traditionalism in these circumstances may be protective for mental health as making acculturative steps leaves individuals at risk of losing social support, and being identified as deviant in society is risky for emotional stability and mental health. This was how we explained the mental health advantage of young Bangladeshi girls in East London, if they had traditional identities when this was based on their clothing choices (Bhui and Hotopf, 1997; Bhui et al., 2008b). At key points of developmental transition, such consistency and clarity of identity may strengthen resilience.

Table 10.1 provides unpublished data from a study of Punjabi and English primary care attendees, and contrasts profiles of somatic complaints on the Bradford somatic inventory (Mumford, 1991; Mumford et al., 1991). This instrument assesses symptoms expected in

South Asian subjects, based on pilot work among Pakistani and English women. The range of symptoms is demonstrated by our work on Punjabi and English people in South London, showing the prevalence of these somatic symptoms in people with and without case status (recognised as having a common mental disorder on the clinical interview schedule, CIS-R; Lewis *et al.*, 1992). Although the symptoms are all found in each group, they can be more common in one or other group. Specific somatic complaints have been mapped onto particular cultures, for example, 'nervios' and 'brainache' among Mexican Americans; sinking heart, feeling hot and gas among Indians (Ahmed and Bhugra, 2007).

The management of somatic symptoms: a specialist cognitive behavioural therapy approach

The central practice of cognitive behavioural therapy is the collaborative construction of a shared understanding or formulation of the problem with which the patient is presenting. This may seem immediately problematic when the patient presents with a commitment to a non-psychological explanation of their difficulty. However, when a patient is presented with the therapist's alternative but individually adapted perspective, irrespective of the degree of emphasis on physical complaints, this may be experienced as empowering and information giving.

Case study

D is a 32-year-old mother of a 5-year-old son who has lived in the UK since the age of 3 years. She was diagnosed with postnatal depression when her son was 3 months old and shamefully describes her paranoid and odd behaviour across a 6-month period. She is referred to psychotherapy for help with anxiety, low mood and interpersonal difficulties; however, her assessment appointment is dominated by talk of somatic ailments including lack of energy, limb weakness and concern that the physical strain of childbirth has left her with an undiagnosed condition. She describes a westernised upbringing in a multicultural borough of London in which her peers were a mixture of African, white and mixed race as well as Bengali. On marriage she moved to live with her husband and mother in law in Tower Hamlets which she described as much more like 'back home'. Her distress and fearfulness post-birth have been attributed by her mother in law, and to a lesser extent by her husband, to the work of mischievous Jinn; her vulnerability to Jinn arising because of the perceived immoral behaviour of her mother.

How does she make sense of this acute period of illness? Is she a suitable candidate for a talking therapy?

In actual fact she does very well when given an opportunity to review her experience of a severe mental health crisis and to think about her own explanation in the context of her developmental experience and the ongoing sense of constraint and fearfulness. She experiences fear living with a highly critical and doubting elder woman. The therapy involves psychoeducation regarding the postnatal crisis and the physiology of anxiety and the role of avoidance in its maintenance. Within a cognitive behavioural framework she is encouraged to look at the different perspectives around her non-critically. She could not tolerate overt criticism of her mother in law's perspective but with support was able to develop and trust more her own perspective. Behavioural experiments encouraged her to seek conversation and develop openness with a more similar peer group at work which strengthened her tolerance at home and eased the strain. Somatic preoccupations diminished in line with the strengthening of her confidence in her psychological robustness. A lifespan developmental context for her own thoughts, feelings and behaviours was helpful in challenging her fears that she was mad or under the influence of Jinn (her mother in law's perspective).

Conclusions

The work in this chapter is predicated on the clinician/therapist being able to enquire about unusual beliefs and forms of identity with which they are unfamiliar. Understanding the individual's culture of origin, some history about their migration experience, the environment both in their home country, in their particular developmental context and in their new home all become important. Understanding their identity and their explanations for their predicament are all essential parts of a therapeutic alliance and trust. Being understood as a form of engagement needs to precede the delivery of interventions, and even then trust has to be sustained by an authentic attempt to address problems perceived by the patient to be important. This may mean the therapist has to spend more time on psychoeducation and social interventions prior to delivering a psychological intervention. The cultural formulation has been described in DSM-IV as a method of assessing identity, illness perceptions, transference and counter-transference and making adaptations to the overall care process. The use of this formulation as a guide to, rather than template for, communication and exploring the patient's perspectives is recommended as part of the assessment. There are now many structured tools that permit the assessment of explanatory models and illness perceptions, and identity. Perhaps we should be using these in routine practice alongside outcome measures.

Key points

- Extended assessment periods for somatic presentations with perceived non-psychological mindedness; this permits some psychoeducational work prior to judgements about suitability
- Understand the role of somatic complaints and the reasons why these may be presented
- Consider the cultural formulation as a form of enquiry
- Model and encourage individual flexible perspective-taking and set out the costs and benefits of thinking in particular ways and holding onto specific sets of beliefs
- Use behavioural experiments
- Consider issues of authority; for example, ensure that the therapist is convinced by their model and has created a relationship of trust and non-invasiveness, and an invitation to take part in a therapy that is not oppressive
- CBT for bodily symptoms can be used at metacognitive and behavioural levels
- Cultural practices and social interventions may be used by psychotherapists as a form of engagement and can increase the sense of benevolence; the patient's help-seeking is a route to empowerment and benefit rather than dependence.

References

Ahmed, K., Bhugra, D. (2007). Depression across ethnic minority cultures: diagnostic issues. *World Cultural Psychiatry Research Review*, 2, 47–56.

Beliappa, J. (1991). Illness or distress. *Alternative Models of Mental Health*. London: Confederation of Indian Organisations.

Bhui, K., Hotopf, M. (1997). Somatization disorder. *British Journal of Hospital Medicine*, **58**(4), 145–9.

Bhui, K. S., McKenzie, K. (2008). Rates and risk factors by ethnic group for suicides within a year of contact with mental health services in England and Wales. *Psychiatric Services* **59**(4), 414–20.

Bhui, K., McKenzie, K., Rasul, F. (2007). Rates, risk factors and methods of self harm among minority ethnic groups in the UK: a systematic review. *BMC Public Health*, 7, 336.

Bhui, K., King, M., Dein, S., O'Connor, W. (2008a). Ethnicity and religious coping with mental distress. *Journal of Mental Health*, **17**(2), 141–51.

Bhui, K., Khatib, Y., Viner, R. *et al.* (2008b). Cultural identity, clothing and common mental disorder: a prospective school-based study of white British and Bangladeshi adolescents. *Journal of Epidemiology and Community Health*, **62**(5), 435–41.

Gillam, S. (1990). Ethnicity and the use of health services. *Postgraduate Medical Journal*, **66**(782), 989–93.

Gillam, S. J., Jarman, B., White, P., Law, R. (1989). Ethnic differences in consultation rates in urban general practice. *British Medical Journal*, **299**(6705), 953–7.

Gupta, V., Johnstone, L., Gleeson, K. (2007). Exploring the meaning of separation in second-generation young South Asian women in Britain. *Psychology and Psychotherapy*, **80** (Pt 4), 481–95.

Helman, C. G. (1991a). The family culture: a useful concept for family practice. *Family Medicine*, **23**(5), 376–81.

Helman, C. G. (1991b). Limits of biomedical explanation. *Lancet*, **337**(8749), 1080–3.

Kirmayer, L. J. (2007). Psychotherapy and the cultural concept of the person. *Transcultural Psychiatry*, **44**(2), 232–57.

Kirmayer, L. J., Robbins, J. M., Paris, J. (1994). Somatoform disorders: personality and the social matrix of somatic distress. *Journal of Abnormal Psychology*, **103**(1), 125–36.

Kirmayer, L. J., Groleau, D., Looper, K. J., Dao, M. D. (2004). Explaining medically unexplained symptoms. *Canadian Journal of Psychiatry*, **49**(10), 663–72.

Krause, I. B. (1989). Sinking heart: a Punjabi communication of distress. *Social Science and Medicine*, **29**(4), 563–75.

Kumari, N. (2004). South Asian women in Britain: their mental health needs and views of services. *Journal of Public Mental Health*, **3**(1), 30–8.

Lewis, G., Pelosi, A. J., Araya, R., Dunn, G. (1992). Measuring psychiatric disorder in the community: a standardized assessment for use by lay interviewers. *Psychological Medicine*, **22**(2), 465–86.

McKenzie, K., Bhui, K., Nanchahal, K., Blizard, B. (2008). Suicide rates in people of South Asian origin in England and Wales: 1993–2003. *British Journal of Psychiatry*, **193**(5), 406–9.

Mumford, D. (1991). The Bradford somatic inventory. *Nursing Times*, **87**(38), 52–3.

Mumford, D. B., Bavington, J. T., Bhatnagar, K. S. *et al.* (1991). The Bradford somatic inventory. A multi-ethnic inventory of somatic symptoms reported by anxious and depressed patients in Britain and the Indo-Pakistan subcontinent. *British Journal of Psychiatry*, **158**, 379–86.

Neki, J. S. (1973). Guru-chela relationship: the possibility of a therapeutic paradigm. *American Journal of Orthopsychiatry*, **43**(5), 755–66.

Raleigh, V. S. (1998). Suicide, country of birth and coroner's verdicts. *British Journal of Psychiatry*, **173**, 185–6.

Raleigh, V. S. (2000). High rates of attempted suicide in Asian women, especially at young ages; investigation of precipitating factors. *Psychological Medicine*, **30**(4), 989.

Tseng, W. S. (2001). *Handbook of Cultural Psychiatry*. San Diego, California: Academic Press.

Woollett, A., Marshall, H. (1996). Reading the body: young women's accounts of the meanings of the body in relation to independence, responsibility and maturity. *European Journal of Womens Studies,* 3(3), 199.

Woollett, A., Marshall, H., Nicolson, P., Dosanjh, N. (1994). Asian womens ethnic identity – the impact of gender and context in the accounts of women bringing up children in East London. *Feminism & Psychology,* 4(1), 119–32.

Woollett, A., Dosanjh, N., Nicolson, P. *et al.* (1995). The ideas and experiences of pregnancy and childbirth of Asian and non-Asian women in East London. *British Journal of Medical Psychology,* **68**, 65–84.

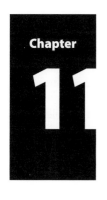

Chapter

11

Cultural bereavement, culture shock and culture conflict: adjustments and reactions

Dinesh Bhugra, Wojtek Wojcik and Susham Gupta

Editors' introduction

When migrants leave their country of origin, it is inevitable that they will leave a number of anchors behind. These may include family, kinship, home, belongings, relationships, friendships and other physical and emotional structures. Depending upon the nature of the migration, preparation for such a move and other factors, the migrant may carry a sense of loss with them. This loss may lead to cultural bereavement, which may be related to some loss of culture, cultural values and norms, especially in the face of adjustment to the new culture. As is to be expected, the response to such a loss will vary from individual to individual and group to group. Another response to the new culture has been described as culture shock, although, again, not every migrant will experience this. Some individuals in the same family may settle down better and quicker compared with others, depending upon the pace of acculturation; this may well contribute to a sense of conflict. In this chapter, the authors highlight some of these factors, especially on the acculturation by and of cultures, rather than simply focusing on individuals. The inter-relationship between cultural bereavement, culture shock and culture conflict needs to be elaborated upon in their impact on individual interactions.

Introduction

One of the key factors in the process of migration is what the individuals carry with them (both in material and emotional terms) and what they leave behind. Depending upon the reasons for migration (whether they are pulled towards the new setting or are pushed out of the old setting), migrants may have time to prepare or may have to leave suddenly. In either case, they will leave certain material, as well as emotional, things behind. The experience of such a loss can take on many connotations. The feelings of loss may be temporary and fleeting or may last for a long time. It is inevitable that the individual's response to the loss will be tempered with a range of other factors.

Following the process of migration and then settling down in the new society, the individual may experience cultural bereavement, culture shock or culture conflict. It is possible that all these may occur at the same time or may do so at different times or not at all. It is likely that cultural shock may occur probably soon after arrival, whereas cultural bereavement may take some time to develop. Cultural conflict is generally

Migration and Mental Health, ed. Dinesh Bhugra & Susham Gupta. Published by Cambridge University Press. © Cambridge University Press 2011.

related to a difficulty between one's own cultural values in comparison with those of the family or the society at large. It is noted in the children of migrants, who may hold values akin to those of the larger society, but these may conflict against the values their parents hold dear.

Healthcare delivery in any system is controlled by the resources made available by the society. In an increasingly smaller globalised world it is imperative that healthcare professionals are aware of these phenomena.

Cultural bereavement

Although grief is often associated with loss, the notion of cultural bereavement arises from an understanding of losses incurred and related to cultural values. Eisenbruch (1990, 1991) described cultural bereavement as the experience of the uprooted person or the group related to loss of social structures, cultural values, identity and an almost unnatural attachment to the past. Working with refugees and attempting to study post-traumatic stress disorder (PTSD), Eisenbruch (1991) noted that such individuals have 'odd' experiences (e.g. being visited by supernatural forces from the past), feeling guilty (for abandoning others and their culture, and perhaps because of their own survival), intrusive images and thoughts of the past with an urge to complete obligations to the dead and feeling preoccupied with anxiety, morbid thoughts and anger. It can be argued that a lot of these symptoms are related to what could be called PTSD. It is worth exploring whether cultural bereavement does occur when people migrate in a planned way. Our conjecture is that it does, but also that managing such experiences becomes easier. However, two other factors must be taken into account. First, whether the individual migrated alone, in which case the sense and degree of loss is likely to be deeper than if they travel in a group and as a family, when they can share their feelings more readily. The second factor is to do with the individual personality and what previous experiences of loss they had and how these were dealt with and managed. Under the circumstances, the individual, if migrating alone, will have a different set of experiences and responses to the loss. The role of the culture in giving colour to the process and expression of bereavement is important. The perceived locus of control of such events (whether the individuals hold themselves responsible or whether the blame is placed on external factors, such as the stars, evil eye, etc.) will also play a role in managing the entire process of bereavement. Western constructs of bereavement may have limited value in explaining expressions of grief in other cultures (Bhugra and Becker, 2005). Therefore, definitions of abnormal grief reactions become culturally influenced and should be treated as such.

Losses experienced

Migrants, whether they choose to migrate voluntarily or involuntarily, will have left family structures, physical belongings, values and perhaps roles behind. Leaving childhood friends, extended family, material possessions, social status, etc. behind will lead to some immediate sense of loss and some loss which may provoke a delayed reaction (Wojcik and Bhugra, 2010). It is inevitable that material possessions may be gathered again, but losses related to friendships, family structures and peers may be more difficult to replace or rebuild. The true impact of the losses can be felt in the short, medium and long terms. The sense of loss may be more acute in the short term, whereas niggling feelings of abandoning social value and cultural support systems may become more evident later on in the post-migration phase. The values an individual places on a loss depend upon a number of factors, and not all individuals will place the same emphasis of loss on similar materials.

Loss can lead to bereavement and it will be helpful to place cultural bereavement in the same context.

Grief and its stages

Davies and Bhugra (2004) point out that various models can be used in our understanding of psychopathology. In this section, we shall attempt to describe in brief various theories related to bereavement. Psychoanalytical and cognitive theories suggest a way forward in our understanding. Kübler-Ross (1969) was a pioneer in palliative care. She described five stages of grief: denial and isolation, followed by anger, bargaining, depression and acceptance. Although these stages were described for dying patients, these same stages are often seen in bereavement. These are not always sequential and often the stages may overlap. When trying to identify depression in such a situation, the clinician must also take into account factors such as job loss, altered roles in the family and financial factors, which were identified by Kübler-Ross (1969). Hope remained a positive emotion during all the processes; related changes in the family also become important. Based on her clinical experience, these stages have entered the public consciousness regarding loss and grief.

Bowlby (1980) described a four-stage mode 1 of loss. These stages include numbness or protest; yearning and searching, disorganisation and despair and, finally, reorganisation. It is easy to see how these stages could be seen in refugees and asylum seekers, but may not be clearcut in other migrants. In his view, a person's environment makes a significant contribution to their psychological development. Bowlby uses attachment theory as a way of conceptualising the propensity of human beings to make strong affectional bonds to particular others, and of explaining many forms of emotional distress and personality disturbances to which unwilling separation and loss give rise (Bowlby, 1980, page 201). Using ethology and control theory, Bowlby suggests that attachment behaviour is conceived as behaviour which focuses on attaining and retaining proximity to another differentiated and preferred individual (conceived as stronger and wiser). Characteristics of attachment theory include specificity, duration, engagement of emotions, ontogeny, learning, organisation and biological function. Virtually all of these can be used as an attachment to one's culture, especially the one in which an individual is born, and therefore the impact of early years is crucial. Loss of such a significant attachment 'figure' is bound to lead to loss and anger at separation. Fear expressed as a result of this loss will lead to anxiety, which may also be influenced by separation anxiety. Although Bowlby argues that parents are crucial attachment figures, our contention is that they cannot be seen in isolation from the culture in which they are born and live.

Psychoanalytical theories of loss and mourning

Freud (1953) described the role of loss in the development of melancholia, but attributed it to unconscious motives and desires. Depressive symptoms related to loss are well described. Internalisation of such feelings leads to depression and externalisation to violence, anger or aggression. Under these circumstances, previous experience of loss, expression of anger and anxiety will continue. As Bowlby (1980) notes, representational models of attachment built in childhood will carry on in adulthood relatively unchanged. Similar processes can be applied to migration and its experiences.

Events that are especially liable to act as stressors for individuals whose attachment patterns are weak thereby lead to anxiety and guilt (Bowlby, 1980). Similar patterns could emerge after moving across cultures. The question that needs to be addressed is – if earlier attachment to culture and figures who are seen as wise and authoritative is weak, does that increase the likelihood of cultural bereavement? Although Bowlby (1980) emphasises that his theories differ from traditional Freudian psychoanalytic theories, it is inevitable that there will be some overlap. Disturbed family functioning and personality development will lead to poor parenting in the younger generation. Leading on from such a model are the concepts of cultural attachment which in some cases may influence acculturation to the new culture and society. Under these circumstances, ambivalent feelings and resentment will also play a role in expression and management of grief and bereavement.

Cognitive models

Cognitive schema dealing with loss will depend upon the cultural context. For example, an inability to perform the rites and rituals following death of a relative will produce feelings of bereavement along with helplessness, which may compound a sense of loss and also a lack of control. In this situation, the symptoms of depression and bereavement will affect each other and any cognitive interventions will have to deal with both. Also, the definitions of abnormal grief reaction will need to be renegotiated in these circumstances. Although the relationship between depression and bereavement is well recognised both in clinical and non-clinical settings, the emphasis on clinical aspects makes the distinction between bereavement and depression often difficult. Partly, this can be attributed to similarity of symptoms, even though intensity may vary. In addition, constructs – both of depression and bereavement – are culturally influenced and need to be taken into account. The importance of these expressions of grief in the cultural context is helpful in determining whether bereavement is abnormal or pathological or not. Risk factors for abnormal grief reaction include history of previous mental health problems, ambivalent feelings towards the deceased, sudden or unexpected death and situations when grieving is not possible.

Bearing these factors in mind, one can begin to see a similar process building up in development of cultural bereavement. Traumatic experiences leading to migration, sudden unplanned extrusion from one culture to another, and ambivalent feelings towards the news will also contribute to this sense of loss. Once in the new culture, individuals may find that their aspirations are not met, which may generate feelings of failure and further ambivalence contributing to the grief reaction. Any model of acculturation and cultural adjustment must take this into account. Grief reaction and bereavement will be associated with anxiety, worry, apprehension and feelings of disorientation. Pseudohallucinations may occur, which may lead to potential misdiagnoses and conflate problems. Clinicians therefore need to be aware of 'normal' feelings of loss and grief before diagnosing these symptoms as abnormal. It is also possible that an individual's self-confidence and self-esteem will change with the stages of adjustment.

Culture shock

Oberg (1960) used culture shock as a term to describe 'shock' experienced by migrants as moving to another culture. Culture shock is said to examine aspects which include stress of moving to a new culture, a sense of loss, confusion in role expectations and self-identity, a sense/feeling of rejection by the new culture, and resulting anxiety and sense of impotence in not being accepted as part of the new culture (Taft, 1977). It is inevitable that levels of social support will shift and change when a migrant moves. Social support is crucial at a number of levels, including acceptance. In societies where support is kinship-based, it is likely that individuals migrating singly may feel more isolated and vulnerable.

Pantelidon and Craig (2006) studied 133 Greek students in London, UK and found that culture shock was related to gender and quality of support, and, although it disappeared with time, increased levels produced higher levels of dysphoria. Diversity of social support networks is crucial in understanding and protecting against culture shock. As females had a higher impact of culture shock, it is likely that the female gender role and gender role expectations play a significant role in experiencing culture shock. Although this study focused on students, it highlights the importance of understanding the impact of two cultures coming together, albeit one at an individual level and the second at a larger level. It is clear that there are some features of culture shock which are in common with cultural bereavement.

Culture conflict

The concept of culture conflict emerges from an interaction of cultural factors between an individual and their within culture and across two cultures (Bhugra, 2004a). In a study of deliberate self-harm in South Asian women and among South Asian adolescents it was found that parents had more traditional attitudes in their cultural identity whereas children were less traditional, thereby creating a tension and what could be termed as culture conflict. A component of such conflict is related to cultural identity (see Bhugra, 2004b for further details). It is inevitable that in some cases cultural and ethnic identity becomes more rigid and problematic. Individuals may choose to cling to their original identity, which may cause tensions with the larger new society but acceptance within their own. These tensions are also related to levels of acculturation. Thus it can be argued that one type of culture conflict may occur within the same culture, between the individual and other members of their culture, and another type will be between the individual and the larger new culture. Each type of these conflicts will differ and will have varying impact and consequences, both on the individual in terms of acculturation itself and on mental illness and disorders. Culture conflict is said to reflect dilemmas faced by an individual in trying to integrate two cultures which may be at extremes of views (Harris and Kuba, 1997; Inman et al., 2001). It is defined as affective and cognitive dissonance arising as a consequence of attempts to assimilate the values and expectations of a new culture (Inman et al., 2001), but the individual may wish to hang onto older values. It is inevitable that these will cause psychological and emotional distress. However, there is a likelihood that not everyone will experience this conflict or that individuals may have other strategies to deal with and protecting themselves against conflict.

In addition to deliberate self-harm (Biswas 1990; Bhugra et al., 1999a; 1999b; 2003), other conditions such as depression and eating disorders (Reddy and Crowther, 2007) have a focus in South Asian females.

Studies have shown that high expressed emotion in the family leads to a relapse of various psychiatric and physical disorders (see review by Bhugra and McKenzie, 2010). It is possible that among ethnic minority families culture conflict may be contributing to high levels of expressed emotion and this avenue needs to be explored further. In addition, such an exploration may lead to intervention strategies which can reduce culture conflict and consequent expressed emotion. Managing culture conflict in a constructive way will also improve an individual's self-esteem and coping strategies in managing transition to the new culture.

To understand culture shock and culture conflict, the role of acculturation and the processes related to it become very important.

Acculturation/assimilation/alienation

Adaptation to a new culture is related to the individuals trying to settle down and modify behaviours and attitudes in response to social expectations. Berry (1976) suggests that adaptation can be of three types – adjustment, reaction and withdrawal. These can be seen as moving towards, moving against and moving away from a stimulus (Berry, 1980). How the majority or new culture deals with migrants and their attitudes both in policy and practice will enable or stifle adjustment. The relationship between the new society and the migrant will influence whether the migrants feel welcomed, settled or rejected. These relationships work on many levels. At a macro level the political, economic and social environment of the new society will influence attitudes and beliefs. At a lesser level, the response of the migrant group within which the individual will react is equally important. A more flexible approach on both sides will encourage a sense of acceptance and belonging which will contribute to adjustment. Equally important are the levels of acculturation which occur at a different pace among groups, families and individuals, and these have major implications for clinical interventions. As an individual moves around in the new society, some aspects of acculturation will occur sooner. For example, a student going to school or university will become acculturated quickly to language and social customs in comparison with an older less educated female who stays at home all day. Thus, levels of acculturation within the entire group also become important.

Acculturation is seen as the process in which individuals and groups from different cultures come into continuous contact with another culture; this leads to changes in one (mostly the minority) culture (Redfield *et al.*, 1936). Berry (1990) points out that such a process needs to be seen at both individual and group levels. He describes varieties of acculturation as assimilation, integration, rejection and deculturation. Assimilation is a result of a gradual coming together by absorbing cultural factors and changing of cultural identity. Anthropologists prefer the term acculturation and sociologists tend to prefer assimilation, whereas both terms have similar meanings. Rejection is where the individuals or groups withdraw from the larger group. Deculturation is characterised by loss of identity and acculturative stress (Berry, 1980). Often deculturation is a reaction to war or sudden invasion. The interactions between the group's cultural identity and the individual's cultural identity will not only lead to culture conflict but will also produce alienation both from one's own group and perhaps also from the larger group. Psychological factors in identity include language, cognitive style, personality, concepts of the self, attitudes and acculturative stress (see Berry, 2007). There is no doubt that with acculturation some of these will change and part of the cognitive dissonance, if it occurs, will contribute to a sense of culture shock, as discussed earlier. Cultural influences on personality development and concepts of the self are very important. This interaction between culture and child development, and subsequently to the development of personality, indicates that cultural mores may influence individual reactions and identity. Following migration, the personality and the notion of the self will need to be seen in the context of developing cultural bereavement, culture conflict and culture shock.

Cultural congruity

Several studies have shown that rates of mental illness are elevated in some migrant groups (see Bhugra, 2004b). In a subsequent paper, Bhugra (2005) proposes that cultural congruity may play a role in understanding these elevated rates. The identity structure analysis includes an appraisal of and current expression of identity and identification as well as the formation and further development of identity (Weinrich, 2003). Multiple types of identities are important.

It has been argued that cultures can be divided into sociocentric and egocentric, as with individuals (Hofstede, 1980/2001; 1984). In egocentric societies, ties between individuals are relatively loose and each individual is supposed to look after themselves or the immediate nuclear family. In collectivist societies, individuals from their birth integrate into kinship-based structures and have very strong in-groups. There is a clear difference between I-consciousness in egocentric societies (where the individual shows autonomy, independence, individual initiative pleasure-seeking and financial independence) in contrast to we-ness seen in collectivist societies. In the latter, collective identity, emotional interdependence, group solidarity and obligations take precedence over the individual. Family interdependence and group identity are important components of sociocentric individuals.

If we take this further, it would appear that egocentric societies and individuals focus on liberalism compared with collectivist societies, which are more likely to be traditional. Collectivist societies focus on the common good; concession and compromise are essential ingredients in developing roles, and group interest and identity are significant. Individualism has shown to have a correlation with higher gross national product (GNP), crime levels, divorce, child abuse and physical and mental illness (Hofstede, 1984). Maercker (2001) noted that traditional values were negatively associated with psychiatric diagnosis. He points out that 15–53% of cross-cultural variance in psychiatric morbidity could be explained by cultural values.

Let us now imagine a sociocentric individual from a sociocentric society migrating to an egocentric society. If surrounded by an egocentric society and individuals, he or she may feel alienated and withdraw themselves. On the other hand, an egocentric individual from a sociocentric society may well settle down very well in an egocentric society. However, if an egocentric individual from a sociocentric society settles down in an egocentric society but is surrounded by a sociocentric community, there may be culture conflict. Thus, an egocentric individual in an egocentric society will have different kinds of stress and this will influence links with egocentric individuals (see Figure 11.1). It is possible that egocentric individuals in sociocentric societies may yield to group norms less than sociocentric individuals in egocentric societies. These interactions must therefore be studied both at individual and group levels.

Racial and cultural congruity become important in understanding where an individual settles down and what kind of response they and their group generate among the larger society. The impact of social attitudes on individuals' self-esteem is well known but what is less clear is whether these attitudes are cushioned by social support or perceived or real alienation. Cultural environments will also influence individual responses.

Social alienation combined with culture shock, bereavement or conflict will push vulnerable individuals towards developing psychiatric disorders. A chronic sense of isolation and alienation may produce chronic difficulties which will influence mental state (Figure 11.2). We do not propose to make large claims on the basis of a dichotomy which is not essentially bipolar, but it is worth thinking about both by clinicians and researchers alike. The concepts of self will be influenced by clinical and cultural factors. Structures in society which maintain and

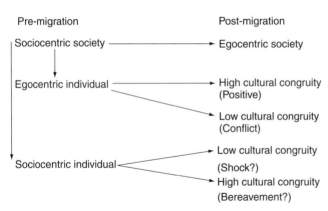

Figure 11.1 Theoretical model linking migration patterns.

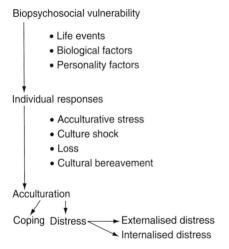

Figure 11.2 Models of vulnerability.

support egocentric or sociocentric societies need to be explored further. With globalisation and industrialisation, it is inevitable that there will be changes in societies. Whether they become fragmented or more egocentric, or create a cognitive dissonance, or they take to the extreme nationalistic views is anybody's guess. Individual personalities, ethnic and cultural identities, religious values and attitudes will all play a role, along with formal education.

Conclusions

The relationship and interaction between cultural bereavement, culture conflict and culture shock needs to be explored further. Although there are common features of experiencing loss and anxiety in all of them it is inevitable that detailed analysis needs to be carried out. Migrants' mental health is often vulnerable to a number of factors, and some chronic factors will play a role in making vulnerable individuals prone to common mental disorders or other psychiatric illnesses. Qualitative and quantitative research will also allow us to explore not only the underlying meaning of these processes, but also how interventions can be developed.

Independence and interdependence of individuals and these relationships with the cultures from which they come and the cultures in which they settle will enable clinicians to understand this distress and vulnerability in the context of cultural identity and cultural congruity. Acculturation itself is fluid and its impact on individuals needs to be explored and understood.

References

Berry, J. (1976). *Human Ecology and Cognitive Style*. New York: Sage.

Berry, J. (1980). Acculturation as varieties of adaptation. In A. M. Padilla, ed. *Acculturation*. Boulder, CO: Westview, 9–26.

Berry, J. (1990). Psychology of acculturation. In R. M. Brislin, ed. *Applied Cross-Cultural Psychology*. Newbury Park: Sage.

Berry, J. (2007). Acculturation and identity. In D. Bhugra and K. S. Bhui, eds. *Textbook of Cultural Psychiatry*. Cambridge: Cambridge University Press.

Bhugra, D. (2004a). *Culture and Self Harm: Attempted Suicide in South Asians in London*. Maudsley Monographs 46. London: Psychology Press.

Bhugra, D. (2004b). Migration and mental health. *Acta Psychiatrica Scandinavica*, **109**(4), 243–58.

Bhugra, D. (2005). Cultural identities and cultural congruency: a new model for evaluating mental distress in immigrants. *Acta Psychiatrica Scandinavica*, **111**(2), 84–93.

Bhugra, D., Becker, M. (2005). Migration, cultural bereavement and cultural identity. *World Psychiatry*, **4**(1), 18–24.

Bhugra, D., McKenzie, K. (2010). Expressed emotion across cultures. In R. Bhattacharya, S. Cross and D. Bhugra, eds. *Clinical Topics in Cultural Psychiatry*. London: RCPsych Publications.

Bhugra, D., Desai, M., Baldwin, D. S. (1999a). Attempted suicide in West London, I. Rates across ethnic communities. *Psychological Medicine*, **29**, 1125–30.

Bhugra, D., Baldwin, D. S., Desai, M., Jacob, K. S. (1999b). Attempted suicide in West London, II. Inter-group comparisons. *Psychological Medicine*, **29**, 1131–9.

Bhugra, D., Thompson, N., Singh, J., Fellow-Smith, E. (2003). Inception rates of deliberate self-harm among adolescents in West London. *International Journal of Social Psychiatry*, **49**(4), 247–50.

Biswas, S. (1990). Ethnic differences in self-poisoning. *Journal of Adolescents*, **13**, 189–93.

Bowlby, J. (1980). *Attachment and Loss*. New York: Basic Books.

Davies, D., Bhugra, D. (2004). *Models of Psychopathology*. London: McGraw-Hill.

Eisenbruch, M. (1990). The cultural bereavement interview: a new clinical research approach for refugees. *Psychiatric Clinics of North America*, **13**, 715–35.

Eisenbruch, M. (1991). From post-traumatic stress disorder to cultural bereavement: diagnosis of Southeast Asian refugees. *Social Science and Medicine*, **33**, 673–80.

Freud, S. (1953). Mourning and melancholia. In *The Standard Edition of the Complete Psychological Works of Sigmund Freud*, *Vol* 14. London: Hogarth Press and Institute of Psycho-Analysis.

Harris, D. I., Kuba, S. A. (1997): Ethnocultural identity and eating disorders in women of colour. *Professional Psychology: Research and Practice*, **28**, 341–7.

Hofstede, G. (1980/2001). *Culture's Consequences: International Differences in Work-Related Values*. Newbury Park, CA: Sage.

Hofstede, G. (1984). *Culture's Consequences: International Differences in Work-Related Values* (abridged edition). Thousand Oaks, CA: Sage.

Inman, A. G., Ladany, N., Constantine, M. G., Morano, C. K. (2001). Development and preliminary validation of the Cultural Values

Conflict Scale for South Asian women. *Journal of Counselling Psychology*, **48**, 17–27.

Kübler-Ross, E. (1969). *On Death and Dying*. New York: Macmillan.

Maercker, A. (2001). Association of cross cultural differences in psychiatric morbidity with cultural values: a secondary analysis. *German Journal of Psychiatry*, **4**, 17–23.

Oberg, K. (1960). Cultural shock: adjustment to new cultural environments. *Practical Anthropology*, **7**, 177–82.

Pantelidon, S., Craig, T. K. J. (2006). Culture shock and social support: a survey in Greek migrant students. *Social Psychiatry and Psychiatric Epidemiology*, **41**, 771–81.

Reddy, S., Crowther, H. (2007). Teasing, acculturation and cultural conflict: psychosocial correlates of body image and eating attitudes among South Asian women. *Cultural Diversity and Ethnic Minority Psychology*, **13**, 45–53.

Redfield, R., Linton, R., Herskovit, M. (1936). Memorandum for the study of acculturation. *American Anthropologist*, **38**, 149–52.

Taft, R. (1977). Coping with unfamiliar cultures. In N. Warren, ed. *Studies in Cross-Cultural Psychology*. London: Academic Press.

Weinrich, P. (2003). Identity structure analysis. In P. Weinrich and W. Sanderson, eds. *Analysing Identity and Cross-Cultural Societal and Clinical Contexts*. Hove: Routledge, 9–76.

Wojcik, W., Bhugra, D. (2010). Loss and cultural bereavement. In D. Bhugra, T. K. J. Craig, and K. S. Bhui, eds. *Mental Health of Refugees and Asylum Seekers*. Oxford: Oxford University Press, 211–23.

Collective trauma

Daya Somasundaram

Editors' introduction

When individuals migrate as a group, especially if such a migration is to escape war or genocide, it is likely that group experiences will also mould individual experiences, individual coping skills and strategies, and individual responses. Those who migrate for educational and economic reasons and do so voluntarily will demonstrate different experiences and responses to migration in comparison with those who migrate involuntarily as a result of political factors. Again, migrants will respond in different ways. Somasundaram describes collective trauma as an under-recognised but salient response to various types of massive traumas resulting from disasters, and representing the negative impact on social processes at the collective level. Such a trauma will be reflected in social networks, relationships, institutions, capital and resources related to social and economic capital. Loss of the existing community and anxieties related to relocation will add to the stress experienced by migrants both at individual and group levels. Consequently, collective trauma will cause individuals to respond in different ways – from alienation, mistrust and deep suspicion to dependence and learned helplessness. Resulting brutalisation of the society and the migrant groups may well influence child and adolescent development toward a pathological direction. Using family and traditional relaxation methods will enable clinicians to deal with such experiences.

Introduction

The bonds to home, soil and village are very powerful. The home provides a sense of protection, safety and sanctuary and helps the identity and closeness of the family. The neighbourhood and community offer the points of reference, and meaning to existence. Great indeed must be the forces that compel a person or their family to leave their home and familiar environment to seek another life in a foreign environment. For some the reasons for migration may not be so drastic. In the modern globalised village, the move from one part of the world to another is a mere transition from an urban city lifestyle to a more or less similar environment. With current facilities for international travel, communication and liberal economic opportunities, the transfer to another city, branch or company may be an easy transition, even a habitual pattern enacted before. This is the skilled migrant category and accounts for the 'healthy immigration effect'. People and families with robust health and personalities, highly motivated and skilled in the ways of the modern world, come for economic reasons, to better themselves or settle down in a hospitable environment. Thus

Migration and Mental Health, ed. Dinesh Bhugra & Susham Gupta. Published by Cambridge University Press. © Cambridge University Press 2011.

skilled immigrants are generally healthier and enjoy a better self-perceived sense of wellbeing than native-born persons. However, the health advantage of skilled migrants erodes over time. Disease patterns may tend to converge to those of the host population (Tse and Hoque, 2006). Well-to-do countries are particularly careful in restricting immigration to mainly skilled workers who would make a positive contribution to economical development. Refugees, asylum seekers and those coming for family reunification show a much poorer health status. For example, in the UK, they are found to suffer from conditions as malnutrition, communicable diseases like tuberculosis, hepatitis and HIV/AIDS; and physical injuries from war and torture, as well as depression, anxiety and post-traumatic stress disorder (PTSD) (Wilkinson, 2007). In Australia, similar psychosocial problems have been reported (Silove, 2007; Somasundaram, 2010).

Although the small numbers of refugees and asylum seekers and those migrating for family reunion appear to form the most vulnerable group compared to voluntary, planned migration of skilled professionals, workers and students, there may be hidden within the latter category many who are migrating due to persecution, threat, violence or trauma but use the regular channels. Thus, if we look at the background factors that would have set the process of migration in motion, an unrecognised but salient force can be called *collective trauma*. Many communities, particularly from poorer already compromised countries around the globe, are exposed to various types of massive traumas that result from disasters, both man-made and natural. In addition to individual level sequelae like PTSD, depression and anxiety (American Psychiatric Association, 1980; 1994), the term collective trauma is being introduced to represent the negative impact at the collective level to the wounding and injury to the social fabric; that is, on the social processes, networks, relationships, institutions, functions, dynamics, practices, capital and resources. The long-lasting impact at the collective level or, as some have called it, tearing in the social fabric (Milroy, 2005), would then result in social transformation (Bloom, 1998) of a sociopathic nature that can be called collective trauma. Collective events and consequences may have more significance in collectivistic communities than in individualistic societies (Hofstede, 2005). The individual becomes embedded within the family and community so much so that traumatic events are experienced through the larger unit and the impact will also manifest at that level. The family and community are part of the self, their identity and consciousness. The demarcation or boundary between the individual self and the outside becomes blurred. For example, because of close and strong bonds and cohesiveness, nuclear and extended families tend to function and respond to external threat or trauma as a unit rather than as individual members (Somasundaram, 2007). They share the experience and perceive the event in a particular way. During times of traumatic experiences, the family will come together with solidarity to face the threat as a unit and provide mutual support and protection. In time, the family will act to define and interpret the traumatic event, give it structure and assign a common meaning, as well as evolve strategies to cope with the stress. Thus it may be more appropriate to talk in terms of family dynamics rather than of individual personalities. There may be some individual variation in manifestation, depending on responsibilities and roles within the family and personal characteristics, while some may become the scapegoat in the family dynamic that ensues. Similarly, communities, the village and its people, way of life and environment provide organic roots, a sustaining support system, nourishing environment and network of relationships. The village traditions, structures and institutions are the foundations and framework for daily life. A person's and family's identity are defined to a large extent by their village or group of origin. Their *collective identity* more or less places the person in a particular sociocultural matrix. The impact of collective trauma on families, extended families, kinship groups, villages and communities includes mass migratory processes as they try to flee from the traumatic ecological context. People try to rebuild their lives in a new environment of safety and opportunity. Individually or as families they may migrate to new places and continue to struggle to bring others across one by one. Those coming from collectivistic societies (Hofstede, 2005) remain bound through organic links to those left behind and feel responsible for their welfare. However, the legacy of collective trauma continues to plague them in their new homes, haunting their settlement process.

Previous field workers have already drawn attention to community level problems caused by disasters. Kai Erikson (Erikson, 1976, 1979) gives a graphic account of collective trauma as 'loss of communality' following the Buffalo Creek disaster in the USA. He and colleagues described the 'broken cultures' in North American Indians and 'destruction of the entire fabric of their culture' owing to the forced displacements and dispossession from traditional lands into reservations, separations, massacres, loss of their way of life, relationships and spiritual beliefs (Erikson and Vecsey, 1980). There was a description of 'cultural bereavement' (see Chapter 6) caused by the loss of cultural traditions and rituals in Indochinese refugees in the US (Eisenbruch, 1991) and collective trauma owing to the chronic effects of war (Somasundaram, 2007). Parker (1977)mentioned the psychosocial and 'relocation stressor' following Cyclone Tracy in Darwin, linking it to the 'sociocultural needs for societal integration and stability'. More recently, a number of discerning workers in the field have been drawing attention to the importance of looking at the family (Ager, 2006; De Jong, 2002; Tribe, 2004; Tribe and Family Rehabilitation Centre Staff, 2004) and cultural dimension (De Jong, 2002, 2004; Landau and Saul, 2004; Miller and Rasco, 2005; Silove *et al.*, 2006) following disasters. Finally, Abramowitz (2005) has given a moving picture of 'collective trauma' in six Guinean communities exposed to war. This chapter attempts to describe the effect of collective trauma on migration and settlement in the host country and various interventions that can be used in such contexts.

Causes

Disasters have an effect not only on individuals (Somasundaram, 1998), but also on their family, extended family, ethnic group, community, village and wider society. Large scale destruction, deaths, injuries and subsequent chaos result in mass displacements, uprooting from familiar surroundings, deprivations of all sorts, insecurity and social disconnection. Social institutions, structures, leadership, connections and relationships, vital community resources and social capital may be irretrievably lost. In addition, during civil conflicts, arbitrary detention, torture, massacres, extrajudicial killings, disappearances, rape, forced displacements, bombing and shelling become common. Whole communities or villages are targeted for total destruction, including their way of life and their environment (Summerfield, 1996). Modern warfare has now become internal; civil wars, where the conflict is more psychological for control of loyalties through intimidation, terror and counter-terror, and the fighting occurs within civilian populations, where 90% of casualties are civilians (Machel, 1996). Apart from wars for complete extermination (that is, genocide), the goal of modern warfare is more for absorption and assimilation into one dominant culture and way of life. The minority is expected to forgo its own culture and identity and merge with or become subservient to the dominant culture. When they try to resist the process, ethnic or civil conflict erupts. Unlike after natural disasters, civil conflict causes community trauma by the creation of a 'repressive ecology' based on imminent, pervasive threat, terror and inhibition that causes a state of generalised insecurity, terror and rupture of the social fabric (Baykai *et al.*, 2004).

Another important casualty in war has been the implicit faith in the world order, and social justice in particular. Those responsible for what may be called war crimes and the worst types of human rights abuses are never punished except for a few recent examples with the International Criminal Court in the Hague and previous tribunals. Few cases of massacres, disappearances, torture, rape, custodial killings and mass graves have been investigated and brought to light. However, impunity prevails in the majority of cases. The victims usually have to bear it in silence, a silence that is often individual as well as collective.

It becomes easy to understand why people, families and communities want to flee such pernicious ecological contexts.

Consequences

The cumulative effect of all these devastating events and ecological contexts on the community can be described as collective trauma. In addition to the sum total of individual traumas, which can in itself be substantial given the widespread nature of the traumatisation due to disaster(s), there are impacts at the supra-individual family, community and social levels that produce systemic changes in social dynamics, processes, structures and functioning. In fact, the psychosocial reactions in the individual may have come to be accepted as a normal part of life. Thus being tense, ever vigilant, readily startled, irritable, having nightmares and poor sleep and experiencing multiple somatic complaints would not be considered unusual in the contexts from which migrants come. However, at the community level, manifestations of extreme experiences can, for example, be seen in the prevailing coping strategies. People have learned to survive under extraordinarily stressful conditions. However, some coping strategies that may have had survival value during intense conflict may become maladaptive after migration and attempts to settle into a host community. For example, people have learned to be silent, uninvolved and to stay in the background, which would have helped in survival. They develop a *deep suspicion* and *mistrust* that may have survival value in intensive, internecine inter- and intra-ethnic group conflict. Similar paranoid attitudes were found after the 9/11 attacks in New York (Aber *et al.*, 2004). Trust is the basic binding glue that keeps communities and societies together – trust in relationships, that they will not be betrayed, that others will fulfil their obligations, responsibilities and undertakings, that their intentions are benign; trust in social structures and institutions, justice, law, values and cultural beliefs, the future; and, finally, trust in themselves, their family and kin. Trust is gradually destroyed by war. This cohesive force is progressively weakened, setting in motion a vicious self-fulfilling cycle, spiralling downwards to increasing suspicion and mistrust. These suspicious attitudes and lack of trust are carried with migrants into the host country and into their attempts to adapt into the society. However, these impede their forming relationships and the trusting, well intended efforts and programmes for them. It goes further, leading to difficulties with their own communities and subcultural practices that would normally be protective and a useful way of settling into a new setting. In fact, usually intra-ethnic group contact and relationships are protective factors, promoting mental health and useful salutogenic social level intervention for acculturation stress among migrants. They thus become socially withdrawn, isolated and marginalised, resisting re-connecting with their own community and wider society.

People learn simply to attend to their immediate needs and survive to the next day. Any involvement or participation carries considerable risk, particularly when there are frequent changes in those in power. The repeated displacements and disruptions of livelihood make people dependent on handouts and relief rations. Similar to Seligman's 'learned helplessness' (Seligman and Groves, 1970), this *dependence* hampers settlement and acculturation. They have lost their motivation for advancement, progress or betterment. There is a general sense of resignation to fate, an ennui. People no longer feel motivated to work, or better their lot. More effort and interest is seen to be spent on obtaining social welfare payments, disability pensions, housing, grants and avoiding language classes or vocational training. After a brief honeymoon period of relief at reaching a safer haven and expectation of better things to come, a deep malaise sets in which is difficult to break.

Another conspicuous collective phenomenon caused by modern war has been the brutalisation of society. Apart from the militarisation of all aspects of life (with the ubiquitous checkpoints, armed men, weapons, checking, barbed wire) and the pervasiveness of the 'gun culture', is the long-term effect on thinking and behaviour patterns. Witnessing the horrifying deaths (including killings) of loved ones, friends or strangers, and seeing many mutilated or dismembered bodies, decaying and bloated remains have saturated the consciousness with death as evidenced by drawings, dreams and poetry. Similarly, watching the destruction of what had been a permanent structure, like a home, or having to abandon ones' home under forced circumstances, appears to result in the perceived collapse of everything secure and strong, particularly in children, who lose the hope for a future. With time, people have become habituated to such scenes and experiences. In a way they become immunised to the worst aspects of the war, able to carry on nevertheless, and attend to immediate survival needs in the midst of the destruction and death, a form of resilience. Migrants from collectivistic communities remain locked into their relationships with extended families and kinship groups, feeling responsible and guilty at leaving them behind in the home, neighbouring or distant country to which they may be displaced. Modern technology keeps the collective trauma alive and immanent in their lives. They maintain close contact through mobile phones, keep abreast with current news through television, the internet, other media and other travellers. In fact, they continue to live more in their home network, undergoing all the uncertainty, insecurity, terror, agony and trauma of those left behind, than in the reality around them in the host country. An adverse event back home has an immediate and immense effect on their family. A parent, sister, brother or child sobbing over the phone haunts them for weeks. They would experience the consequences of a suicide bomb attack in their country of origin being shown on TV as if it was happening to them then and there. All their time, money and effort is spent in trying to bring those left behind across to the host country. The long drawn out visa procedures, unfriendly authorities and common refusal of their applications compound their collective sense of helplessness and futility. Individual level trauma therapy in the host country for the migrant will not get far with this vivid presence of the ongoing trauma.

One worrying development is the adverse personality development in male adolescents and youth. Many have lost a parent or sibling. Grief seems to soon overwhelm them. Further, no ongoing, constructive activities or programmes have been designed and implemented for adolescents and youth. Unemployed and at a loose end, they drift into groups and antisocial activities. Some start abusing alcohol or drugs. Parents and elders in the collectivistic community who were traditionally respected no longer have control. There is considerable intergenerational misunderstanding, clash of values and conflict. Intrafamilial dynamics are also adversely affected, particularly where there is an absence of an adult male, who has usually been killed in the war. These youths have come out of an atmosphere of extreme violence, with many witnessing horrifying deaths of relations, the destruction of their homes and social institutions. They have grown up surrounded by war equipment and paraphernalia, and have personally experienced bombings, shelling, extrajudicial killings and displacement. In view of their potential for constructive activity and commitment to meaningful goals, well designed and appropriate special programmes have to be implemented for migrant youths in the host country. Unfortunately, this is often lacking and they do not fit into mainstream programmes.

Disasters and conflict have a major impact on the functioning family system. From the loss of one or both parents, separations and traumatisation in one member, pathological family dynamics adversely affect family members, particularly children. The cohesiveness and traditional relationships are no longer the same. It is a common complaint that children no longer respect or listen to their elders, including teachers. These changing attitudes may reflect normal patterns in host societies but are abnormal in the collectivistic communities from which the migrants often come. A strong influence has been the contemptuous way elders and community leaders are treated by the authorities and the submissive way in which they have responded. Elders are perceived as being powerless and incompetent in dealing with war and its consequences, as well as with the modern world, its practices, travel and bureaucracy. Elders have also been traumatised by the war, affecting their functioning, relationships and parenting skills. Because of the peculiarities of war, males are more often targeted and are at high risk of being killed, arrested, detained, of disappearing, or becoming involved with the fighting forces. Thus migrants are widows who have lost their husbands due to the war and migrate using humanitarian programmes for women. The effect of the absent father on the family, the widow and the children is immense. The loss of the head of family has a marked impact on family dynamics, producing a vacuum that is difficult to fill, causing disruption and disharmony within the family. The widow has to take on the added burden of the male role in a foreign environment, with poor language and social skills. She has to navigate the family through the difficult migration and settlement process, deal with authorities and look after the day-to-day needs of the family without the usual social support back home. The consequence is often psychological and physical illness in the mother and adverse developmental trajectories in the children.

Interventions

The widespread problem of collective traumatisation and 'loss of communality' following disasters is best approached through family and community level interventions (Somasundaram, 1997; 2007). However, it is difficult to reach the affected community that has been left behind back home or in neighbouring countries to intervene at a collective level. One basic social institution that may be available for intervention is the family. The recommendations for providing 'Culturally Competent Services' in a Royal College of Psychiatrists' publication, is that 'the family is usually the preferred point of intervention. Understanding family structure and dynamics will be helpful in service delivery' (Patel and Stein, 2007). The family is central to 'collectivistic communities'. Families tend to think and act as a unit. There are strict hierarchical roles and obligations that emphasise harmony and support each other during difficulties. The individual submerges his or her individual 'self' within the nuclear and extended family dynamics. Migrating families have to make the transition to the more 'individualistic' system in host mainstream societies of the western world that emphasise emancipation from the family. As a result

> immigrant families experience feelings of social and cultural isolation and struggle to function as family systems, especially when considering gender issues, intergenerational factors, and the process of acculturation and assimilation as related to family dynamics. Moreover, the immigrant families struggle within various ecological social systems outside the family system, including the educational, physical and mental health, economic, and political systems (Kawamoto and Anguiano, 2006).

The family can be a source of support and help in the treatment process of clients as well as a cause of problems. Thus when treating individual clients, there is a need to look at how best to address the family as a unit and find support for them. It is worth noting, however, following the western family therapy model may not always be an effective approach to adopt. Instead, a holistic integrated method, which addresses the various needs and relationships and which has a clear understanding of the family dynamics, identifying and mobilising support systems, could work better. In a supportive family environment, members will recover better and may not need individual treatment as such. It is often helpful to involve the family from the onset, at the time when the initial history is taken and when an assessment takes place, and to explore their viewpoint as well. The family may also sit in with the clients when appropriate in regular sessions. Mothers may be invited to bring their young children with them, and they could play or come and go from the outer room. Family members could be given specific tasks, such as giving medication, as well as being used as co-therapists. At times, difficulties in family dynamics may be observed, assessed and even addressed in these settings. It is important to be aware of the extended family and kinship groups back home that continue to be part of the family system from a distance, influencing the migrant family in a myriad of ways. They may also have to be involved in the therapeutic process, which may include supporting visa applications for some key members to increase the social support for the dysfunctional family. The family may be accessing a variety of health and social services in the host country in their desperation without much benefit, but the arrival of a key member, like a grown up daughter, may stabilise the family dynamics and reduce the need for expensive, but ineffective, services.

Another collective level intervention with migrants could be the use of traditional relaxation methods (Somasundaram, 2010). An international panel of eminent experts identified producing a sense of calming as an important empirically supported intervention principle for post-disaster distress, recommending deep, diaphragmatic breathing, muscle relaxation, yoga and mindfulness techniques drawn from Asian culture and meditation methods (Hobfoll et al., 2007). The benefits of these originally spiritual practices are not confined to producing relaxation. When methods are culturally familiar, they tap into past childhood, community and religious roots and thus release a rich source of associations that can be helpful in therapy and the healing process. Mindfulness and meditation draw upon hidden resources within the individual and open into dimensions that can create spiritual wellbeing and give meaning to what has happened. Traditional relaxation methods can be practised individually as well as at a family, group and community level. Thus, collective level dynamics such as family and community support, redefining of the effects and meaning of events, trauma and narratives, and renewed sense of motivation, hope and purpose could be

Table 12.1 Traditional relaxation methods (Somasundaram, 2002)

Regular repetition of words
Hindu – *Jappa: Pranava mantra, 'OM'*
Buddhist – Pirit or chanting: *Buddhang Saranang Gachchami*
Islam – *Dhikir, Takbir, Tasbih: Subhanallah*
Catholic Christians – *Rosary, prayer beads:* the Jesus prayer (*Jesus Christ have mercy on me*)
Cambodia – *Keatha, angkam: Puthoo*; Vietnam *Mophit*
Scientific – T. M. Benson's relaxation response

Breathing exercises
Pranayamam, Anapana Sati or mindful breathing

Muscular relaxation
Shanthi or Sava Asana, Mindful body awareness, Tai Chi

Meditation
Dhyanam, contemplation, Samadhi, Vipassana

Massage
Aurvedic or Siddha oil massage and the Cambodian, *thveu saasay*

released by using traditional methods in group settings. Traditional relaxation methods from different traditions (Somasundaram, 2002), to be used appropriately depending on the culture and religion of the patient as an adjunct in the overall holistic method of treatment (Somasundaram, 1997), that have been found useful in these settings are given in Table 12.1. They could also be helpful in the situations of cultural bereavement described in Chapter 6 by restoring a feeling of cultural connectedness and meaning.

Although migrants with collective trauma may initially resist attempts at socialisation, it is worthwhile encouraging and organising supportive intra- and inter-group interactions, meetings, cultural celebrations and practices. Religious observations and familiar rituals can re-establish a sense of grounding and inner peace. Self-help, supportive and other types of groups based on similar backgrounds, gender or goals are helpful in ameliorating the effects of collective trauma and re-establish trust, relationships and networks. Women and widows do particularly well in group settings. By sharing and learning from each other, they support each other and can learn new skills like language and vocational training in groups. People who have migrated earlier and adapt successfully to the new culture can act as positive role models and provide leadership. Migrants also find fulfilment in aiding new arrivals by showing them practical tips to cope locally.

Other innovative and flexible approaches may have to be adopted to deal with collective trauma. Issues like war crimes, genocide, mass human rights abuses, torture, rape, extra-judicial killings, disappearances, ethnic cleansing and responsibility for disasters should be addressed to restore feelings of social justice and belief in the world. Some migrants may benefit by becoming witnesses, giving testimony and advocating justice. Participating in programmes for 'healing of memories', 'truth commissions' and 'transitional justice' are ways that migrants can become involved in constructive activities that may help them to deal with their own sense of injustice and collective trauma. Some have joined effective peace, humanitarian, advocacy or help groups working globally or for their country of origin. Some may find meaning in their collective and individual suffering and regain a sense of communality by contributing to the welfare of their, or a more global, group of people in different ways, including their struggle for justice, equality, wellbeing and liberty.

References

Aber, J., Gershoff, E., Ware, A. *et al.* (2004). Estimating the effects of September 11th and other forms of violence on the mental health and social development of New York city's youth: a matter of context. *Applied Development Science*, **8**, 111–29.

Abramowitz, S. (2005). The poor have become rich, and the rich have become poor: collective trauma in the Guinean Languette. *Social Science and Medicine*, **61**, 2106–18.

Ager, A. (2006). What is family? In N. Boothby, A. Strang and M. Wessells, eds., *A World Turned Upside Down – Social Ecological Approaches to Children in War Zones*. Connecticut: Kumarian Press, 38–62.

American Psychiatric Association (1980, 1994). *Diagnostic and Statistical Manual of Mental Disorders* (3rd, DSM III; 4th, DSM IV edn). Washington: APA.

Baykai, T., Schlar, C., Kapken, E. (2004). *International Training Manual on Psychological Evidence of Torture*. Istanbul: Human Rights Foundation of Turkey.

Bloom, S. L. (1998). By the crowd they have been broken, by the crowd they shall be healed: the social transformation of trauma. In R. G. Tedeschi, C. L. Park and L. G. Calhoun (eds) *Posttraumatic Growth: Positive Changes in the Aftermath of Crisis*, Mahwoh, NJ: Lawrence Erlbaum Associates, Inc., 179–213.

De Jong, J. (2002). Public mental health, traumatic stress and human rights violations in low-income countries: a culturally appropriate model in times of conflict, disaster and peace. In J. De Jong, ed. *Trauma, War and Violence: Public Mental Health in Sociocultural Context*. New York: Plenum-Kluwer, 1–91.

De Jong, J. (2004). Public mental health and culture: disasters as a challenge to western mental health care models, the self, and PTSD. In J. Wilson and B. Drozdek, eds. *Broken Spirits: The Treatment of Asylum Seekers and Refugees with PTSD*. New York: Brunner/Routledge Press, 159–79.

Eisenbruch, M. (1991). From post-traumatic stress disorder to cultural bereavement: diagnosis of Southeast Asian refugees. *Social Science and Medicine*, **33**, 673–80.

Erikson, K. (1976). Disaster at Buffalo Creek. Loss of communality at Buffalo Creek. *American Journal of Psychiatry*, **133**, 302–5.

Erikson, K. (1979). *In the Wake of the Flood*. London: Allen Unwin.

Erikson, K., Vecsey, C. (1980). A report to the People of Grassy Narrows. In C. Vecsey and R. Venables, eds. *American Indian Environments – Ecological Issues in Native American History*. New York: Syracuse University Press, 152–61.

Hobfoll, S. E., Watson, P., Bell, C. C. *et al.* (2007). Five essential elements of immediate and mid-term mass trauma intervention: empirical evidence. *Psychiatry*, **70**, 283–315.

Hofstede, G. (2005). *Cultures and Organizations: Software of the Mind*, 2nd edn. New York: McGraw-Hill.

Kawamoto, W. T., Anguiano, R. V. (2006). Asian and Latino immigrant families. In B. B. Ingoldsby and S. D. Smith, eds. *Families in Global and Multicultural Perspective*. Thousand Oaks, California: Sage Publications, 209–30.

Landau, L., Saul, J. (2004). Facilitating family and community resilience in response to major disaster. In F. Walsh and M. McGoldrick, eds. *Living Beyond Loss*. New York: W. W. Norton & Company, 285–309.

Machel, G. (1996). *Impact of Armed Conflict on Children*. New York: United Nations.

Miller, K., Rasco, L. (2005). An ecological framework for addressing the mental health needs of refugee communities. In K. Miller and L. Rasco, eds. *The Mental Health of Refugees: Ecological Approaches to Refugee Mental Health*. New York: Lawrence Erlbaum, 1–64.

Milroy, H. (2005). Australian Indigenous Doctors' Association (AIDA) submissions on the consultative document. *Preventative Healthcare and Strengthening Australia's Social and Economic Fabric*. http://www.nhmrc.gov.au/consult/submissions/_files/52.pdf (accessed July 2010).

Parker, G. (1977). Cyclone Tracy and Darwin evacuees: on the restoration of the species. *British Journal of Psychiatry*, **130**, 548–55.

Patel, V., Stein, G. (2007). Cultural and international psychiatry. In G. Stein and G. Wilkinson, eds. *General Adult Psychiatry*. London: Royal College of Psychiatrists, 782–810.

Seligman, M., Groves, D. (1970). Nontransient learnt helplessness. *Psychonomic Science*, **19**, 191–2.

Silove, D. (2007). Adaptation, ecosocial safety signals, and the trajectory of PTSD. In L. Kirmayer, R. Lemelson and M. Barad, eds. *Understanding Trauma: Integrating Biological, Clinical, and Cultural Perspectives*. Cambridge: Cambridge University Press, 242–58.

Silove, D., Steel, Z., Psychol, M. (2006). Understanding community psychosocial needs after disasters: implications for mental health services. *Journal of Postgraduate Medicine*, **52**, 121–5.

Somasundaram, D. (1997). Treatment of massive trauma. *Advances in Psychiatric Treatment*, **3**, 321–3.

Somasundaram, D. (1998). *Scarred Minds*. New Delhi: Sage Publications.

Somasundaram, D. J. (2002). Using traditional relaxation techniques in minor mental health disorders. *International Medical Journal*, **9**(3), 191–8.

Somasundaram, D. (2007). Collective trauma in northern Sri Lanka: a qualitative psychosocial–ecological study. *International Journal of Mental Health Systems*, **1**, 5.

Somasundaram, D. (2010). Using cultural relaxation methods in post trauma care among refugees in Australia. *International Journal of Culture and Mental Health*, **3**(1), 16–24.

Summerfield, D. (1996). The impact of war and atrocity on civilian populations: basic principles for NGO interventions and a critique of psychosocial trauma projects. *Relief and Rehabilitation Network, Network paper 14*. London: Overseas Development Institute.

Tribe, R. (2004). A critical review of the evolution of a multi-level community-based children's play activity programme run by the family rehabilitation centre (FRC) throughout Sri Lanka. *Journal of Refugee studies*, **17**, 114–35.

Tribe, R. and Family Rehabilitation Centre Staff (2004). Internally displaced Sri Lankan war widows: the women's empowerment programme. *The Mental Health of Refugees: Ecological Approaches to Healing and Adaption*, 161–8.

Tse, S., Hoque, M. E. (2006). Healthy immigrant effect – triumphs, transience and threats. In *Prevention, Protection and Promotion. Proceedings of the Second International Asian Health and Wellbeing Conference*. Auckland: University of Auckland, 9–18.

Wilkinson, G. (2007). Psychiatry in general practice. In G. Stein and G. Wilkinson, eds. *General Adult Psychiatry*. London: Royal College of Psychiatrists, 747–81.

The impact of acculturative stress on the mental health of migrants

Pedro Ruiz, I. Carol Maggi and Anna Yusim

Editors' introduction

Adjustment to the new society and new culture following migration takes a degree of time and effort. Different individuals respond in different ways and the process of acculturation may take many forms. Some of these acculturative processes may well start in the pre-migration phase and may carry on for a long period after migration. Migrants may influence the majority culture, but by and large it is the majority culture which affects the minority one. Individuals from the minority culture and the minority culture itself will change in response to the exposure to the majority culture. In this chapter, Ruiz *et al.* describe the acculturative stress related to migration. The stress occurs as a result of cultural and psychological changes and can lead to mental health problems. The contact between the majority and the minority cultures, and migrants and the majority culture will often lead to some stress – levels of which will vary according to a number of factors. Degrees of pluralism and tolerance in the new society and age, gender, marital status and educational and economic status are individual factors which may influence acculturative stress. Such stress will also increase substance misuse in vulnerable individuals. Ruiz *et al.* recommend that the conceptualisation of stress be integrally related to psychological phenomena. Clinicians who treat migrants must be aware of the impact that acculturative stress can have on migrants and on the new culture.

Introduction

Human migration has existed for centuries. The process of urbanisation by which large numbers of rural populations are able to congregate and settle in small urban areas has also influenced the migration process a great deal. Generally speaking, most processes of migration have a pattern of population movements from rural areas to urban areas. Additionally, this migration process has also happened from continent to continent. This migration process from continent to continent has not always been a voluntary one; for instance, from the 1600s to the 1800s millions of persons were forced to migrate as slaves from Africa to North America. Wars and other types of conflicts, such as religious and language differences, have also led over time to major migration exoduses from country to country or from region to region. On other occasions, poverty has influenced populations to move from poor countries to wealthy countries with the hope of improving their socio-economic conditions. In essence, the human migratory process has prevailed since the Earth was created until the present time; for sure, from 40 000 BC to the present time.

Migration and Mental Health, ed. Dinesh Bhugra & Susham Gupta. Published by Cambridge University Press. © Cambridge University Press 2011.

Table 13.1 Top 10 asylum countries from 2000 to 2002

Countries	Legal refugees (asylum)
Britain	300 000
Germany	240 000
United States	230 000
France	175 000
Canada	120 000
Netherlands	95 000
Belgium	90 000
Austria	90 000
Sweden	70 000
Switzerland	60 000

Table 13.2 Migration within the European Union in 2000

Countries	Immigrants
Italy	181 300
Great Britain	140 000
Germany	105 000
France	55 000
Netherlands	53 000
Sweden	24 400
Greece	23 900
Spain	20 800
Ireland	20 000
Austria	17 300
Belgium	12 100
Portugal	11 000
Denmark	10 100
Luxembourg	3 600
Finland	2 400

Since World War 2, a steady and ongoing migratory process has taken place into the United States. Additionally, since the creation of the European Union, a large migratory process has also taken place into the countries of the European Union, and within the European Union countries as well. For instance, during the period 2000–2002, the top 10 asylum countries in the

Table 13.3 Judgement of host society on migrants

Countries	Agree/accept (%)	Disagree/reject (%)
United States	22	74
Great Britain	33	69
France	32	66
Germany	31	65
Russia	26	72
Turkey	34	61

world were those shown in Table 13.1 (Ruiz, 2004a). Likewise, within the European Union, in the year 2000, the migration process has been as shown in Table 13.2 (Ruiz, 2004a). During the past two decades, an extensive globalisation process has taken place all over the world (Ruiz, in press). This globalisation process has, among other things, greatly impacted the mental health status of many of these migrants because of the role of 'acculturative stress'.

Understanding acculturative stress

The process of globalisation, which has recently affected all regions of the world, has also greatly impacted upon the mental health status of many of these migrants. This has happened in large part via the role of acculturative stress (Berry, 2001, 2005; Group for the Advance of Psychiatry, 1989). When migrants abandon their countries of origin and move to another country, they bring with them not only a desire to improve their socio-economic conditions, but also their languages, religions, traditions and heritages; that is, their 'culture', as well as their 'ethnic' and 'racial' characteristics (Gonzalez *et al.*, 2001; Ruiz, 2004b).

In this context, *culture* could be defined as a set of meanings, behavioural norms and values used by migrants to construct their unique view of their world. These values include language, non-verbal expressions of thoughts and emotions, religious beliefs, moral principles and social relationships (Gonzalez *et al.*, 2001). *Ethnicity* could also be described as a subjective sense of belonging to a given group of persons who have a common origin, and with shared social and cultural values and practices. In this context, *ethnicity* is a component of a person's or a group of persons' sense of 'identity' (Gonzalez *et al.*, 2001). Similarly, *race*, while often perceived as a set of physical, biological and genetic characteristics, is also commonly used by people as a psychosocial concept under which humans have chosen to group themselves based primarily on general physiognomy (Gonzalez *et al.*, 2001).

During the migration and settlement process, the migrants' culture comes into contact with the host society's culture. Most often, this contact leads to conflicts, and these conflicts produce stress for both the migrants and the members of the host society. However, the level of stress is higher among the migrants. This stress is known as 'acculturative stress', which is part of the 'acculturation process'. The differences in cultures between the migrant groups and the members of the host society have been clearly depicted via opinions or judgements by the members of the host society with respect to the migrant groups (Ruiz, 2004a; also see *USA Today*, 13 June 2007). This is reflected in how members of the host society judge and accept or reject newly arrived migrants into their culture (Table 13.3).

Obviously, in the countries described above the majority of the members of the host society tend to reject the full integration of migrant groups from different cultural, ethnic or racial backgrounds into their society (Ruiz, 2004b; see also *USA Today*, 13 June 2007). These cultural differences, which always manifest to a given degree during migration, produce a certain level of acculturative stress as part of the acculturation process. Over time, as the culture of the migrants interface with the culture of the host society or the majority culture, the process of acculturation leads to a series of outcomes. The acculturation process is a dual process of cultural and psychological changes that takes place between two or more cultural groups; some as part of the majority culture, some as part of the minority culture. Most of the time, however, the culture of the host society symbolises or represents the majority culture (Berry, 2005; Group for the Advance of Psychiatry, 1989; Ruiz, 2005).

With respect to the outcomes of the cultural interactions between the members of the migrant groups and the members of the majority/host society, generally speaking, four different types of outcomes can be produced. They are integration, assimilation, separation or rejection and marginalisation (Berry, 2005; Dansen *et al.*, 1988; Group for the Advance of Psychiatry, 1989). All of these outcomes are related to the results of the phases of acculturation and the level of the acculturative stress, among other things. They also begin during the pre-contact period; that is, before the migrant leaves his or her country of origin. They then continue through the contact period between the two countries (the home country and the host country), through the conflict period when both cultures (minority and majority) interface, through the crisis period when the acculturative stress is at its highest level and, finally, through the adaption period vis-à-vis the majority/host society (Berry *et al.*, 1987; Group for the Advance of Psychiatry, 1989; Lazarus and Folkman, 1984; Ward *et al.*, 2001).

The integration outcome, which happens to be the most healthy one on the part of the migrant, takes place when the migrant person retains his or her culture of origin and fosters contacts and interactions with the members of the majority/host society. The assimilation outcome happens when the migrant person rejects or denies his or her culture of origin, while fostering interactions and contacts with the members of the majority or host society. The separation or rejection outcome occurs when the migrant separates or rejects his or her own culture, and also refuses to foster contacts or interactions with the majority/host society. At times, this separation between the migrant and the host society is forced by the host society, thus creating a form of segregation. Finally, the marginalisation outcome occurs when the migrant refuses his or her own culture of origin, while also deciding not to foster contacts or interactions with the majority/host society.

There are, of course, a series of variables that can play a major or minor role in the process of acculturation and, thus in the level of acculturative stress. They are societal, group-related, demographic, sociological and/or psychological and behavioural. The societal variables have to do with the type of society represented by the majority culture of the host society or, for that matter, of the migrant or migrant groups. They relate to the degree of 'pluralism', 'tolerance' and 'racist' qualities prevalent in the host society (majority culture) or the migrant groups (minority culture). The group-related variables, whether they be manifested primarily in the majority/host society's culture or the minority/migrant's culture, relate to touristic variables, temporary worker variables, sojourner variables, immigrant variables or refugee variables. The demographic variables are dependent on age, gender, marital status, level of education, race, ethnicity, religion, climate, urban or rural location, foreign- or host country-born and economic status. In general, younger persons tolerate the impact of migration better, as do persons born in the host country, females, married persons, persons with a high level of education, wealthy persons, and persons with similarities of race, ethnicity, religion, climate and geography between the host society and the migrant group. The other variables that influence the acculturation process include the sociological or psychological variables related to family (maternal/paternal deprivation, childhood traumas/conflicts, etc.), home sickness or separation conflicts, self-identity problems, status of group cohesiveness, generational differences (first generation migrants are at greatest risk), status of network systems, one's sense of power or powerlessness, level of rigidity or flexibility, and prejudices or negative attitudes. In general, all of these sociological and psychological variables apply more to the migrant than to the host society. The behavioural variables are the ones that more traumatically and negatively impact on the migrant groups. They relate to alcohol/drugs use/abuse, accidents, crime, homicide and suicide.

Given the seriousness of the behavioural variables, it is important that we focus on some of them. Hopefully, this will assist the mental health professionals to think about them, give priority to them, and appropriately and promptly intervene with them when necessary.

Acculturation and suicide

In general, the rate of suicide among Hispanic populations tends to be lower than the rate of suicide in other ethnic or racial groups (Delgado and Ruiz, 1985; Ruiz, 1996a, b). Table 13.4 compares the data of Hispanic suicide rates and the suicide rates of other ethnic groups per 100 000 persons based on country rates (Group for the Advance of Psychiatry, 1989).

These data clearly demonstrate that Hispanic countries, such as Mexico and Spain, have a much lower suicide rate per 100 000 persons than non-Hispanic countries. Also, as seen in Tables 13.5 (World Health Organization, 1973) and 13.6 (US Bureau of the Census, 1987), the comparisons of suicide rates per 100 000 persons between Mexico and the United States show that in Mexico the rates of suicide are not only lower overall, but also in terms of male and female suicide rates, as well as for age groups. Additionally, there are not considerable peaks of suicide rates for either males or females in Mexico, while in the United States there are peaks of suicide rates for males in the age group 20–24 (27.4) and again in age groups 55–64 (28.6), 65–74 (35.3) and 74–84 (57.1). For females, the peaks in the United States are in the age groups 45–54 (9.0), 55–64 (8.4) and 74–84 (7.0). Additionally, if we compare the suicide rates per 100 000 for Mexican Americans and the US population of El Paso and

Table 13.4 Suicide rates per 100 000 persons

Mexico	1.7
Spain	4.1
England	8.2
United States	12.5
Canada	14.8
Japan	17.7
Sweden	19.0
Germany	27.0
Austria	24.8

Table 13.5 Suicide rates in Mexico according to age/sex (rates per 100 000 population)

Age group	Total	Male	Female
15–24	1.3	1.9	0.7
25–34	1.2	1.8	0.5
35–44	1.2	2.2	0.3
45–54	1.2	1.9	0.4
55–64	1.4	2.5	0.3
65–74	1.7	3.3	0.1
74 and over	1.6	2.9	0.5
All ages	0.7	1.1	0.3

Adapted from World Health Organization (WHO), 1973.

Table 13.6 Suicide rates in the US according to age/sex (rates per 100 000 population)

Age group	Total	Male	Female
15–19	10.0	17.3	4.1
20–24	15.6	27.4	5.2
25–34	15.2	25.4	6.4
35–44	14.6	23.5	7.7
45–54	15.6	25.1	9.0
55–64	16.7	28.6	8.4
65–74	18.5	35.3	7.3
74–84	24.1	57.1	7.0
All ages	12.3	21.5	5.6

Adapted from US Bureau of the Census, 1987.

Denver, as depicted in Tables 13.7 (Hatcher and Hatcher, 1975) and 13.8 (Ruiz, 1996b), we can see that as the Mexican Americans become more acculturated as a result of settling in Denver, their rates of suicide become similar to the rates of the US general population for both males and females. In El Paso, however, the rate of suicide for Mexican Americans is higher than the rate of suicide for Mexicans in Mexico (7.0 versus 0.7). However, the rate of suicide for the US general population living in El Paso is much higher than even the suicide rate for the general US population (15.6 versus 11.7). This may be due to the fact that, contrary to the majority US population, in El Paso the majority population is Mexican American. In other words, the role of acculturative stress or the process of acculturation of El Paso is higher among the US general population because this population is much smaller in

Table 13.7 Suicide rates in El Paso, Texas (rates per 100 000 population) from 1970 to 1972.

Mexican American	7.0
White	15.6
US population	11.7

Adapted from Hatcher and Hatcher, 1975.

Table 13.8 Suicide rates in Denver, Colorado (rates per 100 000 population) from 1970 to 1975

	Total	Male	Female
Mexican American	12.9	22.4	4.4
US population	12.7	18.9	6.8

Adapted from Loya, F. *Increases in Chicano Suicide, Denver, Colorado, 1960–1975 – What Can Be Done?* University of California, Los Angeles, California: Neuropsychiatric Institute.

El Paso than the Mexican American population. The Mexican American population is about 500 000 (or 77%) of the total population of El Paso, while all other ethnic groups in El Paso, including the US general population (white) represents the minority population, forming only 23% of this population (Hatcher and Hatcher, 1975; US Bureau of the Census, 2000).

As previously discussed, the role of acculturative stress and acculturation is a major one insofar as suicidal behaviour is concerned. As previously demonstrated, this is true for either Mexican Americans or the US general population (white), depending on which of the two happens to play the role of the minority population.

In another study, covering the suicide rates during the period 1976–1980 of five south-western states with proximity to Mexico (Arizona, California, Colorado, New Mexico and Texas), it has been shown that, over time, as the acculturation process makes its impact on the migrant or minority population, the rates of suicide per 100 000 persons, as well as the suicide peaks and rates for males and females, begin to approach the rates of the majority/host society (Smith *et al.*, 1985). Again, this study demonstrates that the acculturation process negatively impacts the Hispanic migrant population who settled in the US (Table 13.9).

Acculturation and substance use/abuse

Substance use/abuse is another behavioural variable related to the process of acculturation and to the negative impact of acculturative stress on migrant/minority populations as they interact and have contact with the majority/host society. In a comparative study focusing on the use of substances of abuse (Pumariega *et al.*, 1992), it was demonstrated that the rates of use/abuse of substances between the ages of 11 and 19 in a Mexican population was 1.79% while for a Mexican American population it was 11.69%. In this study, it was also shown that the Mexican group of adolescents spent 24–37% of time watching television or listening to the radio and 12.90% with friends, while the Mexican American population spent 40.52%

Table 13.9 Suicide rates during the period 1976–1980 in five south-western states* (rates per 100 000 population)

Age group	White			Hispanic		
	Total	Male	Female	Total	Male	Female
0–14	0.5	0.7	0.2	0.2	0.3	0.1
15–19	11.9	18.6	5.6	9.0	14.8	3.4
20–24	23.3	37.4	9.7	18.7	33.1	5.4
25–29	24.6	36.4	12.2	16.0	26.4	6.1
30–39	22.6	30.7	14.4	14.7	23.8	6.2
40–49	24.8	31.0	18.6	12.2	18.2	6.5
50–59	26.4	34.4	18.9	11.8	19.8	4.7
60–69	26.7	40.9	14.8	11.7	20.0	4.4
70 and over	32.8	63.2	13.7	14.2	28.0	3.0
Total	19.2	27.5	11.2	9.0	14.6	3.3
Age-adjusted Total	18.5	27.5	10.5	10.5	17.8	4.0

* Arizona, California, Colorado, New Mexico and Texas.
Adapted from Smith *et al.* (1985).

watching television or listening to the radio, and 19.72% with friends. Obviously, the changes in the cultural patterns between the youth in Mexico and the youth in the USA appear to have a negative impact in the use/abuse of substances for the group of Mexican Americans who migrated from Mexico to the USA. With respect to alcoholism, a study examining daily drinking patterns between males in Mexico showed that for first generation Mexican Americans it was 20%, second generation Mexican Americans 21%, and third generation Mexican Americans it was 38%, while for Mexicans it was 13% (Gilbert, 1989). The use of this substance (alcohol) increased over generations and was higher in comparison with Mexicans in Mexico. This pattern mimics the pattern of the US general population, thus depicting the influence of the acculturation process vis-à-vis the Mexican migrant population that settled in the USA.

A similar pattern has also been found with respect to illicit drug use among Puerto Rican youth who reside in Puerto Rico, move to the mainland USA, or are born in the mainland USA to Puerto Rican parents who reside in the mainland USA instead of Puerto Rico (Velez and Ungemack, 1995). For the youth from Puerto Rico the use of illegal drugs was 6%; for those who migrated to the US mainland (New York) it was 17%; and for those who were born in the US mainland (New York) to Puerto Rican parents it was 26%. This study also found that the percentage of non-drug users in Puerto Rico was 48%, while among the Puerto Ricans who migrated to the US mainland (New York) it was 25%, and for the Puerto Ricans who were born in the US mainland it was 19%. Again, this study clearly demonstrates the negative impact of the acculturation process and the role of acculturative stress among the Puerto Rican youth who used drugs before their migration to the US mainland, as well as the group that did not use drugs at all while living on Puerto Rico.

The topic of cultural and cross-cultural psychiatry has received much attention in recent years in highly developed industrialised nations, especially in the USA (Johnson et al., 2003; Munoz et al., 2007; Ruiz, 2000). This has happened not only in psychiatry at large, but also in some areas of psychiatry where issues pertaining to culture, including the role of acculturative stress and acculturation, are very relevant and important; for instance, in the area of alcoholism (Johnson et al., 2003), substance abuse (Lowinson et al., 2005; Ruiz et al., 2007), HIV/AIDS (Fernandez and Ruiz, 2006), mental health disparities (Ruiz and Primm, 2009), comprehensive education (Sadock et al., 2009) and in forensic psychiatry (Tseng et al., 2007).

Clinical implications

As alluded to previously, the field of cultural psychiatry is expanding rapidly and currently encompasses all areas and subspecialties within psychiatry (Fernandez and Ruiz, 2006; Johnson et al., 2003; Lowinson et al., 2005; Munoz et al., 2007; Ruiz et al., 2007; Ruiz and Primm, 2009; Sadock et al., 2009; Tseng et al., 2007). In this context, it is imperative that cultural psychiatry be a part of any modern psychiatric curriculum, training programme, review course or continuing medical education activity. The role, for instance, of language differences in the day-to-day clinical practice of psychiatry has been extensively addressed and substantiated via research efforts and clinical applications (Gomez et al., 1985; Lavel et al., 1983; Marcos et al., 1973a, b). It is additionally relevant in the day-to-day practice of clinical psychiatry, particularly from the point of view of adherence to treatment, quality of care delivery, appropriate diagnostic considerations and the psychosocial aspects and/or approaches vis-à-vis mental illnesses (Kamaldeep and Bhugra, 2007; Ruiz, 1995, 1998, 2007).

Nowadays, the conceptualisation of stress is a necessity in every aspect of life (Dohrenwend and Dohrenwend, 1981), as it is in human health in general (Elliot and Eisdorfer, 1982), and in health and disease in particular (Zales, 1985). In addition, the understanding of stress, as well as its conceptualisation is integrally related to psychological phenomena, as well as neurosciences at large (Andrews et al., 2009). It is, therefore, essential that healthcare practitioners and mental healthcare practitioners, especially psychiatrists, be knowledgeable about the role and influence of stress in health and illness (Albalustri, 2007).

Because of our enhanced understanding of the pivotal role of culture in many aspects of health, mental health and stress, the medical training of physicians is increasingly beginning to encompass a cultural focus. In the USA, the unique characteristics related to 'cultural competencies' are becoming central to the current emphasis of core competencies in the training of psychiatry residents. In this regard, with the increasing importance placed on cultural competence in improving the quality of mental healthcare and eliminating racial/ ethnic disparities nationally and globally, psychiatry residencies are faced with the challenge of training their residents to better appreciate and understand the complex relationship between culture, ethnicity and mental health.

The continued presence of ethnic and racial biases in the health and mental healthcare system of the USA and abroad leads occasionally to misdiagnosis of minority patients (Alegria et al., 2008a; Elwy et al., 2008). The poorer quality of care provided to immigrants and ethnic minorities results from the lack of understanding of many mainstream psychiatrists of ethnopharmacological differences and culturally defined mental health syndromes (Alegria et al., 2008b; Horvitz-Lennon et al., 2009; Lewis-Fernandez and Kleinman, 2006; Ruiz et al., 1999; Tseng, 2004; Varner et al., 1998). For this reason, cultural competency has become an integral part of psychiatric residency training. However, with the increased globalisation of healthcare in general and academic departments of psychiatry in particular, our definition of cultural competency has started to go beyond a focus on a few stereotyped conclusions about the unique features of a particular ethnic group or culture.

The transfer of knowledge regarding the role of culture in health and disease must proceed in a bidirectional fashion (Belkin and Fricchione, 2005). In this context, bidirectionality means that the methods of scientific analysis, delivery of care and identification of illness in the host country and culture can be enhanced to the same degree that they can influence and enhance the methods of migrant or immigrant culture. In such a model, the migrant and host communities reposition themselves as partners in the creation of knowledge and understanding of health, illness and, in particular, mental illness. Approaching medicine and psychiatry in a bidirectional fashion encourages clinicians to challenge their paradigm of illness and nosology of disease, and, in consequence, to test and adapt it based on the diversity of culture, experience and circumstance in the rest of the world. Such bidirectional exchange of knowledge has the potential to transform psychiatric practice and equip it with an appreciation of the impact of culture on health, illness, stress and mental health.

Conclusion

Stress has certainly existed since humans became a part of the universe; additionally, animals have also been known to experience and suffer from stress for centuries. The understanding, however, that stress plays a role in health and in illness is a more recent phenomenon. In this respect, culture has more recently been known to play a major role with respect to protection of health and management of illness. During the past 3–4 decades, the role of acculturative stress has become not only recognised vis-à-vis health and illness, but better understood as well. In this context, mental health and mental illness have been extensively studied and researched in recent years insofar as their role in preserving mental health or managing of mental illness is concerned. In this chapter, we have reviewed the most important aspects of acculturative stress vis-à-vis mental health and mental illness. Hopefully, this chapter will stimulate further attention and priority with respect to acculturative stress from the point of view of clinical care, research efforts and educational perspectives.

References

Albalustri, L. (2007). *Estres y Nuevas Perspectivas en Psicopatologia y Salud*. Buenos Aires, Argentina: Editorial Cientifica Interamericana, S.A.C.I.

Alegria, M., Nakash, O., Lapatin, S. *et al.* (2008a). How missing information in diagnosis can lead to disparities in the clinical encounter. *Journal of Public Health Management and Practice*, **14**(11), S26–S35.

Alegria, M., Chatterji, P., Wells, K. *et al.* (2008b). Disparity in depression among racial and ethnic minority populations in the United States. *Psychiatric Services*, **59**(11), 1264–72.

Andrews, G., Charney, D. S., Sirovalka, P. J., Regier, D. A. (eds) (2009). *Stress-Induced and Fear Circuitry Disorders: Refining the Research Agenda for DSM-V*. Arlington, Virginia, American Psychiatric Association.

Belkin, G. S., Fricchione, G. L. (2005). Internationalism and the future of academic psychiatry. *Academic Psychiatry*, **29**(3), 240–3.

Berry, J. W. (2001). A psychology of immigration. *Journal of Social Issues*, **57**(3), 615–31.

Berry, J. W. (2005). Acculturation: living successfully in two cultures. *International*

Journal of Intercultural Relations,
29, 697–712.

Berry, J. W., Kim, U., Minde, T., Mok, D. (1987).
Comparative studies of acculturative stress.
International Migration Review, **21**,
491–511.

Dansen, P., Berry, J. W., Sartorious, N. (eds)
(1988). *Health and Cross-Cultural
Psychology: Toward Applications.* London:
Sage Publications.

Delgado, A., Ruiz, P. (1985). Suicide and
Hispanic Americans. In P. Pichet,
P. Benner, R. Wolf, R. Thau (eds)
*Proceedings of the VII World Congress
of Psychiatry, Psychiatry: The State of
the Art, Volume 8.* New York: Plenum
Press, 433–7.

Dohrenwend, B. S., Dohrenwend, B. P.
(1981). *Stressful Life Events and Their
Contexts.* New York: Prodist, a Division
of Neale Watson Academic Publication,
Inc.

Elliot, G. R., Eisdorfer, C. (eds) (1982). *Stress and
Human Health: Analysis and Implications,
A Study by the Institute of Medicine/
National Academy of Sciences.* New York:
Springer Publishing Company.

Elwy, A. R., Ranganathan, G., Eisen, S. V. (2008).
Race-ethnicity and diagnosis as predictors
of outpatient service use among treatment
initiators. *Psychiatric Services,* **59**(11),
1285–91.

Fernandez, F., Ruiz, P. (eds) (2006). *Psychiatric
Aspects of HIV/AIDS.* Philadelphia,
Pennsylvania: Lippincott Williams &
Wilkins.

Gilbert, M. J. (1989). *Research Monograph No. 18,
DHHS Publication No. (ADM) 89–1435.*
Washington DC: Government Printing
Office.

Gomez, R., Ruiz, P., Rumbaut, R. D. (1985).
Hispanic patients: a linguo-cultural
minority. *Hispanic Journal of Behavioral
Sciences,* **7**(2), 177–86.

Gonzalez, C. A., Griffith, E. E. H., Ruiz, P. (2001).
Cross-cultural issues in psychiatric
treatment. In G. O. Gabbard (ed.)
Treatment of Psychiatric Disorders, 3rd edn,
Vol. 1. Washington, DC: American
Psychiatric Press, Inc., 47–67.

Group for the Advance of Psychiatry. (1989).
*Formulated by the Committee on Cultural
Psychiatry: Suicide and Ethnicity in the
United States,* Report No. 128. New York:
Brunner/Mazel Publishers.

Hatcher, C., Hatcher, D. (1975). Ethnic group
suicide: an analysis of Mexican-American
and Anglo rates for El Paso, Texas. *Crisis
Intervention,* **6**(1), 2–9.

Horvitz-Lennon, M., Frank, R. G.,
Thompson, W. *et al.* (2009). Investigation
of racial and ethnic disparities in service
utilization among homeless adults with
severe mental illnesses. *Psychiatric Services,*
60(8), 1032–8.

Johnson, B., Ruiz, P., Galanter, M. (eds) (2003).
Handbook of Clinical Alcoholism Treatment.
Baltimore, Maryland: Lippincott
Williams & Wilkins.

Kamaldeep, B., Bhugra, D. (eds) (2007). *Culture
and Mental Health: A Comprehensive
Textbook.* London: Hodder Arnold.

Laval, R. A., Gomez, E. A., Ruiz, P. (1983). A
language minority: Hispanic Americans
and mental health. *The American Journal of
Social Psychiatry,* **3**(2), 42–9.

Lazarus, R. S., Folkman, S. (1984). *Stress,
Appraisal and Coping.* New York: Springer.

Lewis-Fernandez, R., Kleinman, A. (2006).
Cultural psychiatry. Theoretical, clinical,
and research issues. *Transcultural
Psychiatry,* **43**(1), 126–44.

Lowinson, J. H., Ruiz, P., Millman, R. B.,
Langrod, J. G. (eds) (2005). *Substance
Abuse: A Comprehensive Textbook,* 4th edn.
Baltimore, Maryland: Lippincott
Williams & Wilkins.

Marcos, L. R., Alpert, M., Urcuyo, L.,
Kesselman, M. (1973a). The effect of
interview language on the evaluation of
psychopathology in Spanish-American
schizophrenic patients. *American Journal of
Psychiatry,* **130**(5), 549–53.

Marcos, L. R., Urcuyo, L., Kesselman, M.,
Alpert, M. (1973b). The language barrier in
evaluating Spanish–American patients.
Archives of General Psychiatry, **11**(29), 655–9.

Munoz, R. A., Primm, A., Ananth, J., Ruiz, P.
(2007). *Live in Color: Culture in American*

Psychiatry. Monster, Indiana: Hilton Publishing Company, Inc.

Pumariega, A. J., Swanson, J. W., Holzer, C. E., Linskey, A. O., Quintero-Salinas, R. (1992). Cultural context and substance abuse in Hispanic adolescents. *Journal of Child and Family Studies*, **1**(1), 75–92.

Ruiz, P. (1995). Assessing, diagnosing and treating culturally diverse individuals: a Hispanic perspective. *Psychiatric Quarterly*, **66**(4), 329–41.

Ruiz, P. (1996a). Aspectos culturales del suicidio entre los Mexico–Americanos. *Medico Interamericano*, **15**(1), 75–8.

Ruiz, P. (1996b). Suicide and acculturation: a Mexican–American perspective. *Psychline Inter-Transdisciplinary Journal of Mental Health*, **1**(2), 26–8.

Ruiz, P. (1998). The role of culture in psychiatric care. *The American Journal of Psychiatry*, **155**(12), 1763–5.

Ruiz, P. (2000). *Ethnicity and Psychopharmacology*, Vol. 19. Washington, DC: American Psychiatric Press, Inc.

Ruiz, P. (2004a). Psychopathology and migration. In *Psiquiatria 2004, III Symposium Almirall, Volume I*. Barcelona, Spain: Libros de Resumenes, 47–60.

Ruiz, P. (2004b). Addressing culture, race & ethnicity in psychiatric care. *Psychiatric Annals*, **34**(7), 527–32.

Ruiz, P. (2005). La psiquiatria en las minorias etnicas: el ejemplo de los Estados Unidos. In J. Vallejo Ruiloba, C. Leal Cercos (eds) *Tratado de Psiquiatria, Volumen II*. Barcelona, Spain: Ars Medica, 2273–80.

Ruiz, P. (2007). Spanish, English, and Mental Health Services. *American Journal of Psychiatry*, **1642**(8), 1113–35.

Ruiz, P. (in press). Therapeutic skills and therapeutic expectations. In D. Bhugra, T. Craig, K. S. Bhui (eds) *Mental Health of Refugees and Asylum Seekers*. Oxford: Oxford University Press.

Ruiz, P., Primm, A. (eds) (2009). *Mental Health Disparities: Clinical and Cross-Cultural*

Perspectives. Philadelphia, Pennsylvania: Lippincott Williams & Wilkins.

Ruiz, P., Varner, R. V., Small, D. R., Johnson, B. A. (1999). Ethnic difference in the neuroleptic treatment of schizophrenia. *Psychiatric Quarterly*, **70**(2), 163–72.

Ruiz, P., Strain, E. C., Langrod, J. G. (eds) (2007). *The Substance Abuse Handbook*. Philadelphia, Pennsylvania: Lippincott Williams & Wilkins.

Sadock, B. J., Sadock, V. A., Ruiz, P. (eds) (2009). *Kaplan & Sadock's Comprehensive Textbook of Psychiatry*, 9th edn. Philadelphia, Pennsylvania: Lippincott Williams & Wilkins.

Smith, J. C., Mercy, J. A., Warren, C. W. (1985). Hispanic suicide: report for five southwestern states for the years 1976–1980. *Suicide and Life Threatening Behavior*, **1**(1), 14–26.

Tseng, W. S. (2004). From peculiar psychiatric disorders through culture-bound syndromes to culture-related specific syndromes. *Transcultural Psychiatry*, **43**(4), 554–76.

Tseng, W.-S., Griffith, E., Ruiz, P., Buchanan, A. (2007). Culture and psychopathy in the forensic Context. In A. Felthous, H. Sab (eds) *The International Handbook of Psychopathic Disorders and the Law, Volume II: Laws and Policies*. West Sussex: John Wiley & Sons Ltd, 473–88.

US Bureau of the Census. (1987). *Statistical Abstract of the United States, Volume 108*. Washington DC: US Government.

US Bureau of the Census. (2000). *Current Populations Report Series*. Washington DC: US Government.

Varner, R. V., Ruiz, P., Small, D. R. (1998). Black and white patients response to antidepressant treatment for major depression. *Psychiatric Quarterly*, **69**(2), 117–25.

Velez, C. N., Ungemack, J. A. (1995). Psychosocial correlates of drug use among Puerto Rican youth: generational status differences. *Social Sciences and Medicine*, **40**(1), 91–103.

Ward, C., Bochner, S., Furnham, A. (2001). *The Psychology of Cultural Shock*. London: Routledge.

World Health Organization (WHO). (1973). *World Health Statistics Annual, Vital Statistics and Cause of Death*. Geneva: Switzerland.

Zales, M. R. (ed) (1985). *Stress in Health and Disease*. New York: Brunner/Mazel, Publishers.

Migration and mental health of older people

Ajit Shah

Editors' introduction

Migration and settlement post-migration are influenced by the role of gender, age and educational status. Older individuals may migrate as primary migrants or they may migrate to join their children or grandchildren in a new country. The pressures on primary and secondary migrants will vary again depending upon the reasons for migration, their socio-economic and educational status among other factors. In this chapter, Shah uses existing epidemiological data on the elderly to illustrate differences between migrant elders and the native ones. These differences demonstrate that explanatory models and access to care varies across these ethnic groups. Interestingly, high rates of primary care consultation but low prevalence of psychiatric disorders suggest that family factors (different explanations, poor recognition, stigma), primary care factors (poor knowledge of services, symptoms may differ, culturally inappropriate screening tools) and secondary care factors may all play a role in poor diagnosis and subsequent engagement with psychiatric services. Shah proposes that better training and educational campaigns may help in improving diagnosis and assessments as well as engagement with psychiatric services.

Introduction

The relationship between migration and mental health in older people within the context of the UK will be examined in the domains of demography, epidemiology of mental disorders and suicide in old age, access to services and potential ways forward to improve service access. Although this chapter uses the UK as the main frame of reference, many of the issues for migrants are likely to be similar in other countries, and literature from other countries is also considered.

Demographic changes

In the UK, migrants are often referred to as black and minority ethnic (BME) individuals. The proportion of BME individuals over the age of 65 years has progressively increased from 1% in 1981 to 3% in 1991 to 8.2% in the 2001 population census in England and Wales (Shah et al., 2005a; Shah, 2007a); this contrasts with 17% of the indigenous population being over 65 years. Moreover, 7.1% of all elderly individuals in England and Wales were from BME groups in the same 2001 population census. The total number of elderly from all BME groups combined was 531 909. Similar demographic changes have been observed in other countries, including the US (Markson, 2003; Mui et al., 2003). Ninety million people are estimated to live outside their country of birth (Bohning and Oishi, 1995).

Migration and Mental Health, ed. Dinesh Bhugra & Susham Gupta. Published by Cambridge University Press. © Cambridge University Press 2011.

Epidemiology

Mental disorders

There are only a few population-based prevalence studies of mental disorders among BME elders in the UK. A small pilot study, in London, of only 45 subjects, reported a prevalence rate of 34% for dementia in an African Caribbean group compared with 4% in the indigenous white British group (Richards *et al.*, 2000). A population-based study of Indian subcontinent elders in Bradford reported prevalence rates of 7%, 20% and 2% for dementia, depression and anxiety neurosis, respectively (Bhatnagar and Frank, 1997).

A population-based study of Gujarati elders in Leicester reported prevalence rates of 0% and 20% for dementia in the age bands 65–74 years and 75+ years, respectively (Lindesay *et al.*, 1997a). These prevalence figures were not significantly different from the comparison group of indigenous white British elders. The stability of the diagnosis of dementia was confirmed at 27-month follow-up, confirming the accuracy of the original diagnosis of dementia in identified cases (Shah *et al.*, 1998). This study also reported prevalence rates of 22%, 1% and 4% for agoraphobia, simple phobia and panic attacks (Lindesay *et al.*, 1997a); simple phobias were less prevalent among the Gujarati. Although the prevalence of depression was not measured, depression scores were not significantly different between Gujarati and indigenous elders.

A population-based study from Liverpool (McCracken *et al.*, 1997) reported the prevalence of dementia in English-speaking individuals of black African, black Caribbean, black other, Chinese and Asian origin as 8%, 8%, 2%, 5% and 9%, respectively, similar to the 3% found in the indigenous white British population. Prevalence in black Africans and Chinese who did not speak English was 27% and 21%, respectively; these higher figures among non-English speakers may have been an artefact of communication and translation difficulties. The prevalence of depression amongst black African, black Caribbean, Chinese and Asian groups was 19%, 16%, 13% and 15%, respectively (McCracken *et al.*, 1997); these figures are comparable to indigenous elders (Shah, 1992a). Lack of social contact was considered to be an important risk factor for depression (McCracken *et al.*, 1997).

A population-based study in Islington reported the prevalence of dementia in those born in the UK, Ireland, Cyprus, and Africa and the Caribbean as 10%, 3.6%, 11.3% and 17%, respectively (Livingston *et al.*, 2001); living in a residential home, age, being African or Caribbean and years of education were significant predictors of dementia. The prevalence of depression in those born in the UK, Ireland, Cyprus, and Africa and the Caribbean was 18%, 16.5%, 28% and 14%, respectively; needing help with functional activities, being female and subjective ill-health were significant predictors of depression on logistic regression analysis.

Chronic health problems, functional disabilities, housing conditions, low family support, low income and reported need for community services were identified as risk factors for depression in convenience samples of Gujarati, Bengali and Somali elders in London (Silveira and Ebrahim, 1995, 1998a, b).

There are no population-based studies of late onset schizophrenia in BME elderly groups, but an increased rate of new contacts with Old Age Psychiatry Services (OAPSs) by African Caribbean elders was reported in London; the incident contact rate for men and women was 172 and 323 per 100 000 population, respectively (Reeves *et al.*, 2001).

The prevalence of dementia among elders from different BME groups in the UK is generally similar or higher than indigenous elders. The prevalence of depression among ethnic elders, in general, was similar to that among indigenous elders; the main exception was a higher prevalence among those born in Cyprus compared to those born in the UK.

Suicides

Only five studies have examined suicides in BME elderly groups (Dennis *et al.*, 2009; McKenzie *et al.*, 2008; Neeleman *et al.*, 1997; Raleigh *et al.*, 1990; Shah *et al.*, 2009), but three (McKenzie *et al.*, 2008; Neeleman *et al.*, 1997; Raleigh *et al.*, 1990) were part of larger studies of suicide across all age groups. Traditionally, suicide rates were thought not to increase with ageing among migrants from the Indian subcontinent to England and Wales and that the suicide rates were low among the elderly in this migrant group (Raleigh *et al.*, 1990). A more recent unpublished study by the author's group observed an increase in suicide rates with ageing among male migrants from the Indian subcontinent and female migrants from Africa and China in England and Wales. There is evidence that suicide rates may have increased among elderly female migrants from the Indian subcontinent between 1993 and 2003 (McKenzie *et al.*, 2008).

A study examining the methods of suicide used by elderly migrants in England and Wales observed that hanging, strangulation and suffocation, poisoning by drugs, and drowning and submersion were the most frequent methods of suicide in elderly males and females in most migrant groups; suicide by smoke, fire and flames was significantly more frequent in elderly females born in the Indian subcontinent; and suicide by unspecified means was significantly more frequent in elderly males born in Ireland, the Indian subcontinent and western Europe (Dennis *et al.*, 2009). The excess of suicides by smoke, fire and flames (burning) in elderly females born in the Indian subcontinent is consistent with previous reports in younger females of Indian subcontinent origin in England and Wales (Hunt *et al.*, 2003; Prosser, 1996; Raleigh and Balarajan, 1992; Raleigh *et al.*, 1990), younger females in India (Adityanjee, 1986; Bhatia *et al.*, 1987), and female Indian migrants to Israel (Modan *et al.*, 1970). The excess of suicides by burning was only observed in older females in contrast to previous reports of an excess in younger females. This may be a cohort effect because the older victims in the current study are likely to belong to the same cohort as the younger victims in the earlier studies from the 1970s and 1980s. Such a cohort effect may be mediated through the current older generations observing traditional cultural practices. Moreover, the persistence of methods of suicide from the country of birth suggests that it is not directly attributable to migration, although the pressures of migration to a new environment may aggravate this (Raleigh and Balarajan, 1992). The excess of suicide by unspecified means among older males born in Ireland, the Indian subcontinent and western Europe is of concern. Potentially preventable methods of suicide may be hidden behind unidentified methods of suicide. The most frequent methods of suicide in older males and females in most country of birth groups were similar to those observed in the older adult population in England and Wales (Cattell, 1988; Cattell and Jolley, 1995; Dennis *et al.*, 2009; Harwood *et al.*, 2000), and previous studies of younger BME suicide victims in England and Wales (Raleigh and Balarajan, 1992; Raleigh *et al.*, 1990; Hunt *et al.*, 2003). The findings indicate that the same preventative strategies proposed for the indigenous population should be applied to BME groups, including older adults, because the prevalent methods of suicide in the majority of country of birth groups were similar to those in the England and Wales group. However, their implementation should be culturally sensitive and appropriate, and careful consideration should be given to factors related to migration, degree of assimilation and acculturation, fluency in English, religion and culture.

A study comparing suicide rates in elderly migrants in England and Wales to those in their country of origin observed wide variations in standardised mortality ratios for elderly suicides among migrants from different countries compared with those born in England and Wales and in their country of origin (Shah *et al.*, 2009). Moreover, suicide rates either converged/diverged towards/from elderly suicide rates for England and Wales in some migrant groups, with significant divergence in other migrant groups. Furthermore, males aged 75+ years from most migrant groups had higher rates than those born in England and Wales. The general heterogeneity in elderly suicide rates across different migrant groups was observed in the elderly in Australia (Burvill, 1995), and in all ages combined in Australia, Canada, England and Wales, and the US (Burvill, 1998; Burvill *et al.*, 1982; Kleiwer, 1991; Kleiwer and Ward, 1988; Raleigh and Balarajan, 1992).

The convergence of elderly suicide rates in some migrant groups but not in others and the general heterogeneity across different migrant groups may have several explanations. First, the well known methodological difficulties observed in epidemiological research on suicides may be important in this context (Shah and Ganesvaran, 1994). Second, most earlier studies did not specifically study the elderly population. Third, most previous studies are over a decade old, and migration patterns have dramatically changed since then. Fourth, the findings collectively suggest that age and sex may have a differential effect on elderly suicide rates in different migrant groups, as has been observed in cross-national studies of elderly suicides (Shah *et al.*, 2008). Fifth, life expectancy may vary across different migrant groups, and increased elderly suicide rates are associated with increased life expectancy (Shah *et al.*, 2008). Sixth, reasons for migration, the process and the impact of migration, and the degree of acculturation and assimilation with the host culture may vary in different migrant groups (Burvill, 1998; Johansson *et al.*, 1997; Kleiwer, 1991; Kleiwer and Ward, 1988; Shah, 2004). Moreover, the duration in the host country after migration may vary across different migrant groups, and this may influence the degree of acculturation and assimilation (Burvill, 1998; Shah, 2004). Seventh, the prevalence of mental illness in the elderly, particularly depressive illness, varies across different migrant groups in England and Wales (Bhatnagar and Frank, 1997; Livingston *et al.*, 2001; McCracken *et al.*, 1997). Furthermore, some elderly migrant groups (particularly South Asians, including Indian, Pakistani, Bangladeshi and Sri Lankan groups) have poor access to old age psychiatry services in England and Wales (Jagger, 1998; Lindesay *et al.*, 1997b; Rait and Burns, 1997; Shah and Dighe-Deo, 1998). Given that between 63% and 82% of elderly suicide victims have depression (Harwood *et al.*, 2001; Waern *et al.*, 2002), elderly migrants from some groups may be denied the opportunity for identification and treatment of the condition. Eighth, cultural factors, including living in extended families, larger household size, the degree of respect and high esteem offered to the elderly, all of which offer protection against loneliness and despair which otherwise may lead to suicide (Shah, 2009), may vary across different migrant groups. A similar hypothesis has been used to explain high elderly suicide rates in Japan (Shimuzu, 1990; Watanabe *et al.*, 1995), Hong Kong (Yip and Tan, 1998), China (Yip *et al.*, 2000, 2005) and Taiwan (Liu *et al.*, 2006), where the elderly have lost their traditional family role. Finally, socio-economic status and income inequality may vary across different migrant groups, and both these variables are associated with suicide in the elderly (Gunnell *et al.*, 2003; Shah *et al.*, 2008). There is a need to compare the impact of all the variables discussed above in migrant groups with and without convergence towards elderly suicide rates among those born in England and Wales.

Scale of the problem

The two most common mental disorders in old age are dementia and depression. The prevalence of dementia doubles every 5.1 years after the age of 60 years (Hofman *et al.*, 1991; Jorm *et al.*, 1987) and prevalence rates of up to 15% have been reported for depression in the elderly (Shah, 1992a). These observations, the demographic changes and the prevalence of dementia and depression among BME elders being similar or higher than that among indigenous elders, suggest that the absolute number of cases of both dementia and depression will significantly increase in BME groups. One recent study estimated the absolute number of cases of dementia in the BME population to be 11 860 in the UK in 2004 (Kings College London and London School of Economics, 2007). Another study estimated the absolute number of cases of dementia to be between 7270 and 10 786, and of depression to be between 33 559 and 52 980 among BME older people from all groups combined (Shah, 2008a). This anticipated increase in psychiatric morbidity has enormous implications for the design, development and delivery of culturally capable, appropriate and sensitive Old Age Psychiatry Services (OAPSs) for BME elders.

Pathways into care

The pathway to reach secondary care OAPSs encompasses several sequential stages: the first appearance of an illness in the community; consultation with the GP; identification and management of the illness by the GP; referral to secondary care; and identification and management of the illness in secondary care (Goldberg and Huxley, 1991). Elders and their families from several different BME groups, including those from the African Caribbean, Asian, Chinese and Vietnamese groups, are well aware of services provided by GPs (Barker, 1984; Bhalia and Blakemore, 1981; McCallum, 1990). They also have high general practice consultation rates (Balarajan *et al.*, 1989; Donaldson, 1986; Gillam *et al.*, 1989; Lindesay *et al.*, 1997b; Livingston *et al.*, 2002). For example, 70% of Gujarati elders in Leicester had consulted their GP in the preceding month (Lindesay *et al.*, 1997b). However, the prevalence of BME elders in contact with OAPSs is generally low (Blakemore and Boneham, 1994; Jagger, 1998; Lindesay *et al.*, 1997b; Rait and Burns, 1997; Shah and Dighe-Deo, 1998); this has also been observed in other countries like Australia (Hassett and George, 2002).

Possible reasons for this discrepancy

Possible reasons for the discrepancy between high general practice consultation rates and low prevalence in OAPSs, despite the community prevalence of mental illness being similar or higher among BME elders, include the influence of factors related to patients and their families, general practice and secondary care (Shah *et al.*, 2005b). Each is examined in turn, although most potential explanations have not been rigorously examined in research studies.

Patient and family factors

Patients and family members may be unfamiliar with symptoms of mental illness (Adamson, 2001; Bowes and Wilkinson, 2003; Marwaha and Livingston, 2002; Purandare *et al.*, 2007; Wai Yin Chinese Women Society, 2007) as traditionally few BME elders reached old age (Manthorpe and Hettiaratchy, 1993; Rait and Burns, 1997). Consequently they may not recognise symptoms of mental illness and dismiss them as a function of old age (Shah *et al.*, 2005b). This may be further complicated by the requirement of functional impairment in the diagnostic criteria for dementia as there may be different thresholds for functional impairment in different cultures depending on the social roles and cognitive demands placed on the elderly (Pollit, 1996; Zhang *et al.*, 1990). These reasons may be further enhanced if the patient is unable to communicate symptoms of mental illness to family members and the GP because of either lack of appropriate vocabulary or fluency in English (George and Young, 1991; Thomas *et al.*, 2009; Thornton *et al.*, 2009; Shah, 1992b, 1997a, b, 1999; Wai Yin Chinese Women Society, 2007); also, for the same reasons, family members may not be able to communicate their concerns to the GP. Other factors related to patients and family members include: the belief that nothing can be done; lack of awareness of available services (Age Concern/Help the Aged Housing Trust, 1984; Barker, 1984; Bhalia and Blakemore, 1981; Lindesay *et al.*, 1997b; McCallum, 1990); lack of awareness of access procedures for available services (Lindesay *et al.*, 1997b); belief that available services are inadequate, inaccessible and culturally insensitive (Hopkins and Bahl, 1993; Lawrence *et al.*, 2006; Lindesay *et al.*, 1997b); previous poor experience of services (Bowes and Wilkinson, 2003; Lindesay *et al.*, 1997b); and fear of stigma attached to mental illness (Barker, 1984; Livingston *et al.*, 2002; Manthorpe and Hettiaratchy, 1993; Marwaha and Livingston, 2002; Wai Yin Chinese Women Society, 2007). Moreover, patients may choose to consult traditional healers rather than GPs for their mental illness (Bhatnagar, 1997).

General practice factors

High awareness of general practice services, high general practice registration rates (often with GPs from the same ethnic background) and high general practice consultation rates should theoretically enable easier diagnosis and access to OAPSs. Moreover, the statutory offer of an annual physical and mental state examination for those over 75 years (Secretaries of State for Health, Wales, Northern Ireland and Scotland, 1989) and the emphasis on single assessment process and shared care protocols for dementia and depression in the National Service Framework for Older People (Department of Health, 2001) should further facilitate this. However, relatively few BME elders receive the annual physical and mental state examination (Lindesay *et al.*, 1997b), and the number of BME elders over the age of 75 years is small.

Routine GP consultations may not identify mental illness in BME elders for several reasons (Shah *et al.*, 2005b). First, the prevalence of mental illness in those consulting the GP may be low; some possible reasons for this were discussed in the section on 'patient and family factors', above. Second, the severity of the mental illness in those consulting GPs may be lower. Third, symptoms of mental illness (including behavioural and psychological signs and symptoms of dementia, which often precipitates clinical presentation) may be less frequent, less severe or different in BME elders consulting GPs than in indigenous elders (Shah, 2007b). Fourth, data on the clinical presentation, diagnostic features and natural history for mental illness in BME elders are sparse (Haider and Shah, 2004; Patel, 2000; Patel *et al.*, 1998; Shah, 2007b), and individual GPs may see relatively few BME elders with mental illness. Therefore, GPs may lack the clinical experience and expertise and the diagnostic skills needed for BME elders – even psychiatrists experience this difficulty (Lindesay, 1998; Shah, 1999). Fifth, these difficulties may be exaggerated by language and communication difficulties (Patel, 2000), age and gender of the assessor, the context and setting of the assessment, and the attitudes and expectations of the patient and the family (Lindesay, 1998). Sixth, there is a paucity of screening and diagnostic instruments for mental illness in BME elders (Shah and Mackenzie, 2007). The existing screening instruments for mental illness in BME elders have generally been developed in the subject's language. As translated versions of instruments have questions in the subject's language, the clinician cannot directly administer the instrument unless he or she is fluent in the relevant language. Moreover, the clinician cannot solely rely on the interpreter to administer the instrument accurately because the clinician will not be able to ascertain the accuracy of this mode of administration. There are no instruments that the clinician can administer in English and, in turn, the interpreter can administer a predetermined and standardised set of translated questions to the patient. Seventh, bias and prejudice of clinicians can also complicate consultations (Solomon, 1992). Finally, well intentioned family members may withhold information if they feel that it will present the patient in a 'bad light' (Shah, 1997a, b, 1999).

If mental illness is identified by the GP it may or may not be treated. It may not be treated for several reasons, including the belief that nothing can be done, the belief that ethnically sensitive secondary care and social services are not available, previous experience of poor response to referrals made to secondary care and social services, and lack of awareness of procedures for accessing secondary care services (Shah et al., 2005b). If the mental illness presenting to the GP is less severe or, in the case of dementia, it lacks troublesome behavioural and psychological signs and symptoms of dementia, the GP may consider referral to secondary care unnecessary (Shah et al., 2005b). The GP may feel that he or she can communicate with the patient better, particularly if they have the same ethnic background as the patient; up to 70% of Asians in the UK are registered with Asian GPs (Johnson et al., 1983). Also, the GP may wish to refer the patient to secondary care but the patient or the family may be reluctant owing to some of the reasons discussed in the section on 'patient and family factors' above (Shah et al., 2005b).

Secondary care factors

There is a paucity of studies examining BME elders with mental illness in OAPSs, with only three published studies (Bhatkal and Shah, 2004; Odutoye and Shah, 1999; Redelinghuys and Shah, 1997). However, all the factors described in the section on 'general practice factors' above equally apply to secondary care (Shah et al., 2005b).

The gloomy situation may be changing

This gloomy situation of poor access to OAPSs by BME elders is changing in some UK services. In three cross-sectional evaluative studies of two OAPSs in west London, Indian subcontinent origin (Odutoye and Shah, 1999; Redlinghuys and Shah, 1997) and Polish (Bhatkal and Shah, 2004) elders received individual components of health and social services at the same frequency as indigenous elders, and their prevalence in the OAPSs was consistent with the local population demography, suggesting equity of access to the OAPSs. A population-based study of a mixed group of BME elders in Islington reported similar findings for the use of primary care, secondary care and social services resources, but OAPSs were not included (Livingston et al., 2002).

For Indian subcontinent origin elders, the equitable access to OAPSs was despite having more individuals in the household and a greater number of children than indigenous elders; the latter finding has also been observed in Australia (LoGiudice et al., 2001). This suggests that the traditional belief that BME elders are looked after by extended family and do not access services is changing and erroneous. Reasons for this may include: younger family members may have lived in the UK longer than the elders (Barker, 1984); younger family members may lead a culturally different lifestyle, and may have been assimilated into the indigenous culture and adopted cultural practices of the indigenous culture (Shah *et al.*, 2005b); younger family members may work long hours and be busy (Barker, 1984); elders may have migrated contrary to the wishes of younger family members or their own wishes (Silveira and Ebrahim, 1995); there may be family tensions (Boneham, 1989; Silveira and Ebrahim, 1995); and there may be financial hardship. These factors may make it difficult for the extended family to provide support and thereby encourage referrals to services (Redelinghuys and Shah, 1997).

Another reason for improved service access in these three studies may have been the design, development and delivery of OAPSs being culturally capable, appropriate and sensitive. This included the ethnicity of staff members (ranging from secretaries to psychiatrists) reflecting the ethnicity of the local population, employment of bilingual nurses on the wards and in the day hospitals, employment of an Indian community psychiatric nurse to cater specifically for patients of Indian subcontinent origin, and locating the two dementia day hospitals in the heart of the community close to population clusters of Indian subcontinent origin and Polish elders (Hoxey *et al.*, 1999). There are other examples of good practice reported by the Care Services Improvement Partnership's (CSIP) Older People's Mental Health Programme (www.olderpeoplementalhealth.csip. org.uk/mental-health-and-well-being-of-black-and-minority-ethnic-elders/showcase-event-presentations.html).

'Count Me In' census

The recently published findings from the 2008 'Count Me In' census of psychiatric inpatients specifically reported age-standardised admission rates for different BME groups over the age of 65 years (about 10 000) (Commission for Healthcare Audit and Inspection, 2008). The standardised admission ratio, with the total elderly population of England and Wales as the standard population, for those aged 65 years and older in different ethnic groups was: higher in the white Irish, other white, white and black Caribbean, other Asian, black Caribbean, black African and other black groups; lower in the white British and Chinese groups; and there was no difference with the standard population in the white and black African, white and Asian, Indian, Pakistani and Bangladeshi groups. However, there are concerns about this national census. The 'Count Me In' census was undertaken on a single day and, as such, does not measure admission rates; it measures bed occupancy (in other words, it records those patients who were occupying inpatient beds on the specified census day). While the census report refers to admission rates and standardised admission ratios, they are actually referring to bed occupancy rates and standardised bed occupancy ratios. This is because data on all inpatients (and not admissions) were collected on a specified census day. Bed occupancy is a function of the number of admission rates *and* length of stay in hospital after the admission *and* available beds; bed occupancy will be higher if the admission rates are higher and/or the length of stay is longer and/or there are too few beds and the levels of demand push occupancy levels up. Reduced availability of beds may either lead to increased bed occupancy rates if beds belonging to patients on 'leave' are used for admissions or the need for a bed may not be registered if the patient is not admitted owing to lack of available beds.

Several factors may influence admission rates among BME elders. First, the prevalence of mental illness may be higher among BME elders than in the indigenous population. The prevalence of dementia was higher in black Caribbean and black African elders in Liverpool, particularly so in those lacking fluency in English (McCracken *et al.*, 1997), and the prevalence of depression was very high among those born in Cyprus (Livingston *et al.*, 2002), and this may in part account for higher admission rates in these groups. Second, the severity of the mental illness and/or the resultant disability may be greater in BME groups. Mini-mental state examination scores were lower among a community sample of African Caribbean elders compared to the general population (Stewart *et al.*, 2002), suggesting greater cognitive impairment. A small community study, with a high refusal rate, reported that African Caribbean elders, compared to indigenous elders, were more likely to have functional impairment (Richards *et al.*, 1998). Convenience samples have reported higher depression scores in elderly Somalis (Silveira and Ebrahim, 1995). Collectively, these observations may, in part, explain higher admission rates in the black Caribbean and black African groups. Third, the potential risks as a consequence of mental illness may be higher in some elderly BME groups, although there are no data supporting this. Fourth, service components designed to enable patients to remain at home may not be culturally appropriate or sensitive and may lead to admission by default. Fifth, many BME elders do not speak English and a significant number are illiterate in their mother tongue. This will result in diagnostic difficulties (Shah, 2007b) and may lead to higher admission rates for assessment, but if this were true then it should apply equally to all BME groups that lack fluency in English. Finally, there is an absence of matching vocabulary for psychiatric symptoms in some languages spoken by BME elders (Shah, 2007b; Shah and Mackenzie, 2007), and this too may lead to diagnostic difficulties, resulting in admission for assessment.

Following admission, several factors may influence length of stay in hospital. First, assessment may be prolonged if the inpatient clinical team has difficulty in communicating with the patient because of language barriers (Shah, 2007b). Second, the well recognised difficulties in securing professional interpreters may further contribute to delays in completing the assessment and formulation of a treatment plan. Third, there is an absence of matching vocabulary for psychiatric symptoms in some languages spoken by BME elders (Shah, 2007b), and this too may lead to diagnostic difficulties resulting in longer length of admission. Fourth, lack of culturally appropriate and sensitive ward environment, meals and therapeutic activities may also lead to delays in recovery. Fifth, paucity of culturally appropriate and sensitive community services (e.g. day centres) may further prolong length of stay despite the patient being clinically fit for discharge. Finally, it is possible that elders from some BME groups may genuinely respond more slowly to treatment; however, because of a paucity of intervention studies in BME groups and their general exclusion from intervention studies of indigenous elderly populations (Shah *et al.*, 2008), data supporting or refuting this point are absent.

The 'standardised bed occupancy ratio' measured in the census needs to be interpreted cautiously as it may be an artefact of increased length of stay rather than a genuine increase in uptake of inpatient services, and it only represents one component of a comprehensive OAPS. The vast majority of patients are cared for in the community.

Policy context

Over the past decade, the mental health of BME groups has become a national priority in the UK. This has resulted in the publication of a number of detailed governmental reports, guidelines and policies. These can broadly be divided into publications relating to BME mental health in general and those relating to elderly mental health with specific mention of BME groups. The most influential documents have been published directly by the Department of Health or related public bodies, including the National Institute for Mental Health in England (NIMHE), National Institute for Health and Clinical Excellence (NICE), the Healthcare Commission and the Care Services Improvement Partnership (CSIP). Similar policies are being developed in other countries (Shah, 2008b).

The National Service Framework (NSF) for Mental Health (Department of Health, 1999), primarily covering working age adults (16–65 years), was one of the first governmental policy documents to acknowledge ethnic inequalities in mental health service provision. The NSF for Older People (Department of Health, 2001) set standards for the health and social care of older people. This document recognised that 'older people from BME communities need accessible and appropriate mental health services', that assessments may be 'culturally biased', that assumptions are sometimes made about the willingness of families to act as primary carers for their older relatives, and that information about services may not be readily available in an accessible form and tends to rely on translated leaflets and posters. This document emphasised that mental health services should 'take account of the social and cultural factors affecting recovery and support', but made few specific suggestions as to how cultural awareness might be improved among mental health and social care professionals.

Forget Me Not, the Audit Commission's analysis of mental health services for older people in England and Wales (Audit Commission, 2000, 2002), challenged the commonly held erroneous assumption that BME families 'look after their own' and have less need for services. It recognised that services 'may be insensitive to cultural norms and may threaten the carer's well-being if they do not reinforce the carer's role in an appropriate manner.' Despite the extensive recommendations in this report, there was little addressing these issues other than suggesting that information for users and carers is distributed 'in languages and formats that can be understood easily by local people'.

Everybody's Business (Department of Health, 2005a), a service development guide, aimed to build on the service models outlined in the NSF for Older People. Although this guide highlighted the needs of a number of special groups, including those with early onset dementia, learning disabilities and older prisoners, there was no specific reference to BME elders other than mentioning that religious and cultural needs should be taken into account when providing service.

The *Inside Outside* report (National Institute of Mental Health England, 2003) recognised the ethnic mental health inequalities both *inside* and *outside* of services, and that they had not been adequately addressed by existing mental health initiatives such as the NSF for Mental Health and the NSF for Older People. This report outlined key components to eliminate mental health inequalities: ensuring accountability and ownership in relation to BME communities; developing a culturally capable service; setting national standards to improve access, care experience and outcome; and enhancing the cultural relevance of research and development.

Delivering Race Equality in Mental Health Care is a 5-year action plan for achieving racial equality and tackling discrimination in mental health services in England (Department of Health, 2005b). It recommends three building blocks: more appropriate and responsive services – specifically mentioning the improvement of clinical services for groups, including older people, asylum seekers and children; community engagement – aiming to engage communities in planning services; better information – improved monitoring of ethnicity, better dissemination of information and good practice, and a new regular census of mental health patients. The document acknowledged that older people from BME communities face the double jeopardy of old age and ethnic minority status, that they can be marginalised in society and have specific needs. Potential difficulties around communication and particularly written language were highlighted, as was the need for services to provide adequate interpretation facilities.

One of the key principles of care outlined in the NICE clinical guidance on dementia related to diversity (sex, ethnicity, age or religion), with a strong emphasis on 'person centred care' (NICE, 2006). Although there was no mention of specific BME groups, this guidance advocated that the needs and preferences of dementia sufferers relating to diversity must be identified and, where possible, accommodated. There was also recognition of language as a possible barrier to care, with recommendations that interpreters are readily available and that written information is provided in the preferred language and/or an accessible format. The NICE technical appraisal on drugs in the cholinesterase inhibitor category used in the treatment of dementia (NICE, 2007) was found to be unlawful because it breached the Race Discrimination Act. It discriminated against people from different ethnic backgrounds, particularly those whose first language was not English, because it relied heavily on an assessment tool developed in English.

The recently published National Dementia Strategy for England also recognises the importance of ethnicity, culture and religion in the systematic development of services for dementia.

There is clear recognition in these policy documents that BME elders face particular challenges and are especially vulnerable to exclusion, marginalisation and inequality in mental health promotion and mental health service access. Greater understanding of the meanings of mental wellbeing and mental ill-health given by BME elders, their help-seeking preferences and their perceptions of reasons for poor access to mental health services may better enable implementation of these policies and inform development of future policies.

Promotion of access to services: a way forward

What can be done to improve access to OAPSs for BME groups? What can be done to promote the design, development and delivery of culturally capable, appropriate and sensitive OAPSs for this group? How can this be achieved? Several strategies are described below.

Identification of factors which promote service delivery and access

Identification and dissemination of examples of good practice is strongly advocated by governmental initiatives, including the *Delivering Race Equality in Mental Health Care: An Action Plan* (Department of Health, 2005b). There is an urgent need to identify examples of good practice, including OAPSs providing equitable access to BME elders in comparison with indigenous elders. Theoretically, this should be possible as all health and social service providers are now required routinely to collect data on ethnicity of service users (Department of Health, 2005b). In turn, there is an urgent need to examine differences between OAPSs with and without equitable access by BME elders critically, and to identify examples of good practice, less good practice, service gaps and factors that promote equitable access.

Identified examples of good practice pertaining to the whole service and individual components of the service, in turn, need to be widely and rapidly disseminated to policy-makers, service commissioners and service providers in primary and secondary healthcare services and social services. The Department of Health and the NIMHE are ideally placed to achieve this. OAPSs with evidence of less good practice and gaps in service provision and their service commissioners need to consider implementation urgently, albeit with local modification, of the identified models of good practice.

Routinely collected data on ethnicity by local authority and primary and secondary healthcare services (Department of Health, 2005b) and data from the annual national census of psychiatric inpatients (Commission for Healthcare Audit and Inspection, 2008) should also be utilised on an ongoing basis to examine the equity of access to OAPSs by BME elders, discriminatory practices, and the cultural capability, appropriateness and sensitivity of OAPSs. This, in turn, should also guide further improvements to existing services and new service developments.

Service developments

OAPSs for BME elders should be developed in accordance with the NSF for Older People (Department of Health, 2001) and the National Dementia Strategy (Department of Health, 2009). BME elders should have access to all the individual components of the service that are available to indigenous elders. Services for BME elders should be integrated with the existing ethnocentric services because segregated services will lead to marginalisation, fragmentation and inability to compete for scarce funding. Services should be available, accessible, acceptable, culturally capable, appropriate and sensitive, and flexible.

Policy-makers, commissioners and OAPS providers and local authorities should be aware of and maintain a high vigilance pertaining to the demographic changes in the different BME elderly populations, and they should also unequivocally acknowledge the consequent increase in psychiatric morbidity. They should, in collaboration with local elderly BME users and their carers, local voluntary sector groups representing them and the wider BME community, identify the needs of BME elders with mental illness. Such collaborations should also focus on the commissioning, design, development and delivery of culturally capable, appropriate and sensitive OAPSs. Effective models of community engagement that can help achieve these ambitions have been described (Department of Health, 2005b). This can be facilitated further by ensuring that BME elders are adequately represented in the annual patient satisfaction surveys conducted by the Healthcare Commission.

Staff training

Clinicians and managers working in mental health services should receive regular and rigorous formal training in cultural capability, awareness, appropriateness and sensitivity to improve their knowledge, skills and attitudes (Department of Health, 2005b). Moreover, clinicians and managers should receive training in and be familiar with local policies on racial harassment and racial discrimination, and have good working knowledge of legislation relevant to racial discrimination (Centre for Ethnicity & Health, University of Central Lancashire [CEHUCLAN] *et al.*, 2003; Department of Health, 2005b). Furthermore, clinicians and managers should receive training in the ascertainment, recording and monitoring of ethnicity, and the importance of using data on ethnicity to identify discriminatory practices, needs and new service developments (CEHUCLAN *et al.*, 2003; Commission for Healthcare Audit and Inspection, 2008). Also, clinicians and managers should make an effort to become familiar with relevant cultural aspects pertaining to the commoner BME groups in the local area; this can be achieved by establishing good links with local voluntary sector ethnic minority groups and religious leaders (Department of Health, 2005b).

Methods of assessment and communication

The conventional clinical principles of history-taking, mental state examination, physical examination and special investigations should be meticulously followed. Furthermore, a careful and detailed collateral history from other informants like relatives should supplement these assessments (Lindesay, 1998). Some basic rules facilitating an accurate assessment include correction of sensory deficits, explanation of the nature, purpose and duration of the assessment, use of explicit, clear and simple instructions, use of a calm, reassuring and patient approach, and reassurance of confidentiality (Lindesay, 1998).

Assessment is contingent upon good communication between the clinician, the patient and the carer (Jones and Gill, 1998; Shah, 1999), particularly because many BME elders do not speak English (Barker, 1984; Lindesay et al., 1997b; Manthorpe and Hettiaratchy, 1993). Ideally, clinicians assessing BME elders should belong to the same ethnic group or be able to speak the patient's language, but this is often not possible. Bilingual health workers have been used to achieve this (Hoxey et al., 1999), but they are uncommon (Phelan and Parkman, 1995). Therefore, interpretation services are usually required (Phelan and Parkman, 1995; Shah, 1997a, b) and these should always be used at key events, including assessments, reviews, case conferences and discussion with carers (CEHUCLAN et al., 2003). Relatives, non-clinical staff, clinical staff and professional interpreters (with and without special training in mental health) have been used (Phelan and Parkman, 1995; Shah, 1997a, b). However, other than in an emergency, professional interpreters should ideally be used (CEHUCLAN et al., 2003), and this will help to reduce bias and protect confidentiality. Service providers should ensure that interpretation services should be readily available (CEHUCLAN et al., 2003; Department of Health, 2005b).

Clinicians using interpretation services should receive formal training in the use of those services (CEHUCLAN et al., 2003). Professional interpreters, including bilingual workers, should receive formal training in interpretation on mental health issues (CEHUCLAN et al., 2003). Patients and carers should be made aware of the nature and purpose of using the interpreter. The interpreter should be briefed on the nature and purpose of the interview and the types of questions that will be asked. Careful consideration should be given to the gender, the precise dialect and ethnicity of the interpreter (CEHUCLAN et al., 2003). The gender of the interpreter may be important in some ethnic minority groups, like elderly Gujarati women, to establish rapport and facilitate ascertainment of accurate and complete history. This is important as the sex ratio declines with increasing age in most ethnic minority groups. Different dialects of the same language may be spoken (e.g. dialects differ for Greek subjects from mainland Greece and Cyprus), and the interpreter should speak the correct dialect. The ethnicity of the interpreter may also be important in this context. For example, Afghani interpreters may speak both Farsi and Pashto, but there may be difficulties if the precise ethnicity of the interpreter is not matched with that of the patient within the Afghani group. It may be worthwhile conducting a literature search to ascertain information on clinical features and clinical presentation when the clinician is unfamiliar with the culture.

Audiotapes, videos, CDs and diagrammatic representations with figures giving information on management and service-related issues can complement the use of interpretation services and may be particularly helpful for illiterate patients and carers (Lindesay et al., 1997b). Educational videos on dementia have been developed internationally by Alzheimer's Disease International, nationally by the Policy Research Institute into Ageing and Ethnicity and Alzheimers Society, and locally by Alzheimer's Concern Ealing. Additionally, translated versions of all information leaflets should be made available for patients and carers who can read their mother tongue.

For everyday communication on inpatient units, day hospitals, day centres and residential and nursing homes it may not be practical to have an interpreter present, and bilingual workers are uncommon. Therefore, there is an urgent need to develop a manual of translated versions of commonly used key phrases (e.g. 'please come and have breakfast', 'please come and have your medication', 'would you like to go for a walk') together with a paraphrased version in English. Either the patients can read the staff's request or, where patients cannot read their own language, staff can read the paraphrased version to the patient.

Development of screening and diagnostic instruments

There is a paucity of both screening and diagnostic instruments for dementia, depression and other mental disorders for use in BME elders.

The mini-mental state examination (MMSE) (Folstein *et al.*, 1975) has been developed in the UK in Gujarati, Bengali, Punjabi, Hindi and Urdu (Lindesay *et al.*, 1997a; Rait *et al.*, 2000a, b). The abbreviated mental test score (Quereshi and Hodkinson, 1974) has been developed in several Asian languages for use among Gujarati and Pakistani elders and in English for use among African Caribbean elders in the UK (Rait *et al.*, 1997, 2000a, b). The MMSE, selected items from the Consortium to Establish a Registry for Alzheimer's Disease (CERAD) neuropsychological test battery (Morris *et al.*, 1989) and the CAMCOG component of the CAMDEX interview (Roth *et al.*, 1986) have been evaluated in African Caribbean elders in the UK (Richards and Brayne, 1996; Richards *et al.*, 2000). Orientation items of the MMSE, selected items of the CERAD battery and the clock drawing test have been evaluated in African Caribbean elders in the UK and normative data is available (Stewart *et al.*, 2001).

The 15-item geriatric depression scale (GDS-15) (Sheikh and Yesavage, 1986) has been evaluated for use among African Caribbean elders in the UK (Abas *et al.*, 1996, 1998; Rait *et al.*, 1999). Three depression screening instruments, including the GDS-15, brief assessment schedule cards (Adshead *et al.*, 1992) and Caribbean culture specific screen (CCSS) (Abas *et al.*, 1998), have been successfully evaluated against a 'gold standard' diagnosis of depression on the geriatric mental state examination (GMS) (Copeland *et al.*, 1987) in African Caribbean elders in the UK (Rait *et al.*, 1999). All three instruments showed satisfactory sensitivity and specificity in detecting depression in older Jamaicans, with little difference between the three scales. In general, lower cut-off scores have been suggested on some scales, such as the GDS for African Caribbean elders in the UK (Abas *et al.*, 1998). The CCSS was developed a priori by ascertaining terminology used to describe emotional distress (Abas *et al.*, 1996) because African Caribbean elders rarely use the terms 'sad' or 'unhappy' to describe emotional distress, but rather they use other terms, including 'being low spirited', 'fed up' and 'weighed down' (Abas, 1996; Abas *et al.*, 1996, 1998).

The symptoms of anxiety and depression scale (Bedford *et al.*, 1976) was used as a diagnostic instrument for depression in Gujarati, Somali and Bengali elders in London (Ebrahim *et al.*, 1991; Silveira and Ebrahim, 1995), but data on its psychometric properties are not available. The short care interview (Gurland *et al.*, 1984) was used as a diagnostic instrument for depression and dementia in elders born in Cyprus, Africa and the Caribbean living in Islington (Livingstone *et al.*, 2002), but data on its psychometric properties in these groups are not available. The GMS was used to diagnose mental illness in Hindi among Indian subcontinent origin elders in Bradford (Bhatnagar and Frank, 1997), but data on its psychometric properties are not available. However, the concordance between the GMS and clinical diagnosis was high (Bhatnagar and Frank, 1997).

All existing screening and diagnostic instruments for mental illness for ethnic minority elders have generally been developed in the subject's language. As translated versions of instruments have questions in the subject's language, the clinician cannot directly administer the instrument unless he or she is fluent in the relevant language. Moreover, the clinician cannot solely rely on the interpreter to administer the instrument accurately because the clinician will not be able to ascertain the accuracy of this mode of administration. There are no instruments that the clinician can administer in English and, in turn, the interpreter can administer a predetermined and standardised set of translated questions to the patient. There is an urgent need to develop instruments that can be used in this manner in day-to-day clinical practice. Furthermore, development of self-rated screening instruments, like the geriatric depression scale, is problematic in subjects who are unable to read their mother tongue; for this group there is a need to develop interviewer-administered instruments.

Research

It is important not to assume that findings from epidemiological studies from the country of origin of ethnic minority elders are applicable in the UK context because the process of migration, fluency in English, the degree of assimilation and acculturation into the host culture and other environmental changes are likely to influence the findings in the UK. Most published studies from many countries appear not to include ethnic minority groups in their investigation (Shah *et al.*, 2008).

There are only a few population-based prevalence studies of mental illness among the elderly from BME groups and there are no incidence studies. There is also a paucity of studies examining the severity of mental illnesses and the resultant disability, risk factors, natural history of mental illnesses, clinical features and clinical presentation of mental illnesses and issues related to carers. Behavioural and psychological symptoms of dementia, which often lead to clinical presentations, have been poorly studied among ethnic minority elders (Shah and Mukherjee, 2000), although studies are emerging (Haider and Shah, 2004).

Therefore, there is a clear need for more population-based epidemiological studies of prevalence and incidence in different BME groups. These studies should also be designed to examine the severity of mental illnesses and resultant disability, risk factors, natural history of mental illnesses, clinical features and clinical presentation of mental illnesses and issues related to carers, including stress and strain. There is also an urgent need to identify the barriers in the pathway to secondary care pertaining to patients and their families, primary care and secondary care, using Goldberg and Huxley's (1991) model of pathways into care. Identification of these barriers will allow development of intervention strategies to reduce the barriers and these, in turn, should be formally evaluated.

In general, population-based epidemiological studies and studies evaluating the efficacy of interventions for mental illnesses exclude BME elderly groups. Therefore, findings from these studies may not always be applicable to BME elderly groups. It has been recommended that such studies should not exclude subjects on the grounds of ethnicity (Department of Health, 2005b).

Public education campaigns

There is an urgent need for public education campaigns at a local, regional and national level targeting the following areas: the importance of early recognition of symptoms of mental illness in old age; the importance of seeking help early to improve outcome; the availability of effective treatments; improving awareness of available services; strategies to reduce stigma; and the improved treatment of risk factors for some mental disorders, including hypertension (Balarajan, 1996; Ritch *et al.*, 1996), cardiovascular disease (Balarajan, 1996; Ritch *et al.*, 1996) and diabetes (Mather and Keen, 1985; Samanta *et al.*, 1987), which are common in some BME groups and may help in the primary prevention of vascular dementia. These campaigns should be directed at BME individuals of all age groups (including service users and their carers), voluntary sector organisations (including those for ethnic minority groups), traditional healers, clinicians and managers in primary and secondary healthcare and social services, service commissioners and policy-makers.

At a local level such campaigns should be collaborations between primary and secondary care, social services and local authorities, voluntary sector organisations (including those for BME groups), and service users and their carers from BME groups. At a national level such campaigns should be collaborations between key stakeholders, including the Royal College of Psychiatrists, the Royal College of General Practitioners, the British Geriatric Society, the Mental Health Act Commission, the Department of Health and voluntary sector organisations, including the Alzheimers Society and Age Concern. Such multifaceted collaborative efforts have been successful in other public education campaigns for mental health, including the Defeat Depression Campaign from the Royal College of Psychiatrists and the Royal College of General Practitioners. NIMHE is also coordinating a 5-year action plan to tackle stigma and discrimination in mental health (Department of Health, 2005b).

Conclusions

The increase in the BME elderly population, coupled with the prevalence of dementia and depression in this group being similar or higher than in indigenous elders, suggests that the absolute number of cases of both dementia and depression will significantly increase among BME groups. However, despite high general practice consultation rates, ethnic minority elders are poorly represented in OAPSs. This observation may be explained by barriers to the pathways into care related to patients and their families, general practice and secondary care factors. Therefore, a multifaceted approach, as described in the preceding section, is needed to ensure that commissioning, design, development and delivery of culturally capable, appropriate and sensitive services actually occurs to improve access to OAPSs by BME elders. Otherwise this vulnerable group will continue to harbour hidden and untreated psychiatric morbidity.

References

Abas, M. (1996). Depression and anxiety among older Caribbean people in the UK: screening, unmet need and the provision of appropriate services. *International Journal of Geriatric Psychiatry*, **11**, 377–82.

Abas, M., Phillips, C., Richards, M., Carter, J., Levy, R. (1996). Initial development of a new culture-specific screen for emotional distress in older Caribbean people. *International Journal of Geriatric Psychiatry*, **11**, 1097–103.

Abas, M., Phillips, C., Carter, J., Walker, S., Banerjee, S., Levy, R. (1998). Culturally sensitive validation of instruments in older African-Caribbean people living in South London. *British Journal of Psychiatry*, **17**, 249–54.

Adamson, J. (2001). Awareness and understanding of dementia in African/ Caribbean and south Asian families. *Health and Social Care in the Community*, **9**, 391–6.

Adityanjee, D. R. (1986). Suicide attempts and suicide in India: cross-cultural aspects. *International Journal of Social Psychiatry*, **32**, 64–73.

Adshead, G., Cody, D., Pitt, B. (1992). BASDEC: a novel screening instrument for depression in elderly medical inpatients. *British Medical Journal*, **305**, 397.

Age Concern/Help the Aged Housing Trust (1984). *Housing for Ethnic Elders*. London: Age Concern.

Audit Commission (2000). *Forget-Me-Not , Mental Health Services for Older People*. London: Audit Commission.

Audit Commission (2002). *Forget-Me-Not*. London: Audit Commission.

Balarajan, R. (1996). Ethnicity and variation in mortality from cardiovascular disease. *British Medical Journal*, **299**, 958–60.

Balarajan, R., Yuen, P., Raleigh, V. S. (1989). Ethnic differences in general practice consultation rates. *British Medical Journal*, **299**, 958–60.

Barker, J. (1984). *Research Perspectives on Ageing: Black and Asian Old People in Britain*, 1st edn. London: Age Concern Research Unit.

Bedford, A., Foulds, G. A., Sheffield, B. F. (1976). A new personal disturbance scale. *British Journal of Social and Clinical Psychology*, **15**, 387–94.

Bhalia, A., Blakemore, K. (1981). *Elders of the Minority Ethnic Groups*. Birmingham: AFFOR.

Bhatia, S. C., Kahn, M. H., Medirrata, R. P. (1987). High risk suicide factors across cultures. *International Journal of Social Psychiatry*, **33**, 226–36.

Bhatkal, S., Shah, A. K. (2004). Clinical and demographic characteristics of elderly Poles referred to a psychogeriatric service. *International Psychogeriatrics*, 2004, **16**, 351–60.

Bhatnagar, K. S. (1997). Depression in South Asian elders. *Geriatric Medicine*, February, 55–6.

Bhatnagar, K. S., Frank, J. (1997). Psychiatric disorders in elderly from the Indian subcontinent living in Bradford. *International Journal of Geriatric Psychiatry*, **12**, 907–12.

Blakemore, K., Boneham, M. (1994). *Age, Race, and Ethnicity: a Comparative Approach*. Buckingham: Open University Press.

Bohning, W., Oishi, N. (1995). Is international migration spreading? *Migration Review*, **29**, 3.

Boneham, M. (1989). Ageing and ethnicity in Britain: the case of elderly Sikh women in a Midlands town. *New Community*, **15**, 447–59.

Bowes, A., Wilkinson, H. (2003). 'We didn't know it would get so bad': South Asian experiences of dementia and service response. *Health and Social Care in the Community*, **11**, 387–96.

Burvill, P. (1995). Suicide in the multiethnic population of Australia, 1979–1990. *International Psychogeriatrics*, 7, 319–33.

Burvill, P. (1998). Migrant suicide rates in Australia and in the country of birth. *Psychological Medicine*, **28**, 201–8.

Burvill, P., Woodings, T. L., Stenhouse, N. S., McCall, N. S. (1982). Suicide during 1961–1970 of migrants in Australia. *Psychological Medicine*, **12**, 295–308.

Cattell, H. R. (1988). Elderly suicides in London: an analysis of coroner's inquest. *International Journal of Geriatric Psychiatry*, **3**, 251–61.

Cattell, H. R., Jolley, D. (1995). One hundred cases of suicide in elderly people. *British Journal of Psychiatry*, **166**, 451–7.

CEHUCLAN (Centre for Ethnicity & Health, University of Central Lancashire), Mental Health Act Commission and NIMHE (2003). *Engaging and Changing: Developing Effective Policy for Care and Treatment of Black and Minority Ethnic Detained Patients*. www.kc.nimhe.org.uk/index.cfm?fuseactionItem.viewResources.intItemID=12939

Commission for Healthcare Audit and Inspection (2008). *Count Me In 2008*. Results of the 2008 national census of inpatients in mental health and learning disability services in England and Wales. London: Commission for Healthcare Audit and Inspection.

Copeland, J. R. M., Kelleher, M. J., Kellett, J. M. et al. (1976). A semi-structured interview for the assessment of diagnosis and mental state in the elderly. The Geriatric Mental State Schedule. 1. Development and reliability. *Psychological Medicine*, **6**, 439–49.

Dennis, M. S., Shah, A. K., Lindesay, J. (2009). Methods of elderly suicides in England and Wales by country of birth groupings. *International Journal of Geriatric Psychiatry*, **24**(11), 1311–13.

Department of Health. National Service Framework for Mental Health (1999). *National Service Frameworks*. London: Department of Health.

Department of Health. National Service Framework for Older people (2001). *National Service Frameworks*. London: Department of Health.

Department of Health. Everybody's Business (2005a). *Integrated Mental Health Services for Older Adults: A Service Development Guide*. London: Department of Health.

Department of Health. Delivering Race Equality in Mental Health Care. (2005b). *An Action Plan for Reform Inside and Outside Services and the Government's Response to the Independent Inquiry into the* Death of David Bennett. www.dh.gov.UK/assetroot/04/10/07/75/04100775.pdf

Department of Health (2009). *Living Well With Dementia: A National Dementia Strategy*. http://www.dh.gov.uk/en/Publicationsandstatistics/Publications/PublicationsPolicyAndGuidance/DH_094058

Donaldson, L. J. (1986). Health and social status of elderly Asians. A community survey. *British Medical Journal*, **293**, 1079–82.

Ebrahim, S., Patel, N., Coats, M. *et al.* (1991). Prevalence and severity of morbidity among Gujarati Asian elders: a controlled comparison. *Family Practice*, **8**, 57–62.

Folstein, M. F., Folstein, S. E., McHugh, P. R. (1975). 'Mini Mental State': a practical method for grading the cognitive state of patients for the clinician. *Journal of Psychiatric Research*, **12**, 189–98.

George, J., Young, J. (1991). *The Physician In Multicultural Health Care and Rehabilitation of Older People*. In A. J. Squires (ed.) London: Edward Arnold.

Gillam, S., Jarman, B., White, P. *et al.* (1989). Ethnic differences in consultation rates in urban general practice. *British Medical Journal*, **299**, 953–8.

Goldberg, D., Huxley, P. (1991). *Common Mental Disorders: A Biosocial Model*. London & New York: Tavistock & Routledge.

Gunnell, D., Middleston, N., Whitley, E., Dorling, D., Frankel, S. (2003). Why are suicide rates rising in young men but falling in the elderly? – a time–series analysis of trends in England and Wales 1950–1998. *Social Science and Medicine*, **57**, 595–611.

Gurland, B., Golden, R., Teresi, J. A. *et al.* (1984). The short-care. An efficient instrument for the assessment of depression and dementia. *Journal of Gerontology*, **39**, 166–9.

Haider, I., Shah, A. (2004). A pilot study of behavioural and psychological signs of dementia in patients of Indian sub-continent origin admitted to a dementia day hospital in the United Kingdom. *International Journal of Geriatric Psychiatry*, **19**(12), 1195–204.

Harwood, D. M. J., Hawton, K., Hope, T., Jacoby, R. (2000). Suicide in older people: mode of death, demographic factors, and medical contact before death. *International Journal of Geriatric Psychiatry*, **15**, 736–43.

Harwood, D., Hawton, K., Hope, T., Jacoby, R. (2001). Psychiatric disorder and personality factors associated with suicide in older people: a descriptive and case-control study. *International Journal of Geriatric Psychiatry*, **16**, 155–65.

Hassett, A. George, K. (2002). Access to a community old age psychiatry service by elderly from non-English speaking background. *International Journal of Geriatric Psychiatry*, **17**, 623–8.

Hofman, A., Rocca, W. A., Brayne, C. *et al.* (1991). The prevalence of dementia in Europe: a collaborative study of 1980–1990 findings. *International Journal of Epidemiology*, **20**, 736–48.

Hopkins, A., Bahl, V. (1993). *Access to Care for People from Black and Ethnic Minorities*. London: Royal College of Physicians.

Hoxey, K., Mukherjee, S., Shah, A. K. (1999). Psychiatric services for ethnic elders. *CPD Bulletin: Old Age Psychiatry*, **1**, 44–6.

Hunt, I. M., Robinson, J., Bickley, H. *et al.* (2003). Suicides in ethnic minority within 12 months of contact with mental health services. *British Journal of Psychiatry*, **183**, 155–60.

Jagger, C. (1998). Asian elders. An under studied and growing population. *Old Age Psychiatrist*, March (**10**), 8.

Johansson, L. M., Sundquist, J., Johansson, S. E. *et al.* (1997). Suicide among foreign-born minorities and native Swedes: an epidemiological follow-up study of a defined population. *Social Science and Medicine*, **44**, 181–7.

Johnson, M. R. D., Cross, M., Cardew, S. (1983). Inner city residents, ethnic minorities and primary health care. *Postgraduate Medical Journal*, **59**, 664–7.

Jones, D., Gill, P. (1998). Breaking down language barriers. The NHS needs to provide accessible interpreting services for all. *British Medical Journal*, **316**, 1476.

Jorm, A. F., Korten, A. E., Henderson, A. S. (1987). The prevalence of dementia: a quantitative integration of the literature. *Acta Scandinavica Psychiatrica*, **76**, 465–79.

Kings College London and London School of Economics (2007). *Dementia UK. The Full Report*. www.alzheimers.org.uk/ News_and_Campaigns/Campaigning/ PDF/Dementia_UK_Full_Report.pdf

Kleiwer, E. V. (1991). Immigrant suicide in Australia, Canada, England and Wales, and the United States. *Journal of the Australian Population Association*, **8**, 111–28.

Kleiwer, E. V, Ward, R. H. (1988). Convergence of immigrant suicide rates to those in the destination country. *American Journal of Epidemiology*, **127**, 640–53.

Lawrence, V., Banerjee, S., Bhugra, D. *et al.* (2006). Coping with depression in later life: a qualitative study of help-seeking in three ethnic groups. *Psychological Medicine*, **36**, 1375–83.

Lindesay, J. (1998). The diagnosis of mental illness in elderly people from ethnic minorities. *Advances in Psychiatric Treatment*, **4**, 219–26.

Lindesay, J., Jagger, C., Mlynik-Szmid, A. *et al.* (1997a). The mini-mental state examination (MMSE) in an elderly immigrant Gujarati population in the United Kingdom. *International Journal of Geriatric Psychiatry*, **12**, 1155–67.

Lindesay, J., Jagger, C., Hibbert, M. J. *et al.* (1997b). Knowledge, uptake and availability of health and social services among Asian Gujarati and white elders. *Ethnicity & Health*, **2**, 59–69.

Liu, H., Wang, H., Yang, M. (2006). Factors associated with an unusual increase in elderly suicide rate in Taiwan. *International Journal of Geriatric Psychiatry*, **21**, 1219–21.

Livingston, G., Leavey, G., Kitchen, G. *et al.* (2001). Mental health of migrant elders – the Islington study. *British Journal of Psychiatry*, **179**, 361–6.

Livingston, G., Leavey, G., Kitchen, G. *et al.* (2002). Accessibility of health and social services to immigrant elders: the Islington study. *British Journal of Psychiatry*, **180**, 369–74.

LoGiudice, D., Hassett, A., Cook, R., Flicker, L., Ames, D. (2001). Equity of access to a memory clinic in Melbourne? Non-English speaking background attenders are more severely demented and have increased rates of dementia. *International Journal of Geriatric Psychiatry*, **16**, 327–34.

Manthorpe, J., Hettiaratchy, P. (1993). Ethnic minority elders in Britain. *International Review of Psychiatry*, **5**, 173–80.

Markson, E. W. (2003). *Social Gerontology Today. An Introduction*. Los Angeles: Roxbury Publishing.

Marwaha, S., Livingston, G. (2002). Stigma, racism or choice. Why do depressed ethnic elders avoid psychiatrists. *Journal of Affective Disorders*, **72**, 257–65.

Mather, H., Keen, M. (1985). The Southall diabetes survey: prevalence of known diabetes in Asians and Europeans. *British Medical Journal*, **291**, 1081–4.

McCallum, J. A. (1990). *The Forgotten People: Carers in Three Minority Communities in Southwark*. London: Kings Fund Centre.

McCracken, C. F. M., Boneham, M. A., Copeland, J. R. M. et al. (1997). Prevalence of dementia and depression among elderly people in black and ethnic groups. British Journal of Psychiatry, 171, 269–73.

McKenzie, K., Bhui, K., Nanchahal, K., Blizard, B. (2008). Suicide rates in people of South Asian origin in England and Wales: 1993–2003. British Journal of Psychiatry, 193, 406–9.

Modan, B., Nissenkorn, I., Lewkowski, S. R. (1970). Comparative epidemiological aspects of suicide and attempted suicide in Israel. American Journal of Epidemiology, 91, 393–9.

Morris, J., Heyman, A., Mohs, R. et al. (1989). The consortium to establish a registry for Alzheimer's disease (CERAD). Part 1. Clinical and neuropsychological assessment of Alzheimer's disease. Neurology, 39, 1159–65.

Mui, A. C., Kang, S., Chen, L. M., Domanski, M. D. (2003). Reliability of the GDS for use among elderly Asian immigrants to the USA. International Psychogeriatrics, 15, 253–71.

National Institute of Clinical Excellence (2006). Dementia. London: NICE Guidelines.

National Institute of Clinical Excellence (2007). Donepezil , galantamine, rivastigmine and memantine for the treatment of Alzheimer's disease. NICE technological appraisal guidance 2 (amended). London: NICE.

National Institute of Mental Health England (2003). Inside Outside- Improving mental health Services for Black and Minority Ethnic Communities in England. London: NIMHE.

Neeleman, J., Mak, V., Wessely, S. (1997). Suicide by age, ethnic group, coroner's verdict and country of birth. A three-year survey in inner London. Bristish Journal of Psychiatry, 181, 463–7.

Odutoye, K., Shah, A. K. (1999). The clinical and demographic characteristics of ethnic elders from the Indian sub-continent newly referred to a psychogeriatric service. International Journal of Geriatric Psychiatry, 14, 446–53.

Patel, N. (2000). Care for ethnic minorities: the professionals' views. Journal of Dementia Care, Jan/Feb, 26–27.

Patel, N., Mirza, N. R., Lindblad, P., Amstrup, K., Samaoli, O. (1998). Dementia and Minority Ethnic Older People. Managing Care in the UK, Denmark and France. Lyme Regis: Russel House Publishing Limited.

Phelan, M., Parkman, S. (1995). Work with an interpreter. British Medical Journal, 311, 555–7.

Pollit, P. (1996). Dementia in old age: an anthropological perspective. Psychological Medicine, 26, 1061–74.

Prosser, D. (1996). Suicide by burning in England and Wales. British Journal of Psychiatry, 168, 175–82.

Purandare, N., Luthra, V., Swarbrick, C., Burns, A. (2007). Knowledge of dementia among South Asian (Indian) older people in Manchester, UK. International Journal of Geriatric Psychiatry, 22, 777–81.

Quereshi, K. N., Hodkinson, H. M. (1974). Evaluation of a ten-question mental test in institutionalised elderly. Age & Ageing, 3, 152–7.

Rait, G., Burns, A. (1997). Appreciating background and culture: the south Asian elderly and Mental Health. International Journal of Geriatric Psychiatry, 12, 973–7.

Rait, G., Morley, M., Lambat, I., Burns, A. (1997). Modification of brief cognitive assessments for use with elderly people from the South Asian sub-continent. Ageing & Mental Health, 1, 356–63.

Rait, G., Burns, A., Baldwin, R. et al. (1999). Screening for depression in African-Caribbean elders. Family Practice, 16, 591–5.

Rait, G., Burns, A., Baldwin, R. et al. (2000a). Validating screening instruments for cognitive impairment in older south Asians in the United Kingdom. International Journal of Geriatric Psychiatry, 15, 54–62.

Rait, G., Morley, M., Burns, A. et al. (2000b). Screening for cognitive impairment in older African-Caribbeans. Psychological Medicine, 30, 957–63.

Raleigh, V. S., Balarajan, R. (1992). Suicide and self burning among Indians and west Indians in England and Wales. British Journal of Psychiatry, 161, 365–8.

Raleigh, V. S., Bulusu, L., Balarajan, R. (1990). Suicides among immigrants from the Indian subcontinent. *British Journal of Psychiatry*, **156**, 46–50.

Redelinghuys, J., Shah, A. K. (1997). The characteristics of ethnic elders from the Indian subcontinent using a geriatric psychiatry service in west London. *Ageing & Mental Health*, **1**, 243–7.

Reeves, S. J., Sauer, J., Stewart, R., Granger, A., Howard, R. (2001). Increased first contact rates for very late onset schizophrenia-like psychosis in African and Caribbean born elders. *British Journal of Psychiatry*, **179**, 172–4.

Richards, M., Brayne, C. (1996). Cross-cultural research into cognitive impairment and dementia: some practical experiences. *International Journal of Geriatric Psychiatry*, **11**, 383–7.

Richards, M., Abas, M., Carter, J. *et al.* (1998). Social support and activities of daily living in older Afro-Caribbean and white UK residents. *Age & Ageing*, **27**, 252–3.

Richards, M., Brayne, C., Dening, T. *et al.* (2000). Cognitive function in UK community dwelling African Caribbean and white elders: a pilot study. *International Journal of Geriatric Psychiatry*, **15**, 621–30.

Ritch, A. E. S., Ehtisham, M., Guthrie, S. *et al.* (1996). Ethnic influence on health and dependency of elderly inner city residents. *Journal of the Royal College of Physicians London*, **30**, 215–20.

Roth, M., Tym, E., Mountjoy, C. Q. *et al.* (1986). CAMDEX: a standardised instrument for diagnosis of mental disorder in the elderly with special reference to the early detection of dementia. *British Journal of Psychiatry*, **149**, 698–709.

Samanta, A., Burden, A. C., Fent, B. (1987). Comparative prevalence of non-insulin dependent diabetes mellitus in Asian and White Caucasian adults. *Diabetes Research and Clinical Practice*, **4**, 1–6.

Secretaries of State for Health, Wales, Northern Ireland and Scotland (1989). *Working for Patients*. London, HMSO.

Shah, A. K. (1992a). *The Prevalence and Burden of Psychiatric Disorders. A Report to the Department of Health*. London: Institute of Psychiatry.

Shah, A. K. (1992b). The burden of psychiatric disorders in primary care. *International Review of Psychiatry*, **4**, 243–50.

Shah, A. K. (1997a). Interviewing mentally ill ethnic minority elders with interpreters. *Australian Journal on Ageing*, **16**, 220–1.

Shah, A. K. (1997b). Straight talk. Overcoming language barriers in diagnosis. *Geriatric Medicine*, **27**, 45–6.

Shah, A. K. (1999). Difficulties experienced by a Gujarati psychiatrist in interviewing elderly Gujaratis in Gujarati. *International Journal of Geriatric Psychiatry*, **14**, 1072–4.

Shah, A. K. (2004). Ethnicity and common mental disorders. In D. Meltzer, T. Fryers, R. Jenkins (eds) *Social Inequalities in the Epidemiology of Common Mental Disorders. Maudsley Monograph 44*. East Sussex: Psychology Press 171–223.

Shah, A. K. (2007a). Demographic changes among ethnic minority elders in England and Wales. Implications for development and delivery of old age psychiatry services. *International Journal of Migration, Health and Social Care*, **3**, 22–32.

Shah, A. K. (2007b). Can the recognition of clinical features of mental illness at clinical presentation in ethnic elders be improved? *International Journal of Geriatric Psychiatry*, **22**, 277–82.

Shah, A. K. (2008a). Estimating the absolute number of cases of dementia and depression in the black and minority ethnic elderly population in the UK. *International Journal of Migration, Health and Social Care*, **4**, 4–15.

Shah, A. K.. (2008b). Do socio-economic factors, elderly population size and service development factors influence development of specialist mental health programme for older people. *International Psychogeriatrics*, **20**, 1238–44.

Shah, A. K.. (2009). The relationship between elderly suicide rates, household size and family structure: a cross-national study. *International Journal of Psychiatry in Clinical Practice*, **13**(4), 253–8.

Shah, A. K., Dighe-Deo, D. (1998). Elderly Gujaratis and psychogeriatrics in a London psychogeriatric service. *Bulletin of the International Psychogeriatric Association*, **14**, 12–13.

Shah, A. K., Ganesvaran, T. (1994). Suicide in the elderly. In E. Chiu, D. Ames (eds) *Functional Psychiatric Disorders of the Elderly*. Cambridge: Cambridge University Press, 221–44.

Shah, A. K., MacKenzie, S. (2007). Disorders of ageing across cultures. In D. Bhugra, K. Bhui (eds) *Textbook of Cultural Psychiatry*. Cambridge: Cambridge University Press, 323–44.

Shah, A. K., Mukherjee, S. (2000). Cross-cultural issues in the measurement of behavioural and psychological signs and symptoms of dementia (BPSD). *Ageing & Mental Health*, **4**, 244–52.

Shah, A. K., Lindesay, J., Jagger, C. (1998). Is the diagnosis of dementia stable over time among elderly immigrant Gujaratis in the United Kingdom (Leicester)? *International Journal of Geriatric Psychiatry*, **13**, 440–4.

Shah, A. K., Oommen, G., Wuntakal, B. (2005a). Cultural aspects of dementia. *Psychiatry*, **4**, 103–6.

Shah, A. K., Lindesay, J., Nnatu, I. (2005b). Cross-cultural issues in the assessment of cognitive impairment. In A. Burns, J. O'Brien, D. Ames (eds) *Dementia*. London: Hodder Arnold. 147–64.

Shah, A. K., Doe, P., Deverill, K. (2008). Ethnic minority elders: are they neglected in published geriatric psychiatry literature. *International Psychogeriatrics*, **20**, 1041–45.

Shah, A. K., Dennis, M., Lindesay, J. (2009). Comparison of elderly suicide rates amongst migrants in England and Wales with their country of origin. *International Journal of Geriatric Psychiatry*, **24**, 292–9.

Sheikh, J. A., Yesavage, J. (1986). Geriatric Depression Scale (GDS). Recent findings and development of a shorter version. *Clinical Gerontologist*, **5**, 165–73.

Shimuzu, M. (1990). Depression and suicide in late life. In K. Hasegawa, A. Homma (eds) *Psychogeriatrics: Biomedical and Social Advances*. Amsterdam: Excerpta Medica, 330–4.

Silveira, E., Ebrahim, S. (1995). Mental health and health status of elderly Bengalis and Somalis in London. *Age & Ageing*, **24**, 474–80.

Silveira, E., Ebrahim, S. (1998a). Social determinants of psychiatric morbidity and well-being in immigrant elders and whites in east London. *International Journal of Geriatric Psychiatry*, **13**, 801–12.

Silveira, E., Ebrahim, S. (1998b). A comparison of mental health among minority ethnic elders and whites in east and north London. *Age & Ageing*, **27**, 375–83.

Solomon, A. (1992). Clinical diagnosis among diverse populations: a multicultural perspective. *Family in Society: The Journal of Contemporary Human Services*, June, 371–7.

Stewart, R., Richards, M., Brayne, C. *et al.* (2001). Cognitive function in UK community-dwelling African Caribbean elders: normative data for a test battery. *International Journal of Geriatric Psychiatry*, **16**, 518–27.

Stewart, R., Johnson, J., Richards, M., Brayne, C., Mann, A. and Medical Research Council Cognitive Function and Ageing Study (2002). The distribution of Mini-Mental State Examination scores in older UK African-Caribbean population compared to MRC CFA study norms. *International Journal of Geriatric Psychiatry*, **17**, 745–51.

Thomas, P., Thornton, T., Shah, A. K. (2009). Language, games and interpretation in psychiatric diagnosis: a Wittgensteinian thought experiment. *Journal of Medical Humanities*. **35**, 13–18.

Thornton, T., Shah, A. K., Thomas, P. (2009). Understanding, testimony and interpretation in psychiatric diagnosis. *Medicine, Healthcare and Philosophy*. **12**, 49–55.

Waern, M., Runeson, B. S., Allebeck, P., *et al.* (2002). Mental disorders in elderly suicides: a case control study. *American Journal of Psychiatry*, **159**, 450–5.

Wai Yin Chinese Women Society (2007). *Report of the Community Led Research Project*

Focussing on: The needs of Chinese Older People with Dementia and their Carers. Preston: University of Central Lancashire.

Watanabe, N., Hasegawa, K., Yoshinaga, Y. (1995). Suicide in later life in Japan: urban and rural differences. *International Psychogeriatrics*, 7, 253–61.

Yip, P. S. F., Tan, R. C. E. (1998). Suicides in Hong Kong and Singapore: a tale of two cities. *International Journal of Social Psychiatry*, **44**, 267–79.

Yip, P. S. F., Callanan, C., Yuen, H. P. (2000). Urban/rural and gender differentials in suicide rates: East & West. *Journal of Affective Disorders*, 57, 99–106.

Yip, P. S. F., Liu, K. Y., Hu, J., Song, X. M. (2005). Suicide rates in China during a decade of rapid social change. *Social Psychiatry and Psychiatric Epidemiology*, **40**, 792–8.

Zhang, M., Katzman, R., Salmon, D. *et al.* (1990). The prevalence of dementia and Alzheimer's disease in Shanghai, China: impact of age, gender, and education. *Annals of Neurology*, **27**, 428–37.

Chapter 15

Migration and its effects on child mental health

Nisha Dogra, Khalid Karim and Pablo Ronzoni

Editors' introduction

Children may well be primary migrants in that they may be running away from one situation, especially in times of war, or they may be trafficked. Unaccompanied children may well have the additional burden of being obliged to prove their age, which will create further stress. Travelling with the family as dependents, children and adolescents may respond to migration as a new exciting adventure and may adjust quicker and better than older migrants. Migration will most certainly affect children's adjustment and socialisation. Within the context of migration there will be additional factors related to changes in family structures and expectations. In this chapter, Dogra *et al.* provide an overview of the impact of migration on children and the family, especially as childhood is socially constructed and culturally influenced. The value and the role of children varies across cultures. Their stages of development will significantly influence their migration experiences. In addition, the stress on the family may worsen if different members of the family acculturate at a different pace; children may become more proficient in the new language and be asked to translate and interpret for the older members of the family, whose linguistic proficiency may be problematic. Educational and adjustment factors may affect children and adolescents disproportionately. A consensus on definitions, access to services and educational policy will prove helpful to children and to their families, as well as to service providers.

Introduction

In this chapter the effects of migration on child mental health are considered. We begin by clarifying how terminology will be used and the focus of the chapter. While acknowledging that there are different types of migrants (for example, economic migrants, refugees and asylum seekers) who may be affected in different ways, the purpose of this chapter is to provide an overview of these circumstances on children's mental health. This chapter does not provide a sociological or historical perspective about migration except to highlight specific issues that are relevant to children's mental health. In thinking about the impact of child mental health, factors that need to be kept in mind, such as the meaning of childhood, are highlighted but are not discussed in detail. The impact of migration on children's mental health, educational attainment and their socialisation are considered, as the three issues often influence each other. In considering child mental health, parenting and how this can be affected by migration is considered. It is well recognised that parenting and family life are

Migration and Mental Health, ed. Dinesh Bhugra & Susham Gupta. Published by Cambridge University Press. © Cambridge University Press 2011.

significant factors in child mental health. Our focus is largely on migration from one country to another but rural to urban migration is also discussed as this is a major issue for many developing countries. The chapter concludes with some suggestions for future work.

Definition of child migrants

There is no single definition of exactly what defines a child migrant. As will be evidenced by some of the literature discussed in this paper, the term migrant is often used to mean those who move for economic reasons, those who are forced to move (asylum seekers) or refugees (where the reason may be practical as opposed to political; for example, victims of natural disasters and war). Child migrants are usually accompanied by adults but there are increasingly a greater number of unaccompanied refugee minors and this brings additional demands on the host country as these children are more vulnerable. This chapter will not focus on the debates around definitions but will, as already mentioned, provide an overview.

Relevant factors to consider in thinking about child mental health

We will not enter the debate on children and their place in society except to highlight that the very notion of childhood is socially constructed and influenced by culture. The value and treatment of children therefore varies across different societies, as will the degree of choice and involvement that children have in their experience of migration.

The other issue that needs to be highlighted with respect to children is that their stage of development may significantly influence their migration experience. In some ways younger children are more adaptable as they will, if migrating with their families, be giving up less of their social world as compared to adolescents. However, younger children are also more dependent on parents and may struggle if their parents struggle. Children may also struggle to share their distress with their parents as they are often sensitive to parental distress and do not wish to exacerbate it. Huemer *et al.* (2009) found that some studies also found younger children to be more vulnerable, which, given dependence on adults, is perhaps unsurprising. Development will also be a factor in how much children may understand about their experience and the changes it brings for them.

Preschool children who experience trauma or separation may respond by showing the problems of anxious attachment. School-aged children may become withdrawn while adolescents may show destructive behaviour. Vuorenkoski *et al.* (1998) discussed migration as being an initially short-term stressor but, depending on the coping mechanisms available and characteristics of migration, it can have either positive or negative effect to the mental wellbeing of the child. Poor adaptation to the new circumstances may manifest itself through decline in physical and/or mental health. Vuorenkoski *et al.* (1998) found that boys who moved before puberty had more psychiatric symptoms than controls both for initial migration and for when the family returned to the country of origin. Girls who moved before puberty were best adapted. Moving away during puberty was more difficult for those returning to the country of origin. Migration appears to be more of a challenge during puberty. This may be related to cultural expectations that adolescents should cope and/or of peer relationships being broken. Children may not share their parents' desires to return to the country of origin.

Conceptualisation of mental health

The conceptualisation of mental health varies from culture to culture and factors other than culture (for example, education and socio-economic factors) may also influence the understanding of mental health and/or illness. In some contexts somatisation of psychological distress is more usual. However, it is important to bear in mind that groups are rarely homogeneous. For migrants that do not speak the host country language, utilisation of services may depend on the use of interpreters, which brings its own set of issues. The way people think about mental health will influence what services they access and the types of treatments they are likely to accept. This is not discussed further in this paper.

Can experiences of migration be generalised from one context to another?

Before discussing the process of migration, we need to consider whether the experiences of migration from one context can be generalised to another context. The historical contexts can be important in how the host country views the migrants and the responsibilities it may take in helping them to settle down. Reviewing the literature and generalising from it can be difficult as the issues may be very particular to specific situations or contexts. Much of the US literature, for example, refers to Mexican migrants into the USA. The issues are not always relevant to other contexts such as migration to Europe from former colonies, or from Europe to Canada, Australia, New Zealand and even the USA. These contexts bring their own issues.

The relationship between migrants and the host country can be very different and the patterns of migration may also vary. For example, the UK and France have different groups which have migrated from former colonies, whereas Germany acquired a large Turkish community. Western European countries have also acquired migrant communities from eastern Europe. To the lay public, migration often implies those that are different to look at and this perspective may be influenced by the media reporting on immigration issues. Immigration evokes strong feelings especially when there is economic hardship. During these times migrants may face increased risk of hostility and discrimination.

There is also quite a lot of literature from Australia which had a policy of mandatory detention of unauthorised migrants. This attracted both national and international concern (Mares and Jureidini, 2004). It is also difficult not to be aware of the Australian 'all white' immigration policies of the early 1970s. In some ways Australia leads on some of the legislation in equal opportunities but how this translates into practice given some of the contexts is unclear. So, in considering the impact of migration on children's mental health, the historical and social contexts need to be borne in mind.

The process of migration

Carballo and Mboup (2005) highlight that the twentieth century saw fundamental changes in the ways in which countries inter-relate and migration as part of this change brings with it a number of challenges, including health-related issues.

Migration usually results either from an active choice made by adults or a family or it may be enforced for economic or other related reasons (such as availability of work). Migration implies a degree of choice as opposed to the position of asylum seekers or refugees who may have even less control over their circumstances.

Migration by its very nature means families or parts of the family leaving somewhere that is home and familiar and moving to somewhere that is different (and thereby 'foreign') and potentially hostile. It is therefore hardly surprising that it is important to consider cultural key issues.

All migrants leave behind a great deal to enable them to forge better lives for themselves, their children and families. The pressures on children may therefore be considerable. Children are affected by migration when:

- The family is separated either by one or both parents migrating and leaving the children behind with other family members
- They migrate with their parent or parents
- They migrate with other family members
- They migrate alone and are unaccompanied
- They live in areas with high levels of migration with the issues that this brings.

Any of these contexts may also apply to refugees in that they may be refugees with their families or be alone as refugees.

Some people move with the intention of settling and beginning new lives. Others move with the intention of staying long enough to earn sufficient money before returning home. Others may migrate illegally and therefore be unsupported through their employment. Migrants may find that their children prefer to see the new country as home so plans to return home may never materialise. The country of origin may take on an idealised version, especially if there are struggles in the new environment.

Pottinger and Williams Brown (2009), in discussing Caribbean migration (mostly to the USA or Canada), describe different types of migration, including:

- Seasonal migration (where parents migrate for periods of months at a time to work in a host country)
- Serial migration (either one or both parents migrate with the intention of sending for the rest of the family at a later date)
- Parental migration (parents migrate for a defined period or indefinitely, but the longer term plan does not involve having the children leave the home country)
- Family migration (the family migrates together).

Another type of migration is where children are sent to live with relatives in other countries for their education. These are contexts that are less likely to apply to refugees, but even in these situations the family may elect to send particular members of the family ahead of others if circumstance so dictates.

Economic factors may dictate the type of migration that happens, and family migration may only be possible when there are the financial resources to do this. If the family migrates together, parents arriving in a new country may have less access to support for childcare than back in their country of origin.

Children tend to adjust reasonably quickly unless they or their loved ones experience trauma directly. Adversity does not appear to cause lasting effect on adaptive behaviours unless important adaptive systems such as cognition and parenting are compromised prior to, or as a result of, the adversity (Masten, 2001).

Carballo and Mboup (2005) argue that the interaction between health and migration is complex and is influenced by the socio-economic and cultural background of migrants, their previous health history and the nature and quality of access to healthcare before migration. It is then further influenced by the circumstances and process of migration itself as well as factors related to the new environment.

The impact of migration on families

The impact of migration on families as a whole may be difficult to assess as family functioning itself is a variable in how migrant children adapt to the migration process. For example, Patino *et al.* (2005) found that there was a relationship between family dysfunction and migration in the development of psychosis in children and adolescents. As the authors point out, it may be that psychosis itself caused the family dysfunction that they measured. It may also be that migration increased stress for the family, leading to dysfunction and/or psychosis. It is also important to note that dysfunction was measured using a 'western' perspective. In this scenario, each factor of family dysfunction, adapting to migration and psychosis is likely to be influenced by a complex interplay of the other factors and many others, so separating each out can be very difficult.

Beckerman and Corbett (2008) highlight that the process of migration in itself means that parents and children need to navigate their place in two cultures as a minimum (the culture of origin and the new culture). Each party may have a different sense of belonging to the culture of origin and this may set up the family for conflict, as may different rates of adaptation and different expectations. The discrepancy between children and parents may lead to increased stress and a lack of family cohesion (Farver *et al.*, 2002).

Migration may also mean that there is power reversal in the family, especially if children acquire language skills that parents are lacking. Children may have more power as they are better placed to communicate with the wider community and this responsibility may be inappropriate. The family may also have redistribution of roles to suit their new environment, leading to changes that have implications as to how it functions. Families may also face stress with the move from rural to urban environments as parents may find their parenting compromised as they struggle to make sense of a perhaps more threatening environment. There may also be a loss of extended family and community support, meaning that parents are either unsupported or have to make use of more formal support systems as fewer informal systems exist for them.

Families may also hide their struggles as children and parents may not want each other to know that they are not managing in an attempt to protect others. Families that migrated because of family dysfunction are unlikely to fare better in a new environment unless some other stressors are reduced because of the migratory experience.

However, families may also become more cohesive as a unit if they work together to adapt to their new environment. Family that do this appropriately are unlikely to become inter-dependent and isolated from the wider community. It is likely that the reasons for migration and socio-economic status are important factors in the stress that migration brings.

The impact of migration on children's lives when separated from their families

Interestingly, there is little research in this area and most of the following section is based on clinical experiences of young people. The lack of research may also suggest that these types of migrants are less visible or the migration more informal. Parents who migrate without their children will usually arrange for surrogate caregivers (usually extended families). These caregivers may or may not be familiar to the children. Some will no doubt provide appropriate alternative parenting while others may not. However, children may not understand the reasons for their parents leaving and feel abandoned by them. These feelings may stay with the child into adulthood as there may be no real opportunity to deal with them. It can be difficult to maintain meaningful contact and develop appropriate relationships, especially if the children are left when young. Older siblings may find themselves taking on responsibility for younger siblings. If the situation is not clearly explained, and sometimes even if it is, children may build up false expectations that they will soon join their parents and may struggle to continue with the life they actually have. When children eventually join their parents they may have grown accustomed to life without them and act out their anger at having been abandoned. This is more likely to be the case if their alternative care was difficult. Even children who were well cared for can struggle with the reunion and struggle to adapt, especially if the reunion is around adolescence when they are making sense of who they are. Children may come from prosperous areas in their country of origin and then be placed in hostile council estates in the new country. In addition to adjusting to their family context they also have to deal with arriving into a new environment which presents its own challenges. The reunion may not live up to expectations as both parties may have developed idealised views of the other. Conflict is likely in these circumstances.

Leaving children behind will also impact on parents and even though rationally they may know they have acted in their children's interest, they can be guilt-ridden. When they are reunited guilt and a wish to make up for the separation may mean their parenting is compromised and they indulge the child.

The issues would be similar for children separated when they are sent to another country for their longer term interests. Children in both contexts may keep maltreatment hidden as they may fear for their safety but also may not want to feel they have let down their parents. It may not be until the children are well into adulthood and perhaps have children of their own that some of these issues are identified and/or resolved.

Overview of the research findings

Stevens and Vollebergh (2008) highlight that for several reasons research in this area is of variable quality. Often the terminology used is unclear and the sample groups studied vary hugely. There was a strong emphasis on impact of self-identified ethnic or racial group membership on mental health, largely led by US perspectives. The authors argued that not all self-identified ethnic minorities are migrants and that not all migrants continue to identify with their original ethnic background. They concluded that both higher and lower levels of problem behaviour were found but that it is hard to make any firm conclusion. Here we will present some of the data but it is important to bear in mind that comparison of studies is also difficult. Carballo and Mboup (2005) also comment on the paucity of quality and/or comparable data.

No difference between migrants and non-migrant groups

Vollebergh et al. (2005) did not find higher rates of mental health problems in migrant children. However, immigrant parents reported more problems in their daughters than non-immigrants. Teachers perceived lower levels if internalising, social and thought problems but higher externalising problems in immigrant girls. However, the study took place in Holland and the immigrant children were mostly Muslim so the cultural mismatch may influence expectations.

Higher levels of problems in migrant groups

Holling *et al.* (2008) undertook a large national German survey and found migration status to be an important variable, as were age, gender and socio-economic status. Younger children, lower socio-economic status and migration were related to more psychopathological problems, with overall prevalence rates similar to other studies. Externalising problems appeared to be the main issue in the migrant sample. Emotional problems did not appear to be moderated by migration status, which may be because there is no difference or because there is a culturally related assessment bias for non-reporting. There is an assumed homogeneity in the non-migrant and migrant samples.

Hovey (2001) reported that 59% of migrant workers' children had one or more psychiatric disorder. The most common disorders were anxiety-related but it was difficult to be sure if they were related to migration or other issues. Hovey also reported greater levels of maltreatment in migrant children and related it to several factors:

- Economic frustration and distress, leading to increased family conflict
- Social and physical isolation, leading to reduced social support and networks
- Poor prenatal care, leading to increased risks.

Hovey also states that many migrant parents have been maltreated as children so may be prone to aggressive parenting styles. It is, however, a huge step to assume that this is the care for many migrant parents.

Van Oort *et al.* (2007) found that internalising problems was a strong predictor for the development of ethnic disparities in educational attainment in migrant Turkish families. They argue that prevention or treatment of internalising problems among Turkish girls will probably contribute to the prevention of educational disparities. First generation labour migrants have a lower socio-economic position than natives in western countries. The argument by Crul and Vermeulen (2003) is that children of migrants grow up poor and remain socio-economically disadvantaged when they grow up. This assumes that migrants make little progress between generations and that parity takes some time. However, attitudes and opportunities to education may be the key. Migrant parents, especially Indian and South Asian parents in the UK, have been stereotyped for pushing their children educationally. Education can be significant in reducing socio-economic disadvantages, as noted by Georgiades *et al.* (2007).

Van Oort *et al.* (2007) found that Turkish migrant adolescents reported more problems than Dutch children. However, the context of being Muslim in Europe after 2001 cannot be ignored.

Von Lersner *et al.* (2008) found that trauma experienced during war and refuge left victims vulnerable and poorly equipped to cope with life in exile. When they returned home (usually under pressure from immigration authorities) they continued to have considerable stress. Although their study related to adults, the findings may be equally applicable to children.

Huemer *et al.* (2009) reviewed mental health problems in unaccompanied minors who were refugees and found that they had higher levels of post-traumatic stress disorder compared to the 'normal' population and accompanied minors. A significant number of refugees are under 18 years of age (44%, and of this 44%, 10% of under the age of 5 years). This is a relevant factor when thinking about services for this group. Despite saying that unaccompanied minors are a diverse group, the authors talk of developing culturally sensitive norms, which seems a rather contradictory position. Girls were in some studies found to be at increased risk of sexual abuse (unaccompanied boys experienced more sexual abuse than boys in general but this was less than for girls).

Lower levels of mental health problems in migrant groups

In an Australian sample, Alati *et al.* (2003) concluded that children of migrants do not differ from comparable children of Australian-born parents in their mental health. In the early years after migration, migrant children showed fewer symptoms of some behavioural problems, but over time these increased to average Australian levels.

Georgiades *et al.* (2007) found that, despite greater socio-economic disadvantage, children living in recent immigrant families had lower levels of emotional/behavioural problems and higher levels of school performance. Living in a neighbourhood with a higher concentration of immigrants was associated with lower levels of problems among immigrant children, but the reverse was true for non-immigrant children. Living in high immigrant areas as an immigrant may provide support whereas in other groups may just indicate socio-economic disadvantage. Xue *et al.* (2005) did not find this in their study.

Factors that influence how migrants settle in their new environment that are likely to be related to the problems faced by children

Political leaning and attitudes towards migrants

Montgomery's (2008) opening paragraph states that 'the immigration of citizens from Third World countries represents a huge social, economic, cultural and ethical challenge to Western societies and will continue to do so within the foreseeable future.' There is a need to 'import' a workforce but with strong ambivalence about investing in helping the migrants to adjust. This is perhaps useful in setting the context of political perspectives about migrants; it does appear as though it is seen as a 'necessary evil'.

Silove *et al.* (2007) outline that the recent influx of asylum seekers from generally poor and non-westernised countries into developed countries has elicited extreme reactions from vocal minority groups opposed to immigration. One only has to look at the rise of the far right in Europe (for example, the Netherlands and the UK). The issue of skin colour is not mentioned by Silove *et al.* (2007), but it is obviously an issue and the issue of racism cannot be ignored.

The problems have been compounded by the increased (real and perceived) threat of terrorism, increasing the hostility towards those that are potentially different. Economic hardship tends to exacerbate the situation as less established migrants may be more vulnerable from its impact. Unemployment may make them especially vulnerable.

Status of residency

Uncertainty about residency status can bring about its own stress. Young people may be under conscious or subconscious pressure to hold on to particular narratives that may strengthen the family case for residency. If one parent has migrated first, the family may face long periods of uncertainty before they can be reunited.

An Australian inquiry into the effect of detention on mental health found that mental distress was common in varying degrees in detained asylum seekers. If these are adults, the distress as well as the context of being detained is likely to impact on parenting. Even though detention centres may be safer than the home they have fled, being detained is likely to bring pressures of its own in an already vulnerable population who may be dealing with previous experience of torture and persecution. They also found that the longer the period of detention the greater the impact on child mental health. Detention is likely to impact on child development but the longer it continues the greater the loss of confidence that the host country is likely to be the sought-after safe haven. The inquiry found that children became institutionalised in the detention centres and suffered from anxiety, distress, bedwetting and self-destructive behaviour. Prolonged uncertainty about residency status is also unlikely to help.

Women and children are more likely to be refugees and may already have suffered significant abuse which is unlikely to be addressed in detention centres. It is also worth noting that children who have been cared for by extended family if their parents migrated may not reveal abuse experienced.

Settling down

Social networks and support

Migrants may be disadvantaged by not having the family and social networks to help them with day-to-day issues. There is often a case made that these communities are in need of highly targeted and specialised services, but that they lack knowledge of existing health and mental health services (McDonald and Steel, 1997). It is unclear if migrants access local services less often because they do not feel they need them or are unaware of them.

Migrants are often forced to go where the work is, and families have little choice about where they choose to settle. They may end up in rural and isolated communities in which they are even more isolated because of their difference. In the UK, it is not unusual in rural areas such as North Wales and Norfolk to find that the only non-indigenous population is medical and/or health staff unable to secure posts at popular hospitals. These individuals may have even less community support than those living in less remote areas.

For children, school may be a protective factor from some of the social adversity but it may also be a significant stressor especially if they are less able to access the curriculum because of language difficulties and/or discrimination. This may be particularly acute for children who may be the focus of attention if they are the only one that is visibly different. There may also be clashes between parental and school expectations of young people. Parents may not be empowered to challenge the school or educational services to secure resources for their child, especially if there are significant learning problems.

As children become older they may experience incongruence between what they experience at home and the wider world. This may set up conflict between them and their families.

Separation from family and the loss of familiar people is often a far greater risk to suffering distress than air raids or bombings (Barnes, 2003). This may be because while the latter is clearly stressful, not knowing about the safety of loved ones may be even more stressful.

Socio-economic disadvantage

Migrants in most countries are socially disadvantaged. How the family adapts may be a key factor. Georgiades *et al.* (2007) stated 'because family dysfunction is higher among recent immigrants versus non immigrant families, it is likely that this resilience works mostly through parenting practices that are more supportive of emotional/behavioural regulation and school performance.'

If migrant children come from families who were relatively wealthy in their country of origin, they may need to make considerable social adjustments, including their social standing in peer groups and the wider community. There is an assumption that migrant children are at risk of mental health problems as they are growing up with two or more, sometimes conflicting, cultural environments, and this exposes children to stress. Mental health problems may themselves leave children at a disadvantage.

Families may also experience a lack of social standing in their new environment. Parents may have had higher status jobs in their country of origin but have to accept lower status jobs in the new country because their qualifications do not have equivalency. They may also find themselves working longer hours and have less time for parenting with less extended family or social support. If the children fail to appreciate the sacrifices parents have made for them there may be considerable family conflict.

Managing discrimination and prejudice

Discrimination and prejudice are significant issues but less touched on in the literature. Migrants often find themselves subject to hostility and this may be reduced in areas where there are high numbers. However, this may mean that they are less able to integrate with local host communities successfully.

Not being able to speak the language of the host country may cause problems with access to appropriate services. Children attending school may be better placed to learn the new language and then find themselves in the uncomfortable position of having to interpret for their parents.

Compounding factors

Children who are asylum seekers or refugees may suffer from conflict exposure prior to migration which is then compounded by the asylum process. Nielsen *et al.* (2008) found, using data reported by teachers, that children who had been seeking asylum for more than 1 year in Denmark had an increased risk of having mental difficulties. Four or more relocations in the asylum system were also associated with a high risk. This is comparable to increased rates of mental health problems in children in local authority care who experience repeated moves.

The Danish data supported that of Steel *et al.* (2004). While detention conditions vary from country to country, both studies found that lengthy detention impacts negatively on mental health. This is likely to be related to increasing institutionalisation and perhaps losing faith. The way that asylum seekers are portrayed and treated is unlikely to help.

Children's psychological health will also be related to their parental mental health. If their parents are anxious or homesick and this becomes chronic, the children may fail to adapt and settle into their new environment.

Parental concerns

Parents may worry about the socialisation of their children; for example, children encountering different moral values in the mainstream society, deterioration of family values and a challenge of their authority. The concerns may be particularly marked for girls, who may be perceived as more vulnerable.

Parents may also be worried about appropriate supervision, especially if both parents work long hours and are not available to the children physically or emotionally.

Parents may also worry about their children's academic progress and be unable to help them as their own education may be limited.

The problems experienced

Children who are migrants or refugees experience the same range of mental health problems that other children do. There is no reason to expect that the rates of disorders that are strongly neurodevelopmental in nature (such as attention deficit hyperactivity disorder or autistic spectrum disorder) will be any greater than any other samples (but note that there is variability in the diagnosis of these between different countries). Children who are traumatised are more likely to suffer from emotional disorders but may present with behavioural difficulties. This is especially likely if they are unable to communicate their distress effectively.

The evidence does not strongly suggest anything specific so in practice while it is useful to be aware of a child's migrant status, it is important not to assume that any problems they experience are because of this or that the status is irrelevant.

Kinzie *et al.* (2006) present the case for treating refugee children as individuals and moving away from the idea that all children in that group need to be managed in the same way. The argument can easily be applied to all migrant groups. If we remember that children's mental health problems mostly have a multifactorial aetiology and we consider migration (and the effects thereof) as part of the whole picture rather than assuming it is the whole picture, we would have a better understanding of the child and their context. This would ensure that any intervention is tailored to their specific need.

Future directions

There is a need to have some consensus about the terminology used to enable better comparisons of migration of different groups and in different contexts. The literature has tended to be dominated by quantitative research, with little focus on children and young people's experiences. It is difficult to be sure that in migrants showing higher rates of mental health problems, how much of a factor migration plays. These children could be high risk groups because of various other factors. The narratives of children and their carers about their experiences and how they met the subsequent challenges might provide rich data which could more meaningfully improve our understanding of their problems and appropriate interventions.

References

Alati, R., Najman, J. M., Shuttlewood, G. J., Williams, G. M., Bor, W. (2003). Changes in mental health status amongst children of migrants to Australia: a longitudinal study. *Sociology of Health & Illness*, **25**, 7, 866–88.

Barnes, D. (2003). *Asylum Seekers and Refugees in Australia: Issues of Mental Health and Well Being*. Sydney: Transcultural Mental health Centre.

Beckerman, N. L., Corbett, L. (2008). Immigration and families: treating acculturative stress from a systemic framework family therapy. *Journal of the California Graduate School of Family Psychology*, **35**(2), 63–81.

Carballo, M., Mboup, M. (2005). *International Migration and Health*: a paper prepared for the Policy Analysis and Research Programme of the Global Commission on International Migration. Global Commission on International Migration.

(http://www.gcim.org/attachements/TP13.pdf, accessed 26 June 2009).

Crul, M., Vermeulen, H. (2003). The second generation in Europe. *International Migration Review*, **37**(4), 965–86.

Farver, J. M., Narang, S. K., Bhadha, B. R. (2002). East meets west: ethnic identity, acculturation, and conflict in Asian Indian families. *Journal of Family Psychology*, **16**(3), 338–50.

Georgiades, K., Boyle, M. H., Duku, E. (2007). Contextual influences on children's mental health and school performance: the moderating effects of family immigrant status. *Child Development*, **78**(5), 1572–91.

Holling, H., Kurth, B. M., Rothenbeger, A., Becker, A., Schlack, R. (2008). Assessing psychopathological problems of children and adolescents from 3 to 17 years in a nationwide representative sample: results of the German health interview and examination survey for children and adolescents (KiGGS). *European Child & Adolescent Psychiatry*, **17**(Suppl. 1), 34–41.

Hovey, J. D. (2001). Mental health and substance abuse. *Migrant Health Issues Monograph Series*. Buda, Texas: National Center for Farmworker Health, Inc.

Huemer, J., Karnik, N. S., Voelkl-Kernstock, S. et al. (2009). Mental health issues in unaccompanied refugee minors. *Child and Adolescent Psychiatry and Mental Health*, **3**, 13.

Kinzie, J. D., Cheng, K., Tsai, J., Riley, C. (2006). Traumatised refugee children: the case for individualised diagnosis and treatment. *Journal of Nervous and Mental Disease*, **194**(7), 534–7.

Mares, S., Jureidini, J. (2004). Psychiatric assessment of children and families in immigration detention – clinical, administrative and ethical issues. *Australian and New Zealand Journal of Public Health*, **28**(6), 520–6.

Masten, A. S. (2001). Ordinary magic Resilience processes in development. *American Psychologist*, **56**(3), 227–38.

McDonald, B., Steel, S. (1997). *Immigrants and Mental Health: an Epidemiological Analysis.*

Sydney: Transcultural Mental Health Centre.

Montgomery, E. (2008). Long term effects of organised violence on young Middle Eastern refugees' mental health. *Social Science and Medicine*, **67**, 1596–603.

Nielsen, S. S., Norredam, M., Christiansen, K. L. et al. (2008). Mental health among children seeking asylum in Denmark – the effect of length of stay and number of relocations: a cross sectional study. *BMC Public Health*, **8**, 293.

Patino, L. R., Selten, J. P., Van Engeland, H. et al. (2005). Migration, family dysfunction and psychotic symptoms in children and adolescents. *British Journal of Psychiatry*, **186**, 442–3.

Pottinger, A. M., Williams Brown, S. (2009). Understanding the impact of parental migration on children: implications for counselling families from the Caribbean. (www.counselingoutfitters.com/Pottinger.htm, accessed 10 June 2009).

Silove, D., Austin, P., Steel, Z. (2007). No refuge from terror: the impact of detention on the mental health of trauma affected refugees seeking asylum in Australia. *Transcultural Psychiatry*, **44**, 359–93.

Steel, Z., Momartin, S., Bateman, C. et al. (2004). Psychiatric status of asylum seeker families held for a protracted period in a remote detention centre in Australia. *Australian and New Zealand Journal of Public Health*, **28**, 527–36.

Stevens, G. W. J. M., Vollebergh, W. A. M. (2008). Mental health in migrant children. *Journal of Child Psychology and Psychiatry*, **49**(3), 276–94.

Vollebergh, W. A. M., Ten Have, M., Dekovic, M. et al. (2005). Mental health in immigrant children in the Netherlands. *Social Psychiatry and Psychiatric Epidemiology*, **40**, 489–96.

Van Oort, F. V. A., Van der Ende, J., Crijnen, A. A. M. et al. (2007). Ethnic disparities in mental health and educational attainment: comparing migrant and native children. *International Journal of Social Psychiatry*, **53**, 514–25.

Von Lersner, U., Wiens, U., Elbert, T., Neuner, F. (2008). Mental health of returnees: refugees in Germany prior to their state-sponsored repatriation. *BMC International Health and Human Rights*, **8**, 8.

Vuorenkoski, L., Moilanen, I., Myhrman, A. *et al.* (1998). Long term mental health outcome of returning migrant children and adolescents. *European Child and Adolescent Psychiatry*, 7, 219–24.

Xue, Y., Leventhal, T., Brooks-Gunn, J., Earls, F. (2005). Neighbourhood residence and mental health problems of 5–11 year olds. *Archives General Psychiatry*, **62**, 554–63.

Chapter 16

Mental health issues related to migration in women

Prabha S. Chandra

Editors' introduction

Migration will inevitably affect people of different genders in different ways. Women may migrate both as primary and secondary migrants, and their experiences after migration are likely to be different. They may also migrate as part of the family. The challenges and coping strategies will be very different. Furthermore, there may be an expectation from the family for the females to remain the same and behave in the same way, whereas the new society and even the members of the family in the new setting may expect different gender roles. This discrepancy between gender roles and gender role expectations will place an additional burden on the individual. Chandra illustrates the importance of gender in the process of migration by placing it on the centre stage. Her use of feminisation is to denote an increase in the number of females in a given setting – this is not and should not be seen as a sexist term. Mental health determinants for women migrants include risk factors related to unfavourable socio-economic factors as well as gender. Domestic labour has specific issues related to women's mental health. Women are more likely to have higher rates of psychiatric disorders and are also more likely to be carers, thereby experiencing additional stress, of which clinicians must be aware.

The feminisation of migration

Until recently, issues related to migration were considered gender-neutral. However, with rapid mobility across nations, marked changes in economic policies the world over and more women migrating compared to a decade ago, migrant health has taken on a gender dimension.

The United Nations Population Division (2005) estimates for the period 1965–2005 show that there have been almost as many female as male migrants, rising only slightly from 47% in 1960 to 50% in 2005. Nearly two-thirds of the migrant population has settled in developed countries, where the feminisation of migration is slightly higher (52%) than it is in developing regions (46%).

Migration is known to have a differential impact on men and women, although some issues may be common to both. Men and women migrate for different reasons, have different methods of migration and have a great variation in the experience of migration.

Women migrate in three different ways: as primary migrants, i.e. for work or study; as secondary migrants, i.e. accompanying their spouses who are the primary migrants; and, thirdly, as part of family reunification, i.e. when a woman from one country marries a person from another country and moves there.

Migration and Mental Health, ed. Dinesh Bhugra & Susham Gupta. Published by Cambridge University Press. © Cambridge University Press 2011.

While the gender dimension is important in the experience of migration, it must be remembered that the majority of migrations happen because of economic need and also from less developed countries to more wealthy nations. In this sense the migrant is inherently at a disadvantage as they would have not left their home country if it was not for a better life.

It is important to understand that gender in most countries from which migration occur influences the roles and relationships within a family and the role a woman has to play in the community. This gender demarcation in roles causes different health risks. An important aspect is the difference in roles and identities of women in their countries of origin and countries of migration which impacts health and help-seeking behaviours (Bhugra, 2004a). While this is true for all aspects of health, it has particular relevance to mental health. In addition to the above, between-countries migration often results in the woman becoming an ethnic minority in the country of destination.

Recent migrants have been reported to enjoy better health than do the host country populations. This phenomenon, known as the 'healthy migrant effect', is attributed to the various selection processes that labour migrants undergo before arriving at their destination (Razum et al., 2000). However, some time after migration, immigrants' and nationals' health patterns converge and, for some health conditions, such as self-rated health, immigrants fare worse. Alicia Lla'cer et al. (2007) report that this variation in health between the time of migration and a few years after has not been examined with a gender perspective. Also, not much information is available about how mental health fares in the 'healthy migrant' phenomenon at various points of the migration process and the gender-related variations.

Mental health determinants for women migrants

Adjustment to a new country is based on acculturation. Numerous studies have investigated the associations between acculturation strategies and various health-related outcomes (Berry and Sam, 1997). The conceptual framework of acculturation strategies, developed by John W. Berry, describes four types of attitudes. These include integration, assimilation, separation and marginalisation (Berry, 1997). Studies have shown that the associations between these strategies and mental health are to some extent moderated by the characteristics of the cultural groups and the host societies. Some studies have indicated that integration and assimilation are associated with poorer mental health compared to separation and marginalisation. The reasons for these observations are not very clear. Most women who migrate to a different culture would find it difficult to assimilate because they might not be working, they may not be encouraged to socialise because of cultural norms or they may not have the opportunities to do so. The impact of these strategies might also be different between women who are primary migrants compared to those who are secondary migrants.

Predictors of mental health among migrants include variables of both traumatic and non-traumatic character. Several studies have shown that poor social support, economic difficulties, female gender, unemployment, poor sociocultural adaptation, adverse life events after arrival and pre-migration traumatic episodes are associated with mental ill-health (Knipscheer and Kleber, 2006; Schweitzer et al., 2006; Sundquist et al., 2000). Perceived ethnic discrimination has also been shown to predict mental illness among immigrants in some studies (Noh et al., 1999). However, these findings are not always uniform and have shown between-country variations.

Research has revealed that migrants' mental health is dependent on several contextual and individual characters, of which gender forms an important part. Tinghög et al. (2010) divide these factors schematically into three groups:

1. Non-immigrant-specific risk factors of persistent character (e.g. unfavourable socio-economic situation)
2. Non-immigrant-specific risk factors of sudden and traumatic character (e.g. specific types of traumatic episodes, number of traumatic episodes experienced)
3. Immigrant-specific risk factors (e.g. female gender, ethnic discrimination, poor sociocultural adaptation).

Bhugra (2005) emphasises that within the process of migration, it is important to study the premigratory phase, the preparatory phase, the personality of the individual, the amount of social support and network and preparation for the process of migration. Prospective studies that assess these predictors of mental health problems related to migration among women are lacking.

In a cross-sectional Swedish study which addressed this issue and compared mental health among Finns, Iraqis and Irani immigrants it was found that Iraqis and Iranis had a much higher prevalence of anxiety and depression compared to the Finns (Tinghög *et al.*, 2010). The mean values of low wellbeing and depression/anxiety were highest in the Iraqi group, followed by the Iranian group. The study also concluded that factors that predicted poor mental health included non-immigrant-specific factors (i.e. poor economic security, being female, being divorced/widow/widower, poor social network), non-immigrant-specific experiences of traumatic nature (i.e. high number of types of traumatic episodes), and immigrant-specific factors (i.e. poor sociocultural adaptation). Together these factors 'explained' the major part of the markedly higher prevalence of mental ill-health among the Iraqi and Iranian immigrant groups. To be a woman from Iraq appeared to be a risk factor in itself. The authors speculate that this might be because some migrant women experienced an especially high discrepancy between existing gender roles in the two societies.

The mental health of domestic workers in Asia

Women domestic workers in Asia are a specific population who need attention from mental health workers. Rapid economic growth in many Asian and Arab cities and countries (including Hong Kong, Singapore, Malaysia, Kuwait, Dubai and Saudi Arabia) has resulted in the demand for foreign domestic workers (FDWs). The majority of these are women, and the demand for FDWs has been met mainly from the Philippines, Indonesia and Sri Lanka over the past decades, reflecting the poor socio-economic conditions of these countries. FDWs are almost always women who leave their families to take up poorly paid jobs in more prosperous countries to secure a higher income and better future for their families. These FDWs are often marginalised in many ways. They can be discriminated against sexually, racially and socially because of their gender, religion, language and skin colour and employment status in the foreign land. They are often exploited and abused, making them vulnerable to psychiatric problems (Abu-Habib, 1998; Cox, 1997). A few systematic studies are now available from Kuwait (El-Hilu *et al.*, 1990; Zahid *et al.*, 2004) and Hong Kong (Lau *et al.*, 2009) regarding the unique mental health issues in this population.

El-Hilu *et al.* from Kuwait (1990) reported that FDWs were five times more likely to be admitted to a psychiatric hospital compared to local women. Most of these women were admitted with acute reactive psychiatric disorders. More recently, in the same setting it was found that admission rates were 1.86 times higher for FDWs than female Kuwaiti patients (Zahid *et al.*, 2004). Even after 14 years, stress-related psychiatric disorders still predominated, with 'reaction to severe stress' being the most frequent diagnosis. In Kuwait, studies indicate that, among FDWs, a history of medical or psychiatric conditions, poor educational level and language skills, and being a non-Muslim and a Sri Lankan national have been reported to be significant risk factors for psychiatric morbidity (Zahid *et al.*, 2003). Nearly 75% of the patients in the Zahid *et al.* study were from the Indian subcontinent and their education level was also rather low; a quarter were illiterate and 40% had only 4 years or less education. Half of the patients did not speak English or Arabic.

A qualitative study among Ethiopian domestic workers in Kuwait revealed several important aspects of mental health in these migrants (Anbesse *et al.*, 2009). Focus group discussions were used to explore the experiences of Ethiopian female domestic migrants to Middle Eastern countries, comparing those who developed severe mental illness with those remaining mentally well. Prominent self-identified threats to mental health included exploitative treatment, enforced cultural isolation, undermining of cultural identity and disappointment in not achieving expectations. The participants reported trying to counter these risks by affirming their cultural identity and establishing sociocultural supports.

Given below is a description of these four factors that were perceived as being detrimental to mental health (Anbesse *et al.*, 2009).

Exploitation

Almost all of the women described inhumane working conditions, physical and sexual maltreatment, and denial of basic freedoms. Upon reaching their new place of employment, the women spoke of having to cope with impossibly high workloads, long hours and inadequate rest. Once employed in a home, the women could expect to be shared by other families so that their responsibilities would multiply. The women spoke of being exhausted and overwhelmed by what was required of them, and linked this to the development of mental ill-health.

Enforced cultural isolation

Women reported being extremely distressed about being apart from their families and dislocated from ties with Ethiopia. This situation was exacerbated by the restrictions placed by employers on their freedom to move around, meet with other Ethiopians or attend religious worship. On the other hand, most of the women reported being able to adapt easily to the new country's cultural practices and language.

Undermining of cultural identity

Related to the importance of ties to home was the women's powerfully described reactions to any undermining of Ethiopia and its culture.

Disappointed expectations

Many women reported the high expectations they had of themselves and the expectations that their families had of them so that they could improve their lives. They felt that there was a strong pressure on them not to disappoint the families back home. This often resulted in emotional distress.

Determinants of poor mental health among FDWs

Zahid *et al.* (2003), who studied Kuwait housemaids hospitalised for psychiatric problems, found that more than 25% were diagnosed as having a psychiatric problem within a month of arrival. There are several possibilities why women may have more problems in the early

Table 16.1 Predictors of poor mental health among female domestic workers

Low education
Recent arrival
Belonging to certain specific geographical regions
Past history of psychiatric illness
Past physical illness
Previous hospitalisation
Different religion from the new country
The inability to learn a new language
Poor social support
Inadequate social networks

stages of migration: pre-existing mental health problems, language and cultural issues, or the stress related to poor social support as a consequence of moving into a new country.

A detailed social–psychological investigation of 153 Philippino FDWs revealed limited Chinese language proficiency and inadequate bicultural identity integration, leading to high acculturative stress and insufficient psychological adjustment (Chen *et al.*, 2008). As for the symptomatology, Indonesian FDWs were more likely to react with suicidal ideas while Philippinos tended to present with mutism, although not to a statistically significant degree. Indonesian FDWs were also found to have been admitted for mental health problems earlier than the Philippino FDWs. During the course of their psychiatric illness, Indonesian FDWs tended to have prolonged treatments and a longer hospital stay than their Philippino counterparts. This could be explained by the fact that Indonesians are usually younger, less experienced, less educated and less able to communicate in English. As a consequence, their clinical management is more difficult.

Furthermore, they often fail to assert their rights while support from their agents or employers is frequently minimal. Thus, Indonesian FDWs, especially those who are single or unmarried, are more vulnerable.

Studies among domestic workers in Hong Kong reported similar findings (Lau *et al.*, 2009). When psychosocial stressors were analysed, home/family problems came at the top of the list rather than work difficulties. It seems that home/family issues, together with relationship problems that rank second in the stressors, distress female immigrant workers more than the job itself, although work-related problems like abuse or exploitation are more often highlighted and publicised in the media (Table 16.1).

Cultural alienation and mental health – the mental health of South Asian women in Britain

Cultural alienation, a process in which individuals find themselves cut off from their culture, is considered to be a common risk factor for mental health problems. As a result of inadequate socialisation opportunities, women tend to feel more alienated in new cultures.

While they have limited chances of assimilating fully into the new culture, they tend to lead parallel lives, straddling two value systems – one of their country of origin (which is often more traditional) and the other of their new country (which is based more on gender equality). In the UK, South Asian women have been reported to have nearly double the suicide rate of white women (Neeleman *et al.*, 1997; Raleigh and Balarajan, 1992). Regarding attempted suicide, the rate in UK South Asian women is 1.6 times that of white women and 2.5 times that of South Asian men (Bhugra *et al.*, 1999).

Some of the causes attributed to this higher rate of suicide include family disputes over marriage and lifestyle, marital conflict, in-law problems, stigma, unhappy arranged marriages, expectations of submission by women to men and elders, and culture conflict (Bhugra *et al.*, 1999). In a focus group study, Bhugra and Hicks (2000) found that marital violence, unhappiness in family relationships and depression were reported as some of the commonest factors related to suicide attempts among South Asian women.

In a study that compared South Asian women who attempted suicide with those who did not, Bhugra *et al.* (1999) found that those attempting suicide were significantly more likely to have a history of a past psychiatric disorder, more likely to repeat the attempt and more likely to be in inter-racial relationships. They were also more approving if their children wanted to have inter-racial relationships or choose their marriage partners themselves. However, experiences of racial events were not very different between groups, indicating that a racial life event per se is not likely to lead to self-harm. Those attempting suicide were more likely to have changed their religion and spent less total time with their families. Bhugra and Hicks, (2004) report that cultural alienation, from one's culture and from the majority population, can both be risk factors for women migrants.

Postpartum depression among immigrant mothers and barriers to help-seeking

A study of approximately 600 new mothers in Canada indicated that immigrant mothers (who had immigrated within the last 5 years) had five times the risk of exhibiting depressive symptoms in comparison with Canadian-born women (Dennis *et al.*, 2004). An examination of the psychosocial needs of new mothers revealed that recent immigrant women frequently feel overwhelmed and socially isolated in the postpartum period (Katz and Gagnon, 2002). Depending on the disparity between the original and new culture and the circumstances of immigration, the physical, psychological and emotional strain of motherhood may be especially overwhelming for recent immigrant women as they navigate through an unfamiliar healthcare system, often separated from the comfort of traditional postpartum practices and support networks (Barclay and Kent, 1998). Studies among healthcare providers in trying to understand the barriers to care in this specific population have revealed several important barriers to help-seeking. These include both practical and cultural barriers (Teng *et al.*, 2007). Practical barriers included not knowing where and how to access services, and language difficulties. Cultural barriers included fear of stigma and lack of validation of depressive symptoms by family and society. The lack of cultural recognition and open discussion of postpartum depression may lead many recent immigrant women to dismiss or deny their distress. Stigma was identified by the study participants as a multifaceted barrier to care. They felt that stigma prevented some recent immigrant women from initiating service use, not only because of conflict with personal beliefs and values, but also the fear of being alienated by others and bringing shame to the family.

Ahmed *et al.* (2009) interviewed ten immigrant new mothers with diagnosed depression. The aim of the study was to better understand the following among new mothers with depression: (a) experiences and attributions of depressive symptoms; (b) their experiences with healthcare providers and support services; (c) factors that facilitated or hindered help-seeking; (d) factors that aided recovery; or (e) were associated with women continuing to experience symptoms of depression. Many women attributed their depressive symptoms to social isolation, physical changes, feeling overwhelmed and financial worries. They had poor knowledge of community services. Barriers to care included stigma, embarrassment, language, fear of being labelled an unfit mother or the attitude of some staff. Facilitators to recovery included social support from friends, partners and family, community support groups, 'getting out of the house' or personal psychological adjustment.

Healthcare providers and immigrant women

Studies done in Canada and the Netherlands among healthcare providers indicate interesting reports of whether immigrant women prefer or do not prefer a healthcare worker from the same culture. While theoretically one might assume that a healthcare provider from the same culture would be preferable, clients were concerned about being judged by their peers, and perhaps more surprisingly felt that healthcare providers may breach confidentiality, particularly when they shared the same social community. This concern was most forcibly expressed by closely knit and smaller immigrant communities, who often shared social spheres and who may be inter-related. Some mental health providers reported that some immigrant women would request that they be treated by providers from outside their cultural group. It appears hence that preferences about cultural matching, if available, should be discussed with the woman herself without assumptions that she will welcome being treated by someone from her own culture and country.

Assessment and understanding

There may need to be modifications in the way health providers understand mental health experiences of immigrant women. Depression may not be perceived in a similar manner as assumed by western medicine, and women may have more culturally acceptable ways of understanding their experience. This may lead to under-reporting or misrecognition. Studies have shown several barriers to help-seeking, which include: (a) immigrant women face many difficulties accessing mental healthcare owing to insufficient language skills, unfamiliarity/unawareness of services and low socio-economic status; (b) participants identified structural barriers and gender roles as barriers to accessing the available mental health services; (c) the healthcare relationship between healthcare providers and women had profound effects on whether or not immigrant women seek help for mental health problems (O'Mahony and Donnelly, 2007).

Studies in the Netherlands have also indicated that the immigrant women have barriers to seeking mental health services and that Surinamese, Antillean, Turkish and Moroccan women made considerably less use of mental healthcare services than native-born women. On the other hand, immigrant women more frequently used social work facilities and women crisis intervention centres (Ten Have and Bijl, 1999).

Intimate partner violence in immigrant women has been found to be another major risk factor for depression in South Asian women, both in Britain and Canada. Ahmed *et al.* (2009) discuss reasons for a lack of reporting and help-seeking among immigrant women in the context of spousal violence. The usual reasons are stigma, lack of knowledge about available resources, rigid gender roles which include expected silence and loss of social support.

Interventions and preventive services for women

Much of the literature reviewed in this chapter indicates that immigrant women have unique problems that make them vulnerable to psychological distress. This may range from pre-existing mental disorder, traumatic experiences in the countries of origin, lack of preparedness for the change that migration entails, difficulties in assimilation, isolation from otherwise existing social structures and networks, an inability to articulate distress in health settings, lack of knowledge about existing services and poor access to these services.

It is thus evident that prevention should start from the pre-migration stage itself. While in many situations the woman may have no choice but to migrate (secondary migration or family reunification), wherever possible adequate screening and treatment for mental health problems should be part of the preparation process. Among primary migrants, adequate orientation to changes that might be expected, helping with language and cultural skills (particularly among FDWs) and information about agencies that they can seek help from may be effective in preventing at least some mental health problems.

Several agencies and organisations exist for immigrant women in the USA, UK and Canada but invariably women gain knowledge about them only once they have a problem. During a crisis women may not be able to access these agencies effectively (such as when domestic violence escalates or if a woman has postpartum depression). Ideally, information regarding these agencies should be freely available and they should be part of the acculturation process (much as getting one's social security number or health card).

For younger girls and adolescents, school and college programmes with teens and their parents have been used as a way of improving the post-migration experience and maintaining self-esteem (Khanlou et al., 2002). Theatre and dance have also been used to encourage young people to talk about issues such as identity, cultural pride and cultural tradition, and how they can be used to facilitate assimilation into a new culture in a facilitative and educative environment (McCarthy, 2006).

In addition, Hussain and Cochrane (2004) discuss the need for culturally sensitive services within generic health services that take into account the role of alternative and traditional healing. Moodley (1993) makes a distinction between 'separate' and 'sensitive' services and considers the contributions each model can make in meeting the needs of migrant communities. She maintains that 'separate' services fill the gap left by statutory services and mental health services provide care for 'their own'. Alternatively, 'sensitive' services require fundamental changes in the culture of existing monolithic organisations such as the British NHS. However, she emphasises that any attempt to reorientate services has to be backed by the appropriate level of resources. Where more ethnically sensitive services have been developed and where services have attempted to understand and meet the needs of ethnic minority groups, there have been noticeable improvements in the uptake of services as well as compliance with treatment. Bhugra (2004b) has discussed how a simple measure such as an educational pamphlet about depression and suicidality can change perceptions and attitudes to treatment and help-seeking among British South Asian women.

Conclusions

The feminisation of migration is increasing with globalisation and work opportunities. Migration can be both a positive and distressing experience for women. Mental health problems may predate the migration, contributing to additional risk. Differences in the cultural values and traditions of the country of origin and country of migration may also influence mental health among immigrant women. Social supports and networks have been shown to be one of the most important protective factors for mental health, and migration may often adversely affect social networks. Some situations, such as partner violence and the postpartum period, may make women even more vulnerable to mental health problems. Primary migrants with low education and in the context of poverty (such as among FDWs) have an additional risk.

Help-seeking is often delayed owing to several factors, which include lack of knowledge about services, language problems, cultural explanations for psychological distress and the stigma of being diagnosed with a mental disorder in a strange land. In addition, lack of knowledge and sensitivity among healthcare providers regarding the above factors may contribute to further alienation.

Among women, prevention should ideally start before the process of migration and continue in the early stages of moving to a new culture. Information about services should be available, and early detection of mental health problems by sensitive healthcare providers is necessary.

References

Abu-Habib, L. (1998). The use and abuse of female domestic workers from Sri Lanka in Lebanon. *Gender and Development*, 6, 52–6.

Ahmed, F., Druver, N., McNally, M. J., Stewart, D. (2009). Why doesn't she seek help for partner abuse? An exploratory study with South Asian immigrant women. *Social Science and Medicine*, 69, 613–22.

Anbesse, B., Hanlon, C., Alem, A., Packer, S., Whitley, R. (2009). Migration and mental health: a study of low-income Ethiopian women working in Middle Eastern countries. *International Journal of Social Psychiatry*, 55, 557–63.

Barclay, L., Kent, D. (1998). Recent immigration and the misery of motherhood: a discussion of pertinent issues. *Midwifery*, 14, 4–9.

Berry, J. W. (1997). Immigration, acculturation and adaptation. *Applied Psychology: an International Review*, 46, 5–68.

Berry, J. W., Sam, D. (1997). Acculturation and adaptation. In J. W. Berry, M. H. Segall and C. Kagitcibasi (eds) *Handbook of Cross-Cultural Psychology*, Vol. 3, *Social Behavior and Applications*. Boston: Allyn and Bacon.

Bhugra, D. (2004a). Migration and mental health. *Acta Psychiatrica Scandinavica*, 109, 243–58.

Bhugra, D. (2004b). Migration, distress and cultural identity. *British Medical Bulletin*, 69, 129–41.

Bhugra, D. (2005). Cultural identities and cultural congruency: a new model for evaluating mental distress in immigrants. *Acta Psychiatrica Scandinavica*, 111, 84–93.

Bhugra, D., Desai, M. (2002). Attempted suicide in South Asian women. *Advances in Psychiatric Treatment*, 8, 418–23.

Bhugra, D., Hicks, M. H. (2000). *Deliberate Self-Harm in Asian Women: An Intervention Study*. London: Report to the Department of Health.

Bhugra, D., Hicks, M. H. (2004). Effect of an educational pamphlet on help-seeking attitudes for depression among British South Asian women. *Psychiatric Services*, 55, 827–9.

Bhugra, D., Baldwin, D. S., Desai, M., Jacob, K. S. (1999). Attempted suicide in west London. II. Inter-group comparisons. *Psychological Medicine*, **29**, 1131–9.

Chen, S. X., Benet-Martinez, V., Bond, M. H. (2008). Bicultural identity, bilingualism, and psychological adjustment in multicultural societies: immigration-based and globalization-based acculturation. *Journal of Personality*, **76**, 803–38.

Cox, D. (1997). The vulnerability of Asian women migrant workers to a lack of protection and to violence. *Asian and Pacific Migration Journal*, **6**, 59–75.

Dennis, C-L. E., Janssen, P. A., Singer, J. (2004). Identifying women at-risk for postpartum depression in the immediate postpartum period. *Acta Psychiatrica Scandinavica*, **110**, 338–46.

El-Hilu, S. M., Mousa, R., Abdulmalek, H. *et al.* (1990). Psychiatric morbidity among foreign housemaids in Kuwait. *International Journal of Social Psychiatry*, **36**, 291–9.

Hicks, M. H., Bhugra, D. (2003). Perceived causes of suicide attempts by UK South Asian Women. *American Journal of Orthopsychiatry*, **73**(4), 455–62

Hussain, F., Cochrane, R. (2004). Depression in South Asian Women living in the UK: a review of literature with implications for service provision. *Transcultural Psychiatry*, **41**, 253–60.

Katz, D., Gagnon, A. J. (2002). Evidence of adequacy of postpartum care for immigrant women. *Canadian Journal of Nursing Research*, **34**, 71–81.

Khanlou, N., Beiser, M., Cole, E. *et al.* (2002). *Mental Health Promotion Among Newcomer Female Youth: Post-Migration Experiences and Self-Esteem*. Report. Ottawa, ON: Status of Women Canada.

Knipscheer, J. W., Kleber, R. J. (2006). The relative contribution of post-traumatic and acculturative stress to subjective mental health among Bosnian refugees. *Journal of Clinical Psychology*, **62**, 339–53.

Lau, P. W. L., Cheng, J. G. Y., Chow, D. L. Y., Ungvari, G. S., Leung, C. M. (2009). Acute psychiatric disorder in foreign domestic workers in Hong Kong: a pilot study.

International Journal of Social Psychiatry, **55**, 569–76.

Lla'Cer, A., Zunzunegui, M. V., del Amo, J., Mazarrasa, L., Bolumer, F. (2007). The contribution of a gender perspective to the understanding of migrants' health. *Journal of Epidemiology and Community Health*, **61**, 4–10.

McCarthy, P. (2006). *Education Resource Guide. Beneath the Banyan Tree*. Canada: Theatredirect.

Moodley, P. (1993). Setting up services. In D. Bhugra and J. Leff (eds) *Principles of Social Psychiatry*. Oxford: Blackwell, 490–501.

Neeleman, J., Mak, V., Wessely, S. (1997). Suicide by age, ethnic group, coroners' verdicts and country of birth: a three-year survey in inner London. *British Journal of Psychiatry*, **171**, 463–7.

Noh, S., Beiser, M., Kaspar, V., Hou, F., Rummens, J. (1999). Perceived racial discrimination, depression and coping: a study of Southeast Asian refugees in Canada. *Journal of Health and Social Behaviour*, **40**, 193–207.

O'Mahony, J. M., Donnelly, T. (2007). Health care providers' perspective of the gender influences on immigrant women's mental health care experiences. *Issues in Mental Health Nursing*, **28**(10), 1171–88.

Raleigh, V. S., Balarajan, R. (1992). Suicide and self-burning among Indians and West Indians in England and Wales. *British Journal of Psychiatry*, **161**, 365–8.

Raleigh, V. S., Bulusu, L., Balarajan, R. (1990). Suicides among immigrants from the Indian subcontinent. *British Journal of Psychiatry*, **156**, 46–50.

Razum, O., Zeeb, H., Rohrmann, S. (2000). The 'healthy migrant effect' – not merely a fallacy of inaccurate denominator figures. *International Journal of Epidemiology*, **29**, 191–2.

Schweitzer, R., Melville, F., Steel, Z., Lacherez, P. (2006). Trauma, post-migration living difficulties and social support as predictors of psychological adjustment in resettled Sudanese refugees. *Australian and New Zealand Journal of Psychiatry*, **40**, 179–87.

Silove, D., Sinnerbrink, I., Field, A., Manicavasagar, V., Steel, Z. (1997). Anxiety, depression and PTSD in asylum seekers: associations with pre-migration trauma and post-migration stressors. *British Journal of Psychiatry*, **170**, 351–7.

Sundquist, J., Bayard-Burfield, L., Johansson, L. M., Johansson, S.-E. (2000). Impact of ethnicity, violence and acculturation on displaced migrants: psychological distress and psychosomatic complaints among refugees in Sweden. *Journal of Nervous and Mental Disease*, **188**, 357–65.

Ten Have, M., Bijl, R. (1999). Inequalities in mental health care and social services utilisation by immigrant women. *The European Journal of Public Health*, **9**(1), 45–51.

Teng, L., Blackmore, E. R., Stewart, D. E. (2007). Healthcare worker's perceptions of barriers to care by immigrant women with postpartum depression: an exploratory qualitative study. *Archives of Women's Mental Health*, **10**, 93–101.

Tinghög, P., Al-Saffar, S., Carstensen, J., Nordenfelt L. (2010). The association of immigrant- and non-immigrant-specific factors with mental health among immigrants in Sweden. *International Journal of Social Psychiatry*, **56**, 74–9.

United Nations. (2005). Department of Economic and Social Affairs. *Trends in Total Migrant Stock: The (2005) Revision CD-Rom Documentation*. Population Division United Nations, February, 2006. http://www.un.org/esa/population/publications/migration/UN_Migrant_Stock_Documentation_(2005).pdf.

Zahid, M. A., Fido, A. A., Alowaish, R., Mohsen, M. A. M., Razik, M. A. (2003). Psychiatric morbidity among housemaids in Kuwait. III: Vulnerability factors. *International Journal of Social Psychiatry*, **49**, 87–96.

Zahid, M. A., Fido, A. A., Razik, M. A., Mohsen, M. A. M., El-Sayed, A. A. (2004). Psychiatric morbidity among housemaids in Kuwait. *Medical Principles and Practice*, **13**, 249–54.

Migration and LGBT groups

Dinesh Bhugra, Susham Gupta, Gurvinder Kalra and Stephen Turner

Editors' introduction

Lesbians, gays, bisexual and transgender (LGBT) groups are sometimes described as invisible minorities. They may migrate to urban areas or to other countries for the same reasons as others do, but are also likely to do so for other specific reasons, such as heterosexism, homophobia, bi-negativity, persecution or search for therapeutic interventions. In the majority settings often their health and mental health needs get ignored. Negative attitudes of the new society to migration and to alternative sexualities and identities will produce a situation of double jeopardy for LGBT migrants. In this chapter, the authors set the scene relating to heterosexism, homophobia and bi-negativity. This is followed by specific problems related to LGBT migrants, particularly with regard to coming out and acknowledging associated potential difficulties. Conflicts in coming out with oneself and across families, generations and kinship will add to the stress which may cause the individual to migrate. Settling down in the new country will need additional support. In people from countries where homosexuality and homosexual behaviour are illegal and punishable, the trauma associated with migration will need to be resolved. Laws of the new country, which may not be LGBT-sympathetic, will further contribute to the stress experienced.

Introduction

Lesbians, gays, bisexual and transgender (LGBT) individuals have specific problems related to migration, adjustment and acculturation. Even though they are being discussed as a group, the difficulties they face are likely to be heterogeneous. In many an instance, these individuals have migrated seeking refuge to escape persecution because of their sexual identity. LGBT individuals, like others, will experience both 'push' and 'pull' factors related to migration. Push factors in these cases will include negative attitudes of their family, kinship or society, and isolation and expectations of conformity, etc. Pull factors will relate to finding partners, acceptance, anonymity in a big city and possible liberal attitudes. In these days of easy access to the internet and the possibility of relationships, individuals may move to metropolis areas even within the same country. For transgender people, a major pull factor may be to search for surgical and medical intervention, which may not be available in their region or country. Negative attitudes may vary between the four groups. Homophobia or bi-negativity may contribute to reasons for migration, but these attitudes may well face them again when they arrive in the new country.

Migration and Mental Health, ed. Dinesh Bhugra & Susham Gupta. Published by Cambridge University Press. © Cambridge University Press 2011.

In this chapter, the process of coming out and related issues, homophobia and heterosexism and bi-negativity are highlighted. We attempt to link these attitudes with migratory and postmigratory experiences and explore specific issues in managing LGBT individuals.

Extent

The number of LGBT individuals migrating and/or seeking refuge or asylum will vary according to a number of factors.

It is difficult to know the exact numbers of LGBT individuals migrating at any given time, but some figures can be extrapolated to determine numbers. Kinsey *et al.* (1948, 1953), in a milestone classic study, were able to demonstrate that 4% of men and 1–2% of women were exclusively homosexual (see Michaels, 1996 for a detailed discussion). Not withstanding some serious problems in the method and sample selection, even a conservative estimate would indicate that, of 200 million migrants, refugees and asylum seekers worldwide, 10 million may belong to the LGBT group. It is estimated that LGBT individuals may well migrate for the same reasons that others do, but there will be a group who have migrated or sought refuge especially because of their sexual identity. There are specific factors related to sexual identity, such as cultural attitudes, beliefs, values and gender role expectations, which will determine whether individuals actively or passively hide their identity and/or use this in the process of migration or seeking asylum. Individuals will choose when they come out to themselves or others around them, especially if they believe that this may impede or facilitate their chances of emigrating or seeking asylum. Further complicating factors are whether others around the individual are aware of their sexual identity, especially if migration has occurred in a group. Cultural attitudes differ as it has been argued that in Brazil, for example, the distinction between homosexuality, heterosexuality and bisexuality is a recent one (Parker, 1987).

Specific issues

In addition to the usual factors affecting migrants, there are specific complicating factors related to sexual identity. These, combined with gender role and gender role expectations in the culture of origin and differing expectations in the new culture, will generate additional stress. Each LGBT individual should be seen in the context of their culture surrounded by the new culture and the interaction across cultures taken into account in any assessment or management.

Personal attitudes

LGBT individuals may or may not feel comfortable with their own sexual identity, which will be influenced by social, biological and cultural factors. However, individuals may take some time to recognise feelings of sexual attraction within themselves and may take a longer time in coming to terms with this. Religious values may well influence how they deal with these feelings. Individuals may feel same-sex attraction but, owing to the response and attitudes of the community, may not be able to act on it, and therefore may not identify themselves as gay. Seeing oneself as gay is often a political acceptance and acknowledging this is the last stage in coming out. Until that stage, they may not recognise themselves as gay and may see their sexual behaviour as experimental. A distinction needs to be made between sexual attraction, fantasy and sexual behaviour. Sexual fantasies may be hidden and may be culturally influenced. Sexual behaviour will be obvious and may be observed. Individual beliefs and attitudes will vary according to fantasy, attraction and behaviour, and there may be psychological disjunction.

Coming out

Coming out is described as the cultural process of gay existence, whereby the individual rejects the negative connotations (attributed by others and by themselves) of the homosexual label and positively affirming and acknowledging their sexual orientation. This process signifies an event or a series of events acknowledging to themselves in the first instance and then to others, a non-traditional sexual orientation (usually gay or lesbian) (Hanley-Hackenbruck, 1989). Cohen and Stein (1986) define the process of coming out as a complicated developmental process which involves a person's awareness and acknowledgement of homosexual thoughts and feelings at a psychological level.

Stages of coming out

Coleman (1985) described five stages of coming out and also suggested that each stage needs to be completed with the individual feeling at ease with themselves before moving forward. It is inevitable that at each stage various social and cultural factors will play a role in the process. Whether these stages are entirely linear or overlap occurs between them is debatable. Coleman (1985) suggests these stages to be a pre-coming out stage, coming out, exploration, first relationships and identity integration. The pre-coming out stage may last a long time depending upon the attitudes of the culture from which the individual hails. Subsequently, there is the coming out stage, where the individual acknowledges their sexual orientation to others, also called awareness (Hencken and O'Dowd, 1977), signification (Lee, 1977; Plummer, 1975) or identification (Dank, 1971). The median age for this process has been noted to be 13–18 (Jay and Young, 1979; Weinberg and Williams, 1973). Acceptance from a close friend of the family at this stage means more at a personal level than acknowledgement from a stranger. The stage of exploration is when the individuals start to develop their social and interpersonal skills, leading up to a sense of sexual competence and learning that sexual conquests may not help develop self-esteem. The first relationship stage may be even more problematic, especially as there may not be a model to follow and may leave a sense of low self-confidence. Integration is the stage where relationships settle down and are free of mutual distrust and possessiveness. Trenchard and Warren (1984) found that coming out stories had common themes in their sample. Friends were told first and then others, and the family was often the last to be informed. In a small sample of South Asian gay men, Bhugra (1997) found that families and religion played an important role in the process of coming out, especially among Muslims. Parents and work colleagues were often the last to be told, and individuals used different models to hide their sexuality. In the case of males, definitions and patterns of masculinity and relationships between sons and parents play an important role in the process of coming out.

The development of a homosexual identity is dependent upon how the individual attaches specific meanings to the concept of homosexuality and being homosexual (Dank, 1971). The commitment to a homosexual identity may not occur in an environment where the cognitive category of homosexuality does not exist (Davenport-Hines, 1990). Thus the individual and others may use alternative explanations for this.

Immigration and coming out conflicts: in a small sample of immigrants in Canada, Tremble *et al.* (1989) noted that all young people in their sample had experienced conflict while coming out. The parental responses varied from embarrassment, shock, self-blame, blaming the new culture and seeing the sexuality as a western disease. They also noted that these individuals had experienced difficulties in coming out to their families but also found it difficult to settle down in a gay community in the face of discrimination. Not surprisingly, however, they experienced difficulties in reconciling their sexual orientation with their ethnic or racial identity. For the child of immigrant parents, the process of coming out against a backdrop of cultural expectations and mores which may be anti-gay may well be complex and difficult.

On the other hand, on the basis of the sexual identity the individual may reject their own culture entirely. In a small sample of Japanese–Americans, Wooden *et al.* (1983) noted that double identities were important and these often ran in parallel, but Chan (1989) noted that in her sample, lesbians and gay men identified more with their sexual identity than their ethnic one, which may well be another source of tension between them and their families. Facing racism because of their ethnic identity and homophobia as a result of their sexual identity, the individual may feel caught in a double jeopardy. Gay black men often have to make a choice between identifying with the black community or identifying with the gay community (Beame, 1982). The role expectations may be in conflict and one identity may be more politicised than the other. Icard (1986) notes that the gay black male (the same may also apply to other groups) is placed psychologically in a position of triple jeopardy, influenced by society at large, the black community and the gay community. How well any individual copes with these factors and associated stress will be affected by appropriate growth and development and integration of various identities.

Bandura (1977) offers an explanation for self-efficacy to play a central role in analysing changes. Behaviour of the person is influenced by the expectations of the efficacy of their actions as well as what outcomes are expected. Thus, in a behavioural sense our actions are related to the expected outcome.

Efficacy expectations thus include various sources such as performance accomplishments, vicarious experiences, verbal persuasion and emotional arousal. All these are affected by various social expectations. Thus, applied to black and sexual identities, these become more complex (Bandura, 1977).

Core gender identity is defined as the individual's primary identification as male or female, usually a permanent trait determined in childhood. This will be assessed by clinical interview or self-report (Pillard, 1991). Gender role is a set of expectations about how male and female roles pan out and how these roles develop and are carried out. These, according to Pillard (1991), are culturally determined at any given point in time. Pillard (1991) describes sexual orientation as the erotic attraction to one sex or the other – homosexual, heterosexual or bisexual. However, bisexuality does not automatically fit into the middle, and clinicians and researchers need to be aware of this. Masculinity and femininity scales have been used to explore personal values (Table 17.1).

Homosexuality has been reported across history and cultures (Bullough, 1976, 1979; Weinrich and Williams, 1991; Whitam and Mathy, 1986), as has bisexual and transgender behaviour across ages and countries (Bullough, 1974). Bullough (1974) describes cultures as sex-positive or sex-negative. Sex-positive cultures see sex for enjoyment, whereas sex-negative ones see sex for procreation only.

Table 17.1 Masculinity/femininity items (modified from Pillard, 1991)

At times I feel like picking a fight with someone[1]
. . . would rather go to a game than a dance[2]
. . . take a chance alone in a situation where the outcome is doubtful[2]
. . . self-reliant[3]
. . . strong-personality[3]
A wind storm terrifies me[1]
. . . would like to be a nurse[1]
. . . cry easily[2]
. . . yielding[3]
. . . flatterable[3]
. . . eager to soothe hurt feelings[3]

Questions from [1] Gough (1957) California psychological inventory;
[2] Guilford et al. (1978) Guilford–Zimmerman survey; [3] Bem (1981) Bem sex
role inventory.

Homophobia

Homophobia is a term used to describe anti-homosexual feelings related to prejudice and negative attitudes expressed by individuals against gays and lesbians. In a review of the literature, Bhugra (1987) noted that homosexuality has always provoked strong feelings in most societies. Attitudes vary according to age, gender, religion, education and personal contact (see Ahmed and Bhugra, 2010).

Weinberg (1972) used the term homophobia to characterise heterosexuals' dread of being in close quarters with homosexuals as well as homosexuals' self-loathing. Herek (1996) defined heterosexism and homophobia as hostility and prejudice against both homosexual behaviours and gay and lesbian people. Homophobia is not a clinical phobia and implicitly conveys that anti-gay prejudice is an individual clinical entity rather than a social phenomenon rooted in cultural ideologies and intergroup relations (Herek, 1996). It is these intergroup relations which are at the heart of holding heterosexist views which are readily translated against gay migrants, thus making them face double jeopardy.

Herek (1996) argues, that heterosexism is manifested both at cultural and individual levels, and states that, like institutional racism and sexism, it pervades societal customs and institutions operating through a dual process of invisibility and attack. Unlike race or skin colour, homosexuality and homosexual behaviour are not generally visible and as long as they remain so, a veneer of tolerance by society remains. On the other hand, as soon as homosexuals and homosexuality become visible, they are attacked, even by other migrants.

Bernd (2008) found that migrant adolescents in Germany showed more negative attitudes to homosexuality, and that these were related to traditional norms of masculinity and religiosity and personal contacts with homosexuals. Migrant adolescents of Turkish origin had negative attitudes, said to be influenced by religion.

Psychological heterosexism is reflected in the attitudes and behaviours through personal hostility and condemnation of alternative sexualities, and these behaviours may be seen as sinful. Heterosexual men may feel threatened by homosexual men and society may find challenges to masculinity difficult to deal with. As a result of heterosexism, gays and lesbians may be targeted with anger, violence and abuse, both verbal and physical. In the majority of countries around the world such attacks are not seen as part of homophobia or heterosexist behaviour and are not identified as such. Berrill (1992) reported that 44% of respondents had reported violence against them because of their sexual orientation. Attitudes against gays and lesbians are associated with age, gender, education and socio-economic status, religion and living in rural areas. Anti-migrant feelings are also linked with age, gender, educational and economic status. Thus an accumulation of these factors may generate more negative feelings against gay and lesbian migrants. It is also likely that as a result of living in their own cultures, gay and lesbians may carry feelings of internalised homophobia, thereby further complicating the picture both of the migration process and the post-migration adjustment. Hiding one's sexual orientation can cause a painful discrepancy between public and private identities (Herek, 1996).

Hidalgo (2010) notes that, in the USA, attitudes towards both migration and same-sex relationships are increasingly polarised, and these are correlated. If same-sex marriages become a reality, polarisation on both issues is likely to become mutually reinforcing.

Attitudes of the new society

Apart from a few countries where gay men and lesbians have equal age of consent for sex and equal rights with their heterosexual counterparts, most cultures hold a range of attitudes against homosexuality and homosexual behaviour. Heterosexism and homophobia still remain a common feature. However, these attitudes influence social policy and access to healthcare. They are likely to be more negative against gays and lesbians compared with bisexual individuals. Bhugra and de Silva (1998) found, in a group of bisexual individuals in London, that they were attracted both emotionally and sexually both to men and women; however, the prerequisite was emotional attraction rather than sexual. Interestingly, the sexual behaviour among participants was more heterosexual but self-identification varied.

Gays, lesbians and bisexuals are often very selective in coming out to a more distal circle of individuals and this process is likely to be influenced by receiving positive acknowledgement from others who may have responded with acceptance. Increased availability of information and changing social and economic status, e.g. several openly gay and lesbian ministers in government in the UK and elsewhere, have led to some cultures becoming more positive and accepting. There is no doubt that lesbians and gay men are becoming increasingly visible, and contact between the heterosexual majority and individuals with alternative sexualities will reduce negative attitudes and prejudices. Whether positive attitudes trump attitudes to migrants is difficult to ascertain. When LGBT individuals seek sanctuary elsewhere as a result of their sexual identity, they expect acceptance and safety.

Homophobia/heterosexism attitudes have bi-negativity as their counterpart for attitudes against bisexual individuals. Cultural attitudes towards bisexuality and acceptance will differ whether bisexual males or bisexual females are being considered. Combined with attitudes to alternative masculinities and femininities, it is possible that negative attitudes feed into stereotypes and threaten the individual's own level of sexual comfort. Apart from seeing bisexuals as not being able to make their minds up or trying to have their cake and eat it too, the negative attitudes will inevitably force some individuals to hide their sexual identities. Some migrants may feel very vulnerable and therefore will not like the possibility of having their sexual orientation or preference exposed in a public way. Cultures which see sex and sexual activity as a private activity will encourage individuals to be more circumspect of their sexual identity and activity. This 'conflict' between two cultures may add further stress on the individual. Bi-negativity is defined as the stigma faced by bisexual men (Eliason, 2001). Eliason argues that factors related to bi-negativity are not dissimilar from those of homophobia. Age, gender, educational and socio-economic status, those holding traditional views of gender, familiarity with bisexuals, religion and place of residence are all associated with negative attitudes. Thus, self-perceptions of bisexual individuals will influence their world view. Eliason (2001) reported that, of 229 self-identified heterosexual students, 76% had no bisexual acquaintances. Of the sample, 24%, 21% and 14%, respectively, found the idea of bisexual men, homosexual men and lesbians unacceptable. However, 3.5% had had bisexual experiences, and heterosexual men were more hostile in their attitudes, indicating that they may be holding stronger views (perhaps traditional ones) on masculinity.

Bisexuals may see themselves as more acceptable but they are not, and are rejected by heterosexual males and to a lesser degree by heterosexual females. Expected to conform in more traditional settings and persecuted, isolated and alienated in some settings, bisexuals may move to more urban settings where anonymity may be easily available. Some cities gain the reputation of being gay-friendly and will in turn continue to attract more people with alternative sexual identities. Eliason and Raheim (1996) developed a tool to measure attitudes about lesbians, gay and bisexual individuals. Many bisexual females complain that they face more significant prejudice from lesbians than from heterosexuals (Bisexual Anthology Collective, 1995; Weise, 1992). Mohr and Rochlem (1999) noted that heterosexual men rated bisexual men more negatively and that these attitudes correlated with race, religious attendance and political ideology. Part of this negative attitude can be related to stereotypes that bisexual (and homosexual) individuals are less likely to be monogamous, more likely to have sexually transmitted diseases and less able to satisfy their partners sexually (Spalding and Paplau, 1997). Eliason (1997) confirmed this in a study. These findings confirm prejudices and show stereotypes that people hold of sexual minorities. Sexually transmitted diseases, including HIV, are more common among migrants according to Suligoi and Giuliani (1997). In their study from Italy over a four-and-a-half-year period in the early to mid 1990s, these authors found that non-specific urethritis and genital warts were common in North African men, and non-specific vaginitis and latent syphilis were common among women. Compared with an overall prevalence of HIV infection of 50% in the sample, homosexuals from Central South America had a lower rate of 39%. Thus, even among migrants, rates can vary according to the country of origin.

In an interesting paper, Mai and King (2009) emphasised that narratives, practices and understandings of love and sexuality in the context of mobility, belonging and (individual and collective) identities are under-researched. Love is described as a key to the understanding of desire but sometimes individuals can dissociate love from sexual desire, especially when casual sex is involved. Lone migration is described as the essential component of 'new maps of migration' (King, 2002, pages 99–100). The internet has changed the face of sexual attraction and mating with separate multiple identities, and perhaps acts as a potential precursor to mobility (Constable, 2003; Johnson, 2007). Another interesting issue that needs to be explored further is the marriage of convenience to stay in a country, and transnational or inter-racial marriages and their impact on individual identities. Mai and King (2009) point out that it is relatively recently that non-normative experiences of heterosexuality in the Asian migration context are being considered (Huang and Yeoh, 2008; Walsh *et al.*, 2008). Migration itself will influence gender role expectations and in due course this may affect alternative sexual identities.

Another noteworthy observation made by Mai and King (2009) is that sex, love and emotion are interlinked and any of these components will be influenced by migration. They also point out that studies related to migration focus on affective and cognitive aspects rather than emotions.

An understanding of love, sexuality and the role which emotions, sex and love play in collective social formations is important (Mai and King, 2009). A study looking at British migrants to Dubai noted that the individuals negotiate their (emotional) paths in different ways (Walsh, 2009), and it is inevitable that LGBT individuals may also relate in different ways to different groups. From Venezuela, 'transformistas' often migrate to Europe as potential sex workers, sometimes to raise money for surgical interventions (Vogel, 2009). It is not inevitable that this will be the case for every transgendered individual. Among migrants, whether within the same country or across nations, migrants' emotional and sex lives do not receive the attention they deserve, although recently some authors have started looking at these (Ahmad, 2009; Moukarbel, 2009). Depending upon social support systems such as religious networks, LGBT migrants may settle down (Howe, 2007). However, the relationship between love, emotion, sexual behaviour, sexual attraction and sexual fantasy is a complex one and needs to be explored further.

Violence against LGBT groups

In some cases, irrespective of the process of globalisation, or perhaps because of it, countries and cultures go back to more traditional ways of thinking and behaving. This may lead to physical or emotional attacks on sexual minorities who choose to migrate and may end up facing more abuse in the new country. Sexual migration may lead to detachment from the original culture and may yet produce further alienation if the new culture is not accepting of the sexual identity, which may have been the expectation of the migrant. This may further contribute to low self-esteem and alienation not to mention persecution. There are multiple factors involved in that there may be sexual and gender identity, cultural identity and political identity, among others, thereby creating tensions which may prove problematic. The imagined security and safety may end up as a mirage, thereby confusing the migrant. Families may be the source of alienation but may also provide a safe haven from the larger societies and cultures. Visibility of LGBT migrants will influence the attitudes and beliefs of the new society and culture. In turn, non-LGBT migrants may change their views on sexuality after migration (Ahmad, 2003). The attitudes toward LGBT migrants may lead to a welcoming acceptance, a grudging acceptance, entirely neutral response or be negative. The response between the LGBT migrants and the new culture will raise a number of issues for both groups. Clinicians need to be aware of their own feelings and those of the larger group.

Conclusions

LGBT migrants may face problems both as a migrant and as a member of a sexual minority. However, not all LGBT migrants will do so, and the majority will settle down without any difficulties. Support networks and voluntary agencies may prove to be more helpful than statutory services, certainly in adjustment and enabling migrants to settle down. The factors of homophobia and bi-negativity in the society and in mental health services will influence the way in which clinicians respond and how LGBT individuals accept these services. Policy-makers and stakeholders need to be aware of the needs of LGBT patients and provide appropriate, sensitive and accessible services.

References

Ahmad, N. (2003). Migration challenges views on sexuality. *Ethnic and Racial Studies*, **26**, 684–706.

Ahmad, A. N. (2009). Bodies that (don't) matter: desire, eroticism and melancholia in Pakistani labour migration. *Mobilities*, **4**, 309–27.

Ahmed, S., Bhugra, D. (2010). Homophobia: a review. *Sex and Relationship Therapy* (in press).

Bandura, A. (1977). Self efficacy: towards a unifying theory of behavioural change. *Psychological Review*, **84**, 191–215.

Beame, T. (1982). Young, gifted, black and gay: Dr Julius Johnson. *Advocate*, **346**, 25–57.

Bem, S. (1981). *The Sex Role Inventory*. Palo Alto, CA: Consulting Psychologists Press.

Bernd, S. (2008). Attitudes towards homosexuality: levels and psychological correlates among adolescents without and with migration background (former USSR and Turkey). *Zeitschrift für Entwicklungspsychologie und Pädagogische Psychologie*, **40**, 87–99.

Berrill, K. T. (1992). Antigay violence and victimization in the US: an overview. In G. M. Herek and K. T. Berrill (eds) *Hate Crimes: Continuing Violence Against Lesbians and Gay Men*. Newbury Park, CA: Sage, 19–45.

Bhugra, D. (1987). Homophobia: a review of the literature. *Sexual and Marital Therapy*, **2**(2), 169–77.

Bhugra, D. (1997). Coming out by Asian gay men in the United Kingdom. *Archives of Sexual Behaviour*, **26**(5), 547–57.

Bhugra, D., de Silva, P. (1998). Dimensions of bisexuality: an exploratory study using focus groups of male and female bisexuals. *Sexual and Marital Therapy*, **13**(2), 145–57.

Bisexual Anthology Collective (1995). *Plural Desires: Writing Bisexual Women's Realities.* Toronto: Sister Vision: Black Women and Women of Color Press.

Bullough, V. (1976). *Sexual Variance in Society and History*. Chicago: University of Chicago Press.

Bullough, V. (1979). *Homosexuality: A History*. NY: New American Library.

Chan, C. S. (1989). Issues of identity development among Asian-American lesbians and gay men. *Journal of Counseling & Development*, **68**, 16–20.

Cohen, C., Stein, T. (1986). Reconceptualizing individual psychotherapy with gay men and lesbians. In J. Gonsiorek (ed.) *A Guide to Psychotherapy with Gay and Lesbian Clients*. NY: Plenum.

Coleman, E. (1985). Developmental stages of the coming out process. In W. Paul *et al.* (eds) *Homosexuality: Social, Psychological and Biological Issues*. Beverly Hills: Sage, 149–58.

Constable, N. (2003). *Romance on a Global Stage: Pen Pals, Virtual Ethnography and Mail-Order Marriages*. Berkeley, CA: University of California Press.

Dank, B. M. (1971). Coming out in the gay world. *Psychiatry*, **34**, 180–97.

Davenport-Hines, R. (1990). *Sex, Death and Punishment*. London: Collins, 114–16.

Eliason, M. J. (1997). Prevalence and value of biphobia in heterosexual undergraduate students. *Archives of Sexual Behavour*, **26**, 317–26.

Eliason, M. J. (2001). Binegativity: the stigma facing bisexual men. In B. Beenyu and E. Steinman (eds) *Bisexuality in the Lives of Men: Facts and Fiction*. NY: Harrington Park Press, 137–54.

Eliason, M. J., Raheim, S. (1996). Categorical measurement of attitudes about lesbian, gay and bisexual people. *Journal of Gay and Lesbian Social Services*, **4**, 51–65.

Gough, H. G. (1957). *Manual for the California Psychological Inventory*. Palo Alto, CA: Consulting Psychologists Press.

Guilford, J. P., Guilford, J. S., Zimmerman, W. S. (1978). *The Guilford–Zimmerman Temperament Survey*. Orange, NJ: Sheridan Psychological Services.

Hanley-Hackenbruck, P. (1989). Psychotherapy and 'coming out' process. *Journal of Gay and Lesbian Psychotherapy*, **1**(1), 21–40.

Hencken, J. D., O'Dowd, W. T. (1977). Coming out as an aspect of identity formation. *Gay Academic Union Journal: Gai Saber*, **1**, 18–22.

Herek, G. (1990). The context of antigay violence: notes on cultural and psychological heterosexism. *Journal of Interpersonal Violence*, **5**, 316–33.

Herek, G. (1996). Heterosexism and homophobia. In R. P. Cabaj and T. S. Stein (eds) *Textbook of Homosexuality and Mental Health*. Washington DC: APPI.

Hidalgo, D. A. (2010). Reinforcing polarisations: US immigration and the prospect of gay marriage. *Sociological Spectrum*, **30**, 4–29.

Howe, C. (2007). Sexual borderlands: lesbian and gay migration, human rights and the Metropolitan Community Church. *Sexuality Research and Social Policy*, **4**, 88–106.

Huang, S., Yeoh, B. (2008). Heterosexualities and the global(ising) city in Asia. *Asian Studies Review*, **32**, 1–6.

Icard, L. (1986). Black gay men and conflicting social identifies: sexual orientation versus racial identity. *Journal of Social Work and Human Sexuality*, **4**, 83–93.

Jay, K., Young, A. (1979). *The Gay Report*. NY: Summit.

Johnson, E. (2007). *Dreaming of a Mail Order Husband: Russian–American Internet Romance*. Durham, NC: Duke University Press.

King, R. (2002). Towards a new map of European migration. *International Journal of Population Geography*, **8**, 89–106.

Kinsey, A. C., Pomeroy, W. B., Martin, C. E. (1948). *Sexual Behaviour in the Human Male*. Philadelphia, PA: W. B. Saunders.

Kinsey, A. C., Pomeroy, W. B., Martin, C. E. *et al.* (1953). *Sexual Behaviour in the Human Female*. Philadelphia, PA: W. B. Saunders.

Lee, J. A. (1977). Going public: a study in the sociology of homosexual liberation. *Journal of Homosexuality*, **3**, 49–78.

Mai, N., King, R. (2009). Love, sexuality and migration: mapping the issue(s). *Mobilities*, **4**, 295–307.

Michaels, S. (1996). The prevalence of homosexuality in the US. In R. P. Cabaj and T. S. Stein (eds) *Textbook of Homosexuality and Mental Health*. Washington DC: APPI.

Mohr, J. J. and Rochlem, A. B. (1999). Measuring attitudes regarding bisexuality in lesbians, gay male and heterosexual populations. *Journal of Counselling Psychology*, **46**, 353–69.

Moukarbel, N. (2009). Not allowed to love? Sri Lankan maids in Lebanon. *Mobilities*, **4**, 329–47.

Parker, R. (1987). Acquired immuno deficiency syndrome in urban Brazil. *Medical Anthropology Quarterly*, **1**(2), 155–75.

Pillard, R. C. (1991). Masculinity and femininity in homosexuality: inversion revisited. In J. C. Gonsiorek and J. D. Weinrich (eds) *Homosexuality: Research Implications for Public Policy*. Newbury Park, CA: Sage.

Plummer, K. (1975). Homosexual categories: some research problems in the labelling perspective of homosexualitiy. In K. Plummer (ed.) *The Making of a Modern Homosexual*. London: Hutchinson, 53–75.

Spalding, L. R., Paplau, L. A. (1997). The unfaithful lover: heterosexuals' perceptions of bisexuals and their relationships. *Psychology of Women Quarterly*, **21**, 611–25.

Suligoi, B., Giuliani, M. (1997). Sexually transmitted diseases among foreigners in Italy. *Epidemiology and Infection*, **118**, 235–41.

Tremble, B., Schneider, M., Appathurai, C. (1989). Growing up gay or lesbian in a multicultural context. In G. H. Herdt, ed. *Gay and Lesbian Youth*. New York: Haworth Press, 253–66.

Trenchard, L., Warren, H. (1984). *Something to Tell You*. London: London Gay Teenage Group.

Vogel, K. (2009). The mother, the daughter and the cow: Venezuelan transformistas: migration to Europe. *Mobilities*, **4**, 367–87.

Walsh, K. (2009). Geographies of the heart in transnational spaces: love and intimate lives of British migrants in Dubai. *Mobilities*, **4**, 427–45.

Walsh, K., Shen, H., Willis, K. (2008). Heterosexuality and migration in Asia. *Gender Place and Culture*, **15**, 575–9.

Weinberg, G. (1972). *Society and the Healthy Homosexual*. New York: St Martin's Press.

Weinberg, M. S., Williams, C. J. (1973). *Male Homosexuals: Their Problems and Adaptation*. Oxford: Oxford University Press.

Weinrich, J. D., Williams, W. L. (1991). Strange customs: familiar lives: homosexualities in other cultures. In J. C. Gonsiorek and J. D. Weinrich (eds) *Homosexuality: Research Implications for Public Policy*. Newbury Park, CA: Sage.

Weise, E. R. (1992). *Closer to Home: Bisexuality and Feminism*. Seattle: Seal.

Whitam, F. L., Mathy, R. M. (1986). *Male Homosexuality in Four Societies*. New York: Praeger.

Wooden, W. S., Kawasaki, H., Mayeda, R. (1983). Lifestyles and identity maintenance among gay Japanese–American males. *Alternative Lifestyles*, **5**(4), 236–43.

Management, services and training

18 Adapting mental health services to the needs of migrants and ethnic minorities

David Ingleby

Editors' introduction

A significant number of people, irrespective of their symptoms, will seek help from within their social, personal and folk sectors. Only a smaller proportion will approach the professional healthcare sector. To do this, migrants need to be aware of the healthcare system, pathways into care and accessibility of services. Patients and clinicians can work together if there is mutual respect and awareness of the strengths and weaknesses of each other's positions. Often (mental) healthcare services appear to be fragmented, and for a number of reasons patients and their carers find it difficult to navigate these pathways. In this chapter, Ingleby highlights some of the factors at play which influence where and how people seek help. Accessibility of services depends upon a sense of entitlement to these services, which will vary across cultures. In addition, physical accessibility needs to be differentiated from emotional accessibility. Service utilisation tends to increase with the length of time a person has resided in the country, especially related to learning the new language and acculturation. Help-seeking behaviour will depend upon identifying problems and seeking help and the perceived or real barriers which stop help-seeking. Other factors also play a role, such as perceptions of service providers, health literacy and cultural mediation. Quality-of-life, burden-of-care and outcome measures must be taken into account.

Introduction

All over the world, the steady growth of international migration since World War 2 has led to increased cultural, ethnic and linguistic diversity, with over 200 million people now living away from their country of birth. Migration has important consequences for health, but when these are examined it is important to consider not only the first generation but also their descendants, who are not classified as migrants but as ethnic minorities. (Indeed, some health problems may be even greater in later generations than in the first.) For this reason this chapter is about *migrants and ethnic minorities,* or – for the sake of brevity – MEMs.

Migrant status and ethnicity are often linked with inequalities in levels of mental health and the accessibility or quality of the services provided. The two major issues in this field are therefore (1) the nature and prevalence of mental illnesses among MEMs, and (2) the challenge of providing appropriate and accessible mental health services for these groups.

This chapter will focus on the second issue, but we will not be able to ignore the first one completely because questions concerning the nature and prevalence of mental illnesses may

Migration and Mental Health, ed. Dinesh Bhugra & Susham Gupta. Published by Cambridge University Press. © Cambridge University Press 2011.

have important consequences for service delivery. Moreover, inadequate service provision may result in higher rates of illness. However, this chapter will not promote the often-heard argument that the main reason for paying special attention to MEMs is that they have more mental health problems than other groups. In the first place, no such generalisations can be made; secondly, these groups have a right to appropriate and effective services regardless of whether they have any increased vulnerability to mental illness. This is not to deny that health services should respond rapidly to raised levels of illness when they are discovered. But service delivery for MEMs requires above all a *qualitative* change in the way the services are provided, rather than simply a *quantitative* scaling up of existing services. In my view the same applies to the field of 'global mental health', although this issue is outside the scope of this chapter.

It should be noted that the title of this chapter refers to mental health *services*, rather than simply *care*. In the field of transcultural mental healthcare, much attention has been paid to the relation between caregiver and client. However, it is not only the individual caregiver, but also the organisation in which he or she works, that must adapt to new challenges: a 'whole organisation approach' is required (HSE, 2008). Moreover, health systems are not simply concerned with care, but also with prevention, health promotion and health education: the need for improvement in these sectors may be even greater.

The focus of this chapter is on industrialised countries, where the health of MEMs has received increasing attention over the past half century. Much of the pioneering work has been carried out in the traditional 'countries of immigration' (Canada, the USA, Australia and New Zealand). After 1950, however, as the flow of immigrants to European countries started to increase, the topic also began receiving attention in Europe. Early studies related to postcolonial migrants and to the labour migrants who helped to power the postwar European economic boom up to the oil crisis of 1973. After 1973, labour migration to Europe was drastically restricted: most of those immigrating since then have been asylum seekers, family members or marriage partners. During this period the number of descendants of migrants has also steadily risen.

The first international conference on migrant health in Europe was held in 1983 (Colledge *et al.*, 1986). During the 1980s and 1990s, a small band of dedicated researchers and practitioners in several European countries continued to develop the 'state of the art' in this area, without enjoying much support from central government. In the UK, influential books were written by (among others) Littlewood and Lipsedge (1982), Fernando (1991) and Fernando and Keating (1995). It was mainly in the mental health field that American-inspired concepts such as 'cultural sensitivity' or 'cultural competence' first made their appearance in European health systems.

The period since 2000 has seen a dramatic increase in attention for all aspects of MEM health in Europe, and indeed all over the world. More and more countries have adopted national policies on this topic, encouraged by the efforts of intergovernmental agencies. We will return to these policy developments at the end of the chapter.

In this recent work, two fundamental ideas have come to the fore. The first is that only *sustainable, structurally embedded changes in all parts of the health system* are capable of delivering the improvements that are needed. There have been plenty of short-lived, isolated initiatives, but the time for experimentation has passed. The second key notion is that *users have to be involved in the changes that are made*. A much closer relationship needs to be developed between MEM communities and health services, in which these communities come to play an active role as partners.

What is meant by 'appropriate' services?

The provision of 'appropriate' services, i.e. the matching of services to the needs of users, is the main focus of this chapter. Sometimes the concept of 'fit' is used: Pechansky and Thomas (1981) spoke of the 'degree of fit' between health services and their clients. Conversely, to ignore the diversity of users is often derided by critics as a 'one-size-fits-all' approach. Discrimination does not only occur when people who have the same needs are treated differently – it also happens when people with different needs are treated identically.

Historically speaking, the notion that health services should adapt themselves to their users is a relatively new one: traditionally, it was the users who were expected to adapt to the services. After all, medical professionals were the experts who knew what was best for you. However, the increasing emphasis on participation and patients' rights from the 1960s onwards, the rise of consumerism and 'managed care' in the 1980s and 1990s, and the steadily increasing emphasis on 'patient-centred care' have all seriously undermined this notion. Consumerism preached that it was not enough to make people *better;* they also had to be *satisfied* – and the more satisfied they were, the easier it would be to make them better. Managed care was introduced in an attempt to control the spiralling costs of healthcare, particularly within the mental health field. In this approach, services were required to be 'needs-led' or 'demand-driven', i.e. based on the care the client required rather than that which the service provider was accustomed to give. Patient-centred care has steadily gained more supporters since the term was first introduced in 1969 (Saha *et al.*, 2008).

An emphasis on taking users' views seriously about the help they need and the way it should be given is thus not confined to mental health for MEMs, but is found throughout the health system. As a result, there has been considerable progress in improving the 'fit' between services and their users. The problem is that the users in question have been predominantly white and middle class: the needs of other groups have for the most part been ignored.

A shift away from 'top-down' approaches can also be seen in the principles governing international humanitarian aid and development work. Here, the assumption used to be that western agencies knew what people needed and should simply hand out as much of it as donors would pay for. Today, however, aid must be responsive to local values and cultures, sustainable, based on consultation and implemented with the participation of the recipients. A landmark text here is the *Inter-Agency Standing Committee Guidelines on Mental Health and Psychosocial Support in Emergency Settings* (IASC, 2007). These guidelines are not only based on democratic principles, but also on the pragmatic need to use resources as effectively as possible. Perhaps the present chapter can best be summed up as a plea to apply these guidelines not only to mental health in faraway lands, but also closer to home.

Why is partnership particularly important in mental healthcare?

Active participation on the part of the recipient is more important in some types of help than in others. Some interventions, such as fluoridation of the water supply, can be carried out in a 'top-down' way with minimal cooperation from the target group; the treatment will work even if people don't realise they are getting it. Some professionals appear to think that mental illness can be tackled in the same way – and indeed, if treatment were only a question of correcting chemical imbalances in the brain, the quality of one's relationship with the patient would not make much difference to it, although it might affect their willingness to take their medication. However, the field of mental health has always been characterised by a variety of theoretical approaches, ranging from biochemical reductionism to a multidimensional or 'biopsychosocial' approach. Moreover, the notion that patients must themselves work hard at getting better has been prominent in mental healthcare since the introduction of 'moral treatment' at the beginning of the nineteenth century and psychotherapy at the end of it.

Put another way, the more emphasis professionals place on 'illness' rather than 'disease', the more importance they will attach to their relationship with the patient, and the more they will regard themselves as treating the person who has the disease rather than just the disease. This distinction was first introduced by Leon Eisenberg in 1977:

> To state it flatly, patients suffer 'illnesses'; physicians diagnose and treat 'diseases'. Let me make clear the distinction I intend: illnesses are experiences of disvalued changes in states of being and in social function; diseases, in the scientific paradigm of modern medicine, are abnormalities in the structure and function of body organs and systems.
>
> (Eisenberg, 1977, page 11).

Because illness is something that is experienced, the form it takes will be influenced by a patient's situation and culture. This is the core of the problem of healthcare across cultures. Because western health services have been developed to deal with illnesses as they are experienced by western people, they may not be appropriate for tackling illnesses arising in other cultural contexts. In fact, if nothing is done to adapt the services, it is virtually inevitable that this will be the case. This is referred to as 'institutional discrimination', to distinguish it from direct discrimination by individuals: as long as people do not realise it is going on, it could be said to be nobody's fault. However, the situation changes once inequities in healthcare have been brought to light. If no action is taken to remedy them, then the situation changes to one of *active* discrimination. This, unfortunately, is the case in a large number of mainstream healthcare services in the west.

It should not come as a surprise that great differences exist in the way in which people from different countries experience illnesses – indeed, in their readiness to frame their problems in terms of health and illness *at all*. In the first place, the west has left the rest of the world far behind in terms of the level of development of health services. Compared with the amount of money spent per capita on healthcare in the USA, the amount spent in Europe (according to the WHO statistical database) is around 50% – but in most African countries it is less than 1%. Moreover, the level of spending has increased greatly in the last 50 years: the figure for the USA, even after adjusting for inflation, has grown by a factor of eight during this period (Reinhardt, 2002). This spectacular growth in service provision has been accompanied by a commensurate broadening of the concept of health and a lowering of the threshold for treating illnesses. Whether this should be regarded as 'medical imperialism', 'medicalisation', 'psychologisation', or simply the inexorable march of progress, remains of course a contentious issue (BMJ, 2002).

Nowhere are these changes more strikingly demonstrated than in the mental health sector. In large parts of the world, the only mental health provisions that exist are intramural ones – and even these are usually rudimentary. In contrast, outpatient mental health services in western countries underwent a dramatic expansion during the twentieth century and, whereas the authors of the *DSM* in 1952 could make do with 60 categories to cover the whole spectrum of mental illness, their successors in 1994 needed no less than 410. It is therefore no surprise to find that the concept of 'mental illness' in non-western countries is mainly limited to extreme disturbances: so it was, indeed, 100 years ago in the west. Even in Britain, attitudes to mental illness have not kept pace with these dramatic historical changes. For example, the law still requires a person who has had a mental illness at any time in their life to be barred from service as a member of parliament, although this is under review.

Conceptions of 'mental illness', therefore, differ widely in different parts of the world, and this has to be taken into account both in global mental health and in services for migrants and their descendants, whose attitudes are unlikely to be transformed on the spot simply by reading a patient information leaflet. Moreover, there are considerable differences in the frameworks people use to understand mental illness, i.e. in their 'explanatory models' (Kleinman *et al.*, 1978). These models comprise not only notions about aetiology, but also about the severity, prognosis and social or psychological impact of an illness.

Confronted with the diversity of ideas about mental illness, the response of many western professionals is simply to assume that their own ideas are right, and all the others wrong. After all – it is often said – western medicine is based on science, while all other approaches belong to the prescientific era. There is therefore no need to take very seriously the different ways in which people from other cultures understand problematic experience and behaviour. On this view, the only adaptations that have to be made to mental health services concern language barriers and the niceties of intercultural communication.

This attitude dominated multicultural mental healthcare until the rise of the 'new cross-cultural psychiatry' announced by Kleinman in 1977. Unfortunately, it is still surprisingly popular today. Yet the argument against assuming the supremacy of western ideas is not simply that it is arrogant and ill-founded, but that it further increases the gap between services and their users. In other words, even if – despite all the controversies and shifts of scientific opinion – one regards western psychiatry as the unique custodian of objective truth, it is still necessary to pay attention to other views on mental health if one is serious about providing accessible, appropriate services to the people who hold these views.

What is involved in adapting mental health services to the needs of migrants and ethnic minorities?

In this section we will examine firstly the *accessibility* of services, and secondly their *quality*.

Accessibility

'Access' is a complex notion, referring to the ease with which a person who needs help can actually get it (Dixon-Woods *et al.*, 2006; Gulliford, 2009; Gulliford *et al.*, 2002). Its most basic component is the *entitlement* to use health services. In the USA, where MEMs are particularly likely to lack health insurance, this is a major issue – although at the time of writing there is hope that the situation will soon change. Figures from the Migration Policy Institute in Washington (Ku, 2006) show that non-citizen immigrants are more than three times as likely to be uninsured (44%) as native-born citizens (13%). Outside the USA virtually all industrialised countries operate either national health schemes or social insurance schemes, and in Europe MEMs are normally entitled to coverage at the same level as nationals. Exclusions mainly concern undocumented migrants and asylum seekers, for whom entitlements vary widely. For persons lacking entitlement, (mental) health services are often provided by non-governmental organisations (NGOs).

However, there is a lot more to access than entitlement. Problems of accessibility come to light when it emerges that the proportion of those from a given migrant or ethnic group receiving care is lower than would be expected from the size of the group. Of course, such 'under-utilisation' could simply be because of a lower prevalence of problems in the group – but there must also be reason to believe that the need for care is at least as great in that group as in others. In many countries it is indeed found that certain MEM groups do not make as much use of the services as would be expected. Often, service utilisation is found to increase with the length of time a person has resided in the country, and in particular with language learning and acculturation.

Another sign of poor access is when members of particular groups are found to be more likely to enter care at a later stage, when their symptoms are more severe. In the mental health field this is found among Afro-Caribbean men diagnosed as psychotic in the UK; in the Netherlands similar findings have been observed among Moroccans, Antilleans and Surinamers (for a review see Ingleby, 2008). In many cases, the person in question only enters treatment at all because of intervention by the police. For these groups, we can say that the accessibility of locked wards and padded cells is excellent; however, services are not being reached in earlier stages, when they might be more effective.

Many findings in recent years suggest that the most important challenge for mental health services trying to serve MEM communities concerns not the help that is offered, but its accessibility. Let us therefore examine the different components of access in more detail.

Help-seeking behaviour

The first barrier that has to be overcome is that the person – or those around him or her – must *realise* that they need help. Yet, as we saw above, different groups may have widely varying ideas about when one should seek help, and from whom. People whose attitudes were formed in a situation where few services were available will tend to have a higher threshold for seeking help. Moreover, if people do not think help is available, they will try to find a way of ignoring their need for it: this is why estimates of prevalence rates always need to take into account the (perceived) availability of services.

People may have fundamentally different ideas about the *kind* of help they need, depending on the type of explanatory model to which they adhere. To regard emotional problems, difficulties in personal relationships, addictive behaviour or problems at work as manifestations of illness, and to seek help for them from a healthcare professional, is something that westerners have become increasingly accustomed to doing over the past 50–100 years. But many older westerners, as well as people living in developing countries, are more likely to regard them as moral, religious, social or political problems.

Indeed, it is at the stage of identifying problems and seeking help for them that the biggest barriers to accessing mental health services may arise. There may be a large gap between services and MEM users in terms of the explanatory models assumed on each side. Much recent research has focused on health-seeking behaviour and beliefs among MEM populations. For example, Chinese communities are often reported to make less use of mental health services than other groups (cf. Chen and Kazanjian, 2005; Chen *et al.*, 2010; Kung, 2003). The reasons are complex and include practical barriers, but different assumptions about health and illness, mind and body also appear to play an important role.

Nevertheless, one should not regard 'culture' as a closed box within which people are trapped. A static conception of culture, in which health beliefs are regarded as fixed and mutually incompatible, makes 'bridging the gap' between cultures appear an impossible task. But in the dynamic conception of culture, pioneered by Clifford Geertz (1973) and used by most anthropologists today, ideas about health – like any others – are changeable, and seemingly incompatible ideas may be held by one and the same person. Indeed, from the moment the concept of 'explanatory models' was introduced, critics have pointed out that these models are malleable and complex. 'Medical pluralism', in which mainstream western medicine is used alongside traditional or 'alternative' medical systems, is commonplace in both developing and industrialised countries. Williams and Healy (2001) propose that talking about 'exploratory maps' rather than 'explanatory models' would do more justice to the fluidity of peoples' beliefs. The implication is not that conflicts about 'explanatory models' can be ignored; rather, they should not be seen as an insurmountable barrier to providing healthcare across cultures.

At this point it may be helpful to apply the model of acculturation developed by Berry (1997) to beliefs about health. Migrants who trade in their own ideas about health for those current in the host society are demonstrating *assimilation;* those who maintain their beliefs and reject mainstream ones have opted for *separation. Marginalisation* describes the position of those without any clear beliefs about health at all, while *integration* describes the multi-cultural ideal of 'biculturality', combining one's own cultural heritage with the health beliefs and practices of the host country. As with acculturation in the broader sense, these possibilities are to a large extent constrained by the social environment: if only mainstream health-care is available, migrants will have to learn to use it or go untreated. If, on the other hand, such care is hard for them to access, then they probably turn to healers from their own community – or do without. 'Integration', i.e. drawing simultaneously on both sources, is not encouraged in most health services; yet the message of this chapter is that forcing people to assimilate may not result in optimal use of services. The best way to bridge a gap is to start from both sides, which means promoting health literacy in the community at the same time as 'cultural competence' in the services.

Linguistic barriers to access

Next to entitlement, language barriers can present a formidable obstacle to access. Information about services should be offered in whatever languages are necessary to reach potential users, and high quality interpretation facilities must be available. Some governments are keen to require migrants to become fluent in the national language and are therefore ambivalent about supporting language help. However, the idea of withholding information on health from migrants in the hope that it will encourage them to attend language classes seems both implausible and unwise.

Professional interpretation can be provided by telephone services or face to face. However, health service providers often rely heavily on 'informal' interpreters (family members or friends of the patient, or members of staff – including kitchen and cleaning personnel – who happen to speak the language in question). This saves time and money in the short term, but in the long term it may undermine the quality of treatment and even lead to disastrous results. However, even a professional interpreter cannot simply be regarded as a 'translation machine'; it is not just the words that have to be translated, but their meanings, and this requires on the one hand considerable medical knowledge, and on the other an intimate knowledge of the patients' social and cultural context.

The role of 'cultural mediators'

Related to the role of the interpreter, but distinct from it, is the employment of members of MEM communities as 'mediators' or 'consultants'. In Europe, use of this practice is mainly confined to certain countries (in particular the UK, the Netherlands, Belgium, Spain, France and Italy).

Cultural mediators may be employed in a variety of ways. They may work on their own to perform 'outreaching' functions, such as disseminating information within their own community, guiding people to treatment and even carrying out intakes. They may be used as auxiliaries in a treatment situation, to explain medical ideas to the patient and to make the cultural and social context of the patient more understandable to the medical professional, while at the same time acting as interpreter. Such mediators can fulfil an important role in improving access to healthcare and facilitating treatment, but the different modalities of mediation have not yet been fully worked out, while issues of training and professional status are still unresolved.

Health literacy

Another aspect of access concerns knowledge of the health system and the ability to make use of it. A person not only has to realise that they need help: they must know what kind of help is available and how to go about getting it. This requires knowledge of how the health system works and how to make the most effective use of it.

The term 'health literacy' is often used to refer to these skills and knowledge. Obviously, the problem of providing healthcare for people who *literally* cannot read and write in the dominant language is a serious one – but the concept of 'health literacy' is meant to cover a much wider range of competences. The fact that under-use of services is found less often among migrants who have resided in a country for a longer period suggests that acquiring these competences is part of the wider process of acculturation. Integration programmes for immigrants provide an appropriate context for initiatives to stimulate 'health literacy'.

Such initiatives, however – like all health education and health promotion activities – must acknowledge and respect the differing ways in which potential users already think about health matters. In this respect, the term 'health literacy' is badly chosen, because it equates a person who is not well informed about mainstream healthcare and ideas with one who has no ideas at all. But people with different ideas about health are not necessarily 'illiterate': they may simply be reading different 'texts'[1]. If they interpret illness and health in a different framework, it does not mean their heads are empty: their understanding is simply different. One is reminded of the ethnocentric way in which the term 'cultural deprivation' was used in the 1960s to describe groups that did not share white middle class culture.

To access services requires not only knowledge but social skills, and users who are more socially marginalised (and who may also have the greatest need for care) are less well equipped to negotiate the hurdles involved. They are less likely to be able to locate the information they need, or hold their own in a telephone conversation or face-to-face encounter, or negotiate their way past 'gatekeepers'. Such users are often labelled 'hard to reach', but this is simply blaming the user for the inadequacies of the system: typically, little effort has been expended on designing services that will reach them. 'Outreaching' activities are thus essential to improving the accessibility of services for MEM users.

---

[1] The same applies to the concept of 'therapy compliance'. When people do not follow the prescribed treatment because it conflicts with their beliefs, they are not 'ignoring the rules'; they are simply complying with different ones (Tripp-Reimer *et al.*, 2001).

Perceptions of service providers

Even if a person feels they have a mental health problem and wants to have professional treatment for it, they will not seek treatment if they do not trust the available services and have positive expectations of them. Service providers must be perceived as 'user-friendly' and, in particular, 'migrant- and minority-friendly'. Users must feel respected and understood.

If we are to believe the annual reports of the European Fundamental Rights Agency (FRA, 2009), direct discrimination by individuals is encountered relatively seldom in health services. However, there are many more subtle forms of insensitivity which can give an MEM user the feeling that they do not really 'belong'. Some of these problems can be solved if service providers adopt recruitment policies that ensure the staff are representative of the diversity of the population, but this by itself is not enough: the whole organisation must adopt a receptive attitude to MEMs as a matter of policy.

However, relations between mainstream organisations and members of minority communities do not arise in a vacuum. Deeper political or historical factors, such as the legacy of colonialism, may make it harder to build up trust between service providers and MEMs. At the present time, when majority attitudes to cultural diversity in Europe seem to be becoming less tolerant, it is important to realise that tensions in the wider society between MEM communities and the majority do not stop at the door of the service provider. It is no accident that the hardening of attitudes to migrants in the Netherlands has been accompanied by a rise in the popularity of segregated mental health services, in which clients of migrant origin are helped by caregivers with the same background (May and Ingleby, 2008). Against this background it is more important than ever that mainstream health services should actively develop a close working relationship with the communities they serve.

Working closely with communities is not a new idea: it was the main aim of the 'community mental health' approach which was introduced from the 1960s onwards, as well as being a core ingredient of the notion of primary care promoted by the WHO in its 1978 Declaration of Alma Ata. The principle was also incorporated in the *CLAS Standards on Culturally and Linguistically Appropriate Services* issued in 2000 by the US Office of Minority Health (OMH, 2000). Standard 12 prescribes that:

> Health care organizations should develop participatory, collaborative partnerships with communities and utilize a variety of formal and informal mechanisms to facilitate community and patient/consumer involvement in designing and implementing CLAS-related activities.

Bridging the gap between services and the communities they serve means encouraging the *participation* of those communities. In mental health, however, the notion of participation is mainly interpreted as involving users in their own treatment, rather than involving communities in the design of their own services. Moreover, the 'users' are usually considered to be those who are or have been in treatment, rather than the community as a whole. In fact, it may be even more important to involve those who do *not* make use of mainstream services than those who *do*.

NGOs and self-help organisations may play a vital role in bridging gaps between services and their users. Nevertheless, it is essential that these organisations are not regarded as a substitute for mainstream care. Moreover, they must be truly representative of the communities they purport to represent.

of clinicians who then made consensus diagnoses according to *ICD-10* criteria (ibid.: 1543). But those who wrote down the clinical information were *not* operating blind, and if bias exists it is just as likely to occur at this stage as later in the diagnostic process. Clinical descriptions are not objective photographic records: they are judgements made by human beings, intrinsically based on assumptions and interpretations.

Concerning the higher rates of compulsory admissions, studies reviewed by Bhui (2003) showed that black patients are judged to be more dangerous even when their level of pathology is less serious. In fact, a study by Lorant *et al.* (2007) found that the main reason that minority patients are compulsorily admitted is quite simply *the lack of any alternative*. The GAMIAN guidelines for management of patients with serious mental illness (Agius *et al.*, 2005) show how closer involvement of the community can help to anticipate and prevent such crisis situations. When relationships between a community and the health services are as polarised as the above example from the UK suggest, effective partnerships of this kind are starting with a handicap.

The suitability of treatments for different groups

Because research on this topic is relatively undeveloped, we do not know as much as we need to about the differential responsiveness of different groups to particular kinds of treatment and the modifications that may be necessary. One area currently receiving attention concerns psychopharmacology: there is evidence for ethnic differences in the effects and optimal dosage of drugs (Pi and Simpson, 2005).

A more familiar issue is the type of treatment preferred for different groups. In the UK, as we have seen, forcible restraint and isolation are more often used on black male patients, who are also more likely to receive medication (and in higher doses) as well as being less likely to receive psychotherapy (McKenzie *et al.*, 2001; SCMH, 2002). The notion that minority groups are less likely to benefit from psychotherapy is as widespread as it is empirically ill-founded. There is a good case for regarding it as a form of institutional discrimination.

Cultural competence

This term focuses attention not so much on the particular treatment methods that are used, as the *way* in which they are used. In the past 30 years the concept of 'cultural competence' has undergone several shifts.

- First, the emphasis has changed from *knowledge* (in particular, textbook knowledge about other cultures) to *skills* and *attitudes*.
- Second, it is now regarded as much more important to be aware of one's *own* culturally determined presuppositions and biases than to have a store of information about other people's. In any case, the enormous diversity of present-day migration makes the latter an almost impossible aim: in 2001, a survey registered more than 300 languages spoken by London schoolchildren (Baker and Eversley, 2000).
- Third, in the shift to a 'whole organisation approach', cultural competence is now regarded not just as a property of individual health workers but of entire organisations – indeed, of the whole health system.

At the same time, however, there has been a shift away from emphasising 'cultural differences' to a much broader view of the patient's social environment. This recognises the fact that the present social position of MEMs may be more relevant to their health problems than any 'cultural baggage' they may have brought with them from their country of origin.

Conclusion

The adaptation of mental health services for MEMs is a dynamic and fast-growing area which, after many years of neglect, is beginning to be recognised as a priority in many countries. Efforts by intergovernmental agencies such as the World Health Organization, the International Organization for Migration, the Council of Europe and the European Union to put migrant and minority health on the policy agenda are currently gathering strength: major policy documents are due to be issued by both the WHO and the Council of Europe. The main thrust of current EU efforts to promote 'health equity' is directed to the reduction of socio-economic differences, and the same emphasis is found in UK government policy. While the socio-economic dimension is important to an understanding of MEM health, it is important that migration and ethnicity should continue to be regarded as important issues in their own right.

References

Agius, M., Biočina S. M., Alptekin, K. *et al.* (2005). Basic standards for management of patients with serious mental illness in the community. *Psychiatria Danubina*, **17**, 42–57.

Baker, P., Eversley, J. (eds) (2000). *Multilingual Capital*. London: Battlebridge.

Berry, J. (1997). Immigration, acculturation, adaptation. *Applied Psychology: An International Review*, **46**, 5–68.

Bhui, K. (2003). Over-representation of black people in secure psychiatric facilities. *British Journal of Psychiatry*, **178**, 575.

BMJ (2002). Theme issue 'Too much medicine?' *British Medical Journal*, **324** (7342).

Chen A. W., Kazanjian, A. (2005). Rate of mental health service utilization by Chinese immigrants in British Columbia. *Canadian Journal of Public Health*, **96**, 49–51.

Chen, A. W., Kazanjian, A., Wong, H. *et al.* (2010). Mental health service use by Chinese immigrants with severe and persistent mental illness. *Canadian Journal of Psychiatry*, **55**, 35–42.

Colledge, M., van Geuns, H. A. & Svensson, P. G (eds) (1986). *Migration and Health: Towards an Understanding of the Health Care Needs of Ethnic Minorities*. Proceedings of a Consultative Group on Ethnic Minorities (The Hague, Netherlands, November 28–30, 1983). Copenhagen (Denmark), Regional Office for Europe: World Health Organization.

Dixon-Woods, M., Cavers, D., Agarwal, S. *et al.* (2006). Conducting a critical interpretive synthesis of the literature on access to healthcare by vulnerable groups. *BMC Medical Research Methodology*, **6**, 35.

Eisenberg, L. (1977). Disease and illness. Distinctions between professional and popular ideas of sickness. *Culture, Medicine and Psychiatry*, **1**, 9–23.

Fearon, P., Kirkbride, J. B., Morgan, C. *et al.* (2006). Incidence of schizophrenia and other psychoses in ethnic minority groups: results from the MRC AESOP Study. *Psychological Medicine*, **36**, 1541–50.

Fernando, S. (1991). *Mental Health, Race and Culture*. New York: St Martin's Press.

Fernando, S., Keating, F. (1995). *Mental Health in a Multi-Ethnic Society*. London: Routledge.

Fortier, J. P., Bishop, D. (2003). *Setting the Agenda for Research on Cultural Competence in Health Care: Final Report.* Edited by C. Brach. Rockville, MD: US Department of Health and Human Services Office of Minority Health and Agency for Healthcare Research and Quality.

FRA (2009). *Annual Report 2008*. Vienna: European Agency for Fundamental Human Rights. http://fra.europa.eu/fra/index.php

Geertz, C. (1973). *The Interpretation of Cultures*. New York: Basic Books.

Griner, D., Smith, T. (2006). Culturally adapted mental health intervention: a meta-analytic review. *Psychotherapy: Theory, Research, Practice, Training*, **43**, 531–48.

Gulliford, M. (2009). Modernizing concepts of access and equity. *Health Economics, Policy and Law*, **4**, 223–30.

Gulliford, M., Figueroa-Munoz, J., Morgan, M. et al. (2002). What does 'access to health care' mean? *Journal of Health Services Research and Policy*, 7, 186–8.

HSE (2008). *National Intercultural Health Strategy 2007-2012*. Dublin: Health Service Executive (Ireland).

IASC (2007). *IASC Guidelines on Mental Health and Psychosocial Support in Emergency Settings*. Geneva: Inter-Agency Standing Committee (IASC).

Ingleby, D. (2008). *New Perspectives on Migration, Ethnicity and Schizophrenia*. Willy Brandt Series of Working Papers in International Migration and Ethnic Relations 1/08, IMER/MIM, Malmö University, Sweden.

IOM (2003). *Unequal Treatment: Confronting Racial and Ethnic Disparities in Health Care*. Washington: Institute of Medicine.

Kleinman, A. (1977). Depression, somatisation and the new 'cross cultural psychiatry'. *Social Science and Medicine*, 11, 3–10.

Kleinman, A., Eisenberg, L., Good, B. (1978). Culture, illness, and care: clinical lessons from anthropologic and cross-cultural research. *Internal Medicine*, 88, 251–8.

Ku, L. (2006). *Why Immigrants Lack Adequate Access to Health Care and Health Insurance*. Washington: Migration Policy Institute. http://www.migrationinformation.org/ Feature/display.cfm?id=417

Kung, W. W. (2003). Chinese American's help seeking for emotional distress. *Social Service Review*, 77, 110–34.

Littlewood, R., Lipsedge, M. (1982). *Aliens and Alienists: Ethnic Minorities and Psychiatry*. Harmondsworth: Penguin Books.

Lorant, V., Depuydt, C., Gillain, B. et al. (2007). Involuntary commitment in psychiatric care: what drives the decision? *Social Psychiatry and Psychiatric Epidemiology*, 42, 360–5.

May, R., Ingleby, D. (2008). Samen of apart? Geestelijke gezondheidszorg voor allochtonen. [Together or apart? Mental health care for migrants and ethnic minorities.] *Phaxx: kwartaalblad vluchtelingen en gezondheid*, 4/08, 11–13.

McKenzie, K., Samele, C., Van Horn, E. et al. (2001). A comparison of the course and treatment of psychosis in patients of Caribbean origin and British whites. *British Journal of Psychiatry*, 178, 160–5.

OMH (2000). *National Standards on Culturally and Linguistically Appropriate Services (CLAS)*. Washington: US Department of Health and Health Services, Office of Minority Health. www.omhrc.gov/CLAS.

Pechansky, R., Thomas, J. W. (1981). The concept of access: definitions and relationship to consumer satisfaction. *Medical Care*, 19, 127–40.

Pi, E. H., Simpson, G. M. (2005). Cross-cultural psychopharmacology: a current clinical perspective. *Psychiatric Services*, 56, 31.

Reinhardt, U. (2002). How healthy is our health care? *Princeton Alumni Weekly*, April 10 2002. http://www.princeton.edu/~paw/ web_exclusives/plus/ plus_041002Reinhardt.html

Saha, S., Beach, M. C., Cooper, L. A. (2008). Patient centeredness, cultural competence, and healthcare quality. *Journal of the National Medical Association*, 100, 1275–85.

SCMH (2002). *Breaking the Circles of Fear. A Review of the Relationship Between Mental Health Services and African and Caribbean Communities*. London: Sainsbury Centre for Mental Health.

Singh, S. P., Burns, T. (2006). Race and mental health: there is more to race than racism. *British Medical Journal*, 333, 648–51.

Tripp-Reimer, T., Choi, E., Kelley, L. S. et al. (2001). Cultural barriers to care: inverting the problem. *Diabetes Spectrum*, 14, 13–22.

Van de Vijver, F. J. R., Leung, K. (1997). *Methods and Data Analysis for Cross-cultural Research*. Newbury Park, CA: Sage.

Williams, B., Healy, D. (2001). Perceptions of illness causation among new referrals to a community mental health team: 'explanatory model' or 'exploratory map'? *Social Science and Medicine*, 53, 465–76.

Zandi, T., Havenaar, J. M., Limburg-Okken, A. G. et al. (2007). The need for culture sensitive diagnostic procedures. A study among psychotic patients in Morocco. *Social Psychiatry and Psychiatric Epidemiology*, 43, 244–50.

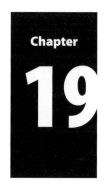

Chapter

19

Intercultural mediation: reconstructing Hermes – the messenger gets a voice

Adil Qureshi, Hilda-Wara Revollo, Francisco Collazos, Jannat el Harrak, Cristina Visiers, María del Mar Ramos and Miguel Casas

Editors' introduction

Cultural competence training deals with making clinicians aware of the need to take cultural factors into account while making assessments, history-taking and planning management. Good clinical practice must be culturally appropriate, taking into consideration factors related to diversity such as culture, religion, gender and sexual orientation. One of the major aspects of cultural awareness training is being aware of how to use interpreters. Sometimes culture brokers are used: these are individuals who belong to a particular cultural group and liaise between their group and the mental health services. Qureshi *et al.* describe the developments of intercultural mediators and advise clinicians on how to use them to the best possible effect. Communication across cultures can be affected by cultural differences but it becomes even more complicated when there is another person present in the therapeutic encounter. Communication occurs at different levels – verbal and non-verbal, through expression of emotions and the use of language. Intercultural mediation involves both message conversion and cultural classification. Thus, clinicians must be aware of its impact in therapeutic encounters and use it appropriately.

Introduction

Despite the increased recognition of the need for preparation of mental health professionals to work with culturally different patients, cultural competence training, generally speaking, remains an objective rather than a reality in most professional preparation programmes (Bhui et al., 2007). Individual cultural competence, even when pertinent training is available, does not guarantee that a clinician will be able to communicate and work effectively with his or her patient. General intercultural awareness, knowledge and skills are not always sufficient, and a clinician may lack specific cultural insight and linguistic competence.

The participation of a third person, trained to facilitate communication, represents a response that is gaining increased acceptance, be it under the rubric of medical interpreter or intercultural mediator, and the like. Despite some differences, all are called upon to 'bridge the linguistic and cultural gap', and implicitly or explicitly, facilitate the therapeutic relationship (Bolton, 2002; Miller *et al.*, 2005). The specific differences between the different roles are ambiguous, with varying degrees of emphasis placed on linguistic and

Migration and Mental Health, ed. Dinesh Bhugra & Susham Gupta. Published by Cambridge University Press. © Cambridge University Press 2011.

cultural interpretation[1]. The specific role that would optimise therapeutic goals, in conjunction with what is realistic, constitutes the focus of this paper. It will be suggested that the conventional notion of the mediator as an 'absent presence' or conduit is untenable for both practical and systemic reasons. Rather, it is argued that this 'third presence' is best conceived of as a 'present presence' that participates as a sort of junior co-therapist following the lead of the clinician.

The thinking in this paper is predicated on our review of existing literature, our clinical experience working with and providing training to intercultural mediators, both in vocational rehabilitation training with the NGO SURT (Associació de donnes per la inserció laboral) as well as in a project of the 'the Caixa' Social and Cultural Outreach Projects and the Catalan Department of Health. Although we initially endorsed the conduit model, we have difficulties working with such a model in the mental health context. In our capacity as trainers and supervisors, we have had many discussions with intercultural mediators who raised some legitimate questions that seriously challenged the received model. Perhaps more poignantly, as clinicians we found that, for all that we attempted to put into practice the absent present model, it simply did not work. Patients would look attentively to the mediator; it was clear that the mediator's presence fundamentally impacted both the therapeutic relationship as well as the dynamic of the session. As this occurred even with the most seasoned and well trained mediators, it was not simply a question of a lack of professional competence. We knew, then, that something had to change. We present below the development of this altered model for intercultural mediation, which, we feel, is consistent with the current literature as well as clinical reality.

Difficulties in intercultural communication

It is not only what the patient says, but how, to whom, under what circumstances, and in whose presence, that influence the actual meaning. Miscommunication can easily occur when each participant believes that he or she understands the other but actually does not, precisely because the message was interpreted in the framework of each participant's cultural context. The potential impact this can have on diagnosis and treatment is considerable. If a mental health professional believes that he or she has correctly understood the patient, the diagnosis can be inaccurate, and thus the treatment inadequate at best and contraindicated at worst.

Free and spontaneous expression in one's mother tongue are not the only aspects that are impeded for the immigrant patient who is not fluent in the local language. Given that the self develops in a specific language, cultural context and environment, its access to memory and expression may vary according to the language used in terms of connotations, richness and attitudes. A person with limited language proficiency could feel inhibited linguistically as well as conceptually and emotionally. Even if the patient is fluent in the language of the clinician, memories, images and ideas that arise could vary linguistically. The fact of being able to choose the language in which treatment is carried out could inspire greater security and confidence in the triadic therapeutic relationship – that is, with the interintercultural mediator and clinician. This is all the more pertinent in mental healthcare given that it is

---

[1] Recognising that some differences exist, for the purposes of this paper, the two – medical interpreter and interintercultural mediator – unless otherwise indicated, will be used interchangeably. For the purposes of brevity, the word 'mediator' will be used in place of 'interintercultural mediator', and in no way should be confused with the conventional mediator role related to conflict management.

precisely through language and the therapeutic relationship that the core of psychotherapeutic work is developed.

Although it is clear that clinician cultural competence can contribute significantly to quality of treatment, there are a number of factors that all too often lie beyond the purview of even the most culturally competent clinician, and it is here that the importance of the intercultural mediator can be seen.

Medical interpretation is increasingly understood to involve more than the literal conversion of a message from one language to another (Hsieh, 2007; Messent, 2003; Tribe and Lane, 2009; Verrept, 2008; also see Chapter 20). Communication itself is far more complex, and operates on a number of different levels. In brief, there is a lot more to communication than the dictionary meaning of the words uttered; 'mere translation' will not suffice to ensure that communication takes place. Communication operates at the non-verbal, affective and contextual levels, and, as applied to interpretation 'involves the fine art and science of translating at the literal, metaphorical, cultural, and nonverbal levels of communication' (Raval and Smith, 2003 page 8).

Intercultural mediation in mental health

The role of the intercultural mediator is traditionally referred to as that of a 'bridge' between cultures, in which communication and, as such, understanding between the culturally different participants is improved while the interference of difference is reduced. Linguistic and cultural interpretation in the triadic interview constitute key functions of the interintercultural mediator in addition to the tasks of informing service users about how to use the healthcare system and to provide cultural orientation to service providers (Beltran, 2001; Collazos et al., 2005; Verrept, 2008). Cultural and linguistic interpretation has been conceptualised, for medical interpreters, with a specific focus on the message and predicated on the 'mail carrier' or 'conduit' model, in which the task of the mediator is to ensure that the message is delivered (Hsieh, 2007; Messent, 2003). Such a model represents a simplification and, indeed, reification of a complex and dynamic process. At the same time, the model can serve as a foundation for understanding the basic functions of the interintercultural mediator in mental healthcare.

The basic function most called upon for use is that of *message conversion*, or linguistic interpretation. In a nutshell, the mediator is simply called upon to convert the message from one language to another. It is understood, however, that this may not be enough; at times literal interpretation is not sufficient, or is indeed counterproductive in those situations in which the meaning of the message is nuanced. The mediator may function as a *message clarifier*, providing not only a literal interpretation but also clarifying the message's meaning given the cultural context. The use of metaphor is perhaps the most straightforward example. If a patient were to say, for example, 'I feel blue', it would be of little help were the mediator to say 'me siento azul', because 'blue' does not have affective significance in Spanish. If the mediator were to *only* provide the metaphoric interpretation, 'me siento triste' without the literal translation, it is possible that important clinical information would be lost, in that it *could* be the case that the patient has some idiosyncratic or indeed psychotic meaning behind his words. Thus it would be optimal were the mediator to say 'I feel blue, which is a metaphor for feeling sad', thus allowing the clinician to make the clinical interpretation.

Finally, there may be times when awareness of the cultural context is necessary to understand what the patient is attempting to communicate, and *cultural clarification* or contextualisation is needed. The words may convey one meaning. Even when their meta-phoric aspects are understood, the context can shift the specific meaning. Thus a patient may respond 'yes' to the question, 'do you understand?' but the specific meaning of the 'yes' can vary given a variety of situational and relational cues. It could also be that the patient explains a situation that is incoherent given the clinician's cultural context; for example, the newly divorced Moroccan woman who asserts that returning to her parent's village is simply not an option. Given the woman's cultural context, such a return is, indeed, untenable. In such cases it will be necessary for the mediator to provide contextual information to enable the clinician to understand. The mediator could explain that in more conservative parts of Morocco, a divorced woman is viewed as a societal outcast and can bring shame to her family, and indeed community, to the extent that she would most likely be overtly and covertly rejected.

Communication and, indeed, behaviour, values, cognition and emotion are highly con-textual. What a person says, how they say it, the references they make, the actions or feelings they describe and their goals and desires are all in part circumscribed by culture and context. Although the mediator can clarify the patient's message, this in itself does not necessarily enable the clinician to understand the patient correctly. Given that a considerable proportion of communication occurs non-verbally, linguistic interpretation and meaning clarification may not be sufficient.

What a patient says may not make sense, or may be misinterpreted because the clinician is not aware of the relationship between the context and the words spoken. Thus it may appear that an African patient is exhibiting psychotic symptoms by their repeated reference to the play of spirits or their active conversations with deceased ancestors, whereas in fact such behaviour is culturally normative. It may be that the patient appears to lack social skills or insight or planning ability. It could be that these perceptions say more about the interpretive filter of the clinician and the medical context than about any 'objective' problem on the part of the patient, although it is possible that the clinical interpretations are correct. At any rate, in such situations the mediator can function as a cultural clarifier to contextualise the situation such that the clinician can better interpret the clinical information provided by the patient. The mediator does not *explain* the culture of the patient (a notion that itself is rather incoherent), nor does the mediator determine if a particular behaviour is indicative of psychopathology. For example, with a sub-Saharan patient who complains about having an animal in his stomach, the mediator might say, 'it can happen that distressed people from sub-Saharan Africa feel that they have an animal in their body'. He or she would *not* say, 'this patient is somatisising, but is not psychotic'.

Following a somewhat different perspective, Rachel Tribe (Tribe and Morrisey, 2004) outlines four models of interpretation that are germane to this discussion. The first is the linguistic mode, which is that of the message converter. The psychotherapeutic or construc-tionist mode is similar to that of the message clarifier in that the literal message takes a backstage to the meaning and feeling of the words. The advocate or community interpreter takes on the role of representing the patient's interests and protecting his or her rights. Finally, the cultural broker–bicultural worker is similar to the cultural clarification role.

The therapeutic relationship and the role of the intercultural mediator

The conventional role of the intercultural mediator is to facilitate communication or bridge the so-called gap between cultures. In the context of mental healthcare the specific role and functions are more demanding and complex (Bolton, 2002; Collazos *et al.*, 2005; Drennan and Swartz, 2002; Miller *et al.*, 2005; Raval and Smith, 2003). The complexity is in large part related to the impact of the intercultural mediator on the psychiatric or psychotherapeutic process. Given the importance of the therapeutic relationship in mental health diagnosis and treatment (Joe *et al.*, 2001; Martin *et al.*, 2000; Norcross, 2002) and given that the development of the therapeutic relationship is more complex in an intercultural context (Blue and Gonzalez, 1992; Paris *et al.*, 2005; Qureshi, 2005), a relevant function of the intercultural mediator, and perhaps the most crucial, is the facilitation of the therapeutic relationship.

The presence of an intercultural mediator in mental healthcare, particularly psychotherapy, can have an impact on the therapeutic relationship. It is not unusual for the patient to 'look to' the mediator as an ally, as a referent, as someone with whom he or she can identify, to the extent that the presence of the mediator, rather than facilitating the therapeutic relationship, detracts from it (Bolton, 2002; Bot, 2005; Miller *et al.*, 2005). Because it is the mediator who speaks the language that the patient understands, even when the clinician maintains eye contact with the patient and addresses her or him directly, even when the mediator instructs the patient to look at the clinician, all too often the primary bond, at least at the outset (see Bolton, 2002), is between the patient and the mediator. It is precisely for this reason that it is recommended by the conduit model that all participants act in such a way as to minimise the protagonism of the mediator (Razban, 2003).

Received wisdom suggests that the optimal role for the mediator is that of an 'absent presence', which is identified as that of the conduit, black-box or robot, 'nonthinking, nonfeeling, and yet highly skilled translation machines' (Hsieh, 2008: p. 1367). The idea is that optimal intercultural mediation is that in which the mediator does nothing more than lend her or his voice, as it were, to the therapist and patient. Taken as such, the role of the mediator is extremely limited, and it is *as if* there are only two bodies in the consulting room.

Such a model is promoted precisely because, in theory, it involves minimal alteration of the standard dyadic therapeutic relationship. Clinician and patient continue the therapeutic work with only a change in voice. At issue is only correct application of mediator technique; if the mediator correctly executes her or his task, the presence of the mediator will not be felt (Razban, 2003).

Although such a model would appear to be optimal, research and experience suggest that it is untenable. Two reasons can be identified: one is that mediators and interpreters generally reject such a passive role represented by their adoption of the 'co-diagnostician role' (Dysart-Gale, 2005; Hsieh, 2008; Miller *et al.*, 2005), and the other is that it defies patterns of human relationship and communication, as systems and contextualist theory makes clear.

Co-diagnostician role

Hsieh (2007, 2008) has written extensively about this very issue, and has developed Davidson's (2002) notion of the 'co-diagnostician', which is defined by interpreters adopting strategies that extend beyond interpreters' functions in bridging the linguistic and cultural difference, and which overlap with providers' responsibilities and functions (Hsieh, 2007: p. 925); Bot (2003) refers to these as 'boundary crossings'.

Through in-depth interviews and clinical observation, Hsieh (2008) found that medical interpreters' performance consistently extended beyond that of the conduit, to the extent that they at times adopted responsibilities proper to the medical staff. In actual practice, then, it would appear that mediators adopt a role that is more active than that prescribed by the conduit model, which more often than not serves to impede or derail the therapeutic process.

A confounding element is that few clinicians are trained to work with mediators, which means that they do not necessarily have a clear idea of what roles and functions they can expect (Tribe and Lane, 2009). In addition, it is not unusual for clinicians to request mediators to, in effect, cover for them (e.g. explain to a patient their treatment; extract from the patient the presenting problem; 'convince' the patient that he or she should trust the clinician and/or treatment). The adoption of the co-diagnostician role is in part a response to the explicit and implicit needs of immigrant patients as identified by the mediator. Indeed, a large part of the complication is role ambiguity, which has at its origin not only a lack of awareness on the part of clinicians but also a lack of training on the part of the mediator and a lack of formal recognition and definition of the latter's professional role. All of this renders a mediator more prone to adopt the co-diagnostician role, more often than not with the best of intentions.

The role of the intercultural mediator in managing 'cultural differences' is complex, and can easily extend into the co-diagnostician role in that the mediator, ostensibly in the interest of cultural sensitivity, alters an aspect of the message. Hsieh cites an interview with an interpreter who discussed the clinician's question 'How many sexual partners do you have?'

> [Providers] ask about sexual contact outside of the marriage, which is really [a] bad question. But, I ask them. It is very *offensive* . . . I said, 'Does your husband go with other women?' . . . In that way, you give responsibility to the husband, because Muslim women are very faithful to their husbands.
> (Hsieh, 2008, p. 1378)

Here the interpreter assumes control over the interview such that the meaning and purpose of the original question is compromised. To some extent, it could be argued that the interpreter adopted the psychotherapist role, in which meaning is given primacy over literal translation, combined with the culture broker role, in which cultural variables are attended to (Tribe and Morrisey, 2004). Unfortunately, in the process, the interpreter engages in cultural reductionism by assuming that simply because the patient is Muslim a question about sexual contact outside of marriage will be offensive, and that Muslim wives are faithful. Perhaps more problematic is that the answer the clinician receives will be the mediator's interpretation of the meaning of the patient's response to a question that is rather different from the original. The real danger is when the mediator assumes such 'control', shifting the meanings without explicitly informing the clinician. At issue here are three related problems that would appear to be germane to the boundary crossings that occur in the co-diagnostician role: (1) the mediator in effect takes control of the session, and (2) changes the content, (3) without informing the clinician, which, individually and especially combined, can have a negative impact on the therapeutic relationship and process.

Process issues can also have an impact on mental health treatment with mediators. In any mediator role, but particularly that of the conduit, the mediator is exposed to bearing the brunt of the patient's emotional expression (Miller *et al.*, 2005; Raval and Smith, 2003), which is not only prejudicial to the mediator but also has an impact on the therapeutic flow in that, in effect, the clinician is 'left out' of the loop. Furthermore, the mediator, who is not, after all, a trained mental health professional, may respond to the emotional charge in a non-professional manner, offering words of encouragement and the like (e.g. 'there, there, things will get better, you will see') that can not only interrupt the therapeutic flow and impede the development of the therapeutic relationship with the clinician, but can also provide the patient with false expectations of improvement at the hands of the mediator. Not only, then, does the patient have expectations that may not be realistic; she or he also situates the locus of change in the mediator.

One of the challenges for the intercultural mediator is that linguistic interpretation may, at times, conflict with the therapeutic relationship. Many patients have a rudimentary command of the language of the mainstream culture, and thus some of the therapeutic interview can be carried out without the intervention of the mediator. It is here that the mediator must have the capacity to determine when the therapeutic relationship has primacy, and when the mediator should withdraw and allow the patient to engage directly with the clinician, in spite of the rather obvious language limitations. There may be moments of, for example, emotional expression, wherein what is important is the relational exchange between the clinician and the patient, and which requires an unmediated process. The mediator who is not sensitive to such a process may conscientiously continue to translate, interfering with the therapeutic process.

Contextualist and systems theory

Another reason that the conduit model is untenable is that, as systems theory makes clear, any change to the system fundamentally alters it (von Bertalanffy, 1968). A system is characterised by the dynamic interactions of its components and the non-linearity of those interactions. Any change in a member of or an addition to the system will have an impact on the other members. There is a circularity and interconnection between all members of the system; therefore, the intercultural mediator in the triadic interview has an effect on all of the participants of the system and conditions the others. Furthermore, the mediator is at the front line of the communication, to the extent that one commentator refers to the mediator as a 'gatekeeper' (Davidson, 2000). The metaphor of a 'bridge' is accurate to the extent that not only does the mediator link the two sides, he or she also resides not as an equal and third point in a triangle, but as the very mechanism that controls the flow of communication between the two participants.

A variety of philosophical and psychological approaches understand human interaction to be both contextual and mutual (Jacobs, 1992; Orange *et al.*, 2001). On the one hand, the specific context of any interaction has an impact. Thus a particular therapist along with a particular patient and particular interintercultural mediator in a particular moment in a particular place combine to create a unique relational dynamic. This suggests that independently of what the mediator does or does not do, her or his presence has an impact on the relational dynamics. The notion of mutuality takes this one step further. Not only does the presence of each participant impact the dynamic, each participant affects each of the others. Thus how the patient shows up, for example, is a function of the particular time and place, as well as her or his reaction to both clinician and mediator.

What all of this suggests is that the role of the mediator in mental healthcare should be reconsidered. The ideal of an absent presence is unrealistic – in effect, it denies the proverbial 'elephant in the room' and suggests that therapy can occur as usual. The danger is that unacknowledged relational dynamics can impact the therapeutic process. Unacknowledged, there is no way, in effect, to regulate between those appropriate and inappropriate boundary crossings such that nothing can be done to alter the situation; no mechanisms are in place that the clinician can use to take charge of these dynamics. An appropriate boundary crossing would be one in which the mediator perceives that one of the participants misunderstands the other owing to different cultural contexts, whereas it would be inappropriate for the mediator to try to calm a patient when expressing emotional distress (Bot, 2003). On the other hand, by conceptualising the role of the mediator as an active participant, under the direction of the clinician, problems can be headed off at the pass.

The junior co-therapist model presented is consistent with the three-person psychology model elaborated by Bot (Bot, 2003; Bot and Wadensjö, 2004). A one-person approach is characterised by an exclusive focus on the psychological processes of the patient, whereas a two-person approach, as exemplified in the relational shift in psychoanalysis, incorporates the person of the therapist into the therapeutic process, predicated on the notion that human beings are fundamentally relational. The three-person approach, then, is one that overtly acknowledges the mediator as part of the therapeutic context. Systemic and contextualist approaches, which underlie the thinking in this paper, have a strong 'here-and-now' orientation, meaning that therapeutic interventions, as appropriate, focus on relational and transferential processes, such as the patient's reaction to the mediator, for example. At the same time, any therapeutic orientation, as well as the psychiatric interview, can benefit from this approach, which, perhaps, is best illustrated when the mediator intervenes to clarify a message or contextualise a situation.

Between the conduit at one extreme and co-diagnostician at the other, we suggest that the junior co-therapist represents the optimal option. In short, a role, midway between that of the conduit or blackbox and that of the co-diagnostician, the junior co-therapist, is optimal. The role involves a minimisation of a distracting presence of the mediator for the therapeutic relationship which is understood to be centred on the link between the clinician and the patient. At the same time, the presence of a third person, as systems and contextualist theory as well as clinical experience demonstrate, indicates the importance of formally recognising the presence of the mediator, including her or him in the session, and allowing a degree of autonomy to initiate appropriate interventions, always under the direction of the clinician. As such, the mediator's presence will be accepted and over the course of the treatment he or she can adopt a degree of initiative, following the clinician's focus such that the primary therapeutic relationship is not compromised. For example, if the mediator perceives that either the clinician or the patient did not understand the other's message, he or she would be free to bring this up to both parties.

Role of the intercultural mediator: not a mail carrier but a junior co-therapist

The presence of an intercultural mediator inevitably affects the therapeutic dyad. Clinical experience demonstrates that more competent mediators have the capacity to read the situation effectively and adapt their participation according to the therapeutic demands. The role of the mediator is not 'fixed' but rather is best conceptualised in the service of communication between patient and clinician and of the therapeutic relationship. All of this makes more or less functional sense in the context of healthcare mediation in general, where the message being communicated is relatively straightforward; the description of symptoms is distinct from the symptoms themselves. In mental health it is often the case that the symptom description is itself symptomatic, and for this reason requires sensitive and intelligent clinical interpretation. Such interpretation, however, is complicated given the cultural variability that can impact how symptoms are presented and described, and it is precisely for this reason that the intercultural mediator is called upon for both linguistic *and* cultural interpretation.

An alternative model for the mental health intercultural mediator is that of a junior co-therapist operating in the context of a three-person psychology, wherein the mediator is not a mere conduit or absent presence but rather an active participant. The mediator is in no way to be confused with the principal clinician; it remains the psychologist or psychiatrist who directs and has responsibility for the patient's treatment. The contribution of the mediator is in the service of the treatment as planned by the clinician. This means that the basic roles as outlined above remain, as does the need for the mediator to adapt to the demands of the specific situation. What changes is the attitude: the mediator forms an active – a present presence – part of the therapeutic triad.

In effect, the proposal is that rather than function as a 'co-diagnostician' in which the mediator can all too easily depart from therapeutically coherent interventions, the mediator functions as a sort of passive agent, a very junior co-therapist who is openly recognised and incorporated therapeutically. The therapist will thus orientate the treatment, capitalising on the mediator's presence. This could take on many forms, including, for example, addressing here-and-now relational issues, role plays pertinent to the patient's therapeutic process, or the sharing of relevant lived experiences. Bot (2003) suggests capitalising on the patient's transference by conceiving of the mediator as a 'blank screen' onto which the patient projects her or his dreams and fantasies. This can be done precisely by exploring these projections in the therapeutic process. In addition, the role of the mediator as an active participant can also facilitate the open incorporation of mediator observations, warnings and the like. Whatever the specifics, however, it must be underscored that it is the clinician who directs the session, with the mediator taking on a supporting role, always following the direction of the former.

Two examples are provided below, drawn from our clinical experience. In the first, the clinician used the mediator to provide a sort of mirroring, such that the patient can get a sense of interpersonal styles that are more or less effective.

> Aisha, a 34-year-old Moroccan woman, was referred to the clinic for depression and a suspected psychosomatic paralysis. One of Aisha's chief issues was her timidity. She frequently lamented that she had few friends, asserting that she was very lonely. She felt that she was simply too shy to meet new people. She was increasingly aware that she was uncomfortable socially and that there was something in her interactions that did not serve her well. On the other hand, she noted that her brother was very effective socially. To explore in greater detail her social interactions, the therapist asked her about her observations of the mediator. What was it that the mediator did? How did she engage with both the patient and clinician? As they explored Aisha's perceptions of the mediator's interpersonal styles, the clinician shifted the focus to differences between the two, and in the process asked both Aisha and the mediator to observe their experience of the other. In the following discussion, in which Aisha received empathic feedback from both mediator and clinician, she was able to get a sense of how her interpersonal style was socially detrimental, and then to identify strategies by which to shift her interactions with others.

In the following example, the clinician wanted to provide the patient with the opportunity to practise as well as experience a conversation with his father. The presence of the mediator meant that the clinician could observe the patient during the process. In addition, the feedback from the mediator concerning his experience of the patient's efforts could appear less contrived than would be the case had the role play been carried out with the clinician.

> Zia, a 26-year-old Pakistani man, felt he had a long overdue conversation with his father. He had been in Spain for 4 years now, and was beginning to like the life here. He had fallen in love with a Spanish woman and was increasingly uncomfortable with the constant

questions about marriage. His mother would frequently tell him about other cousins and relations of his age who had married. She would also tell him about possible brides. He dreaded his upcoming visit as he knew that he would be asked to take tea with various prospects. He was not the slightest bit interested. He was worried about telling his parents, especially his father, that he had no intention of marrying a Pakistani woman, that in fact he was in no rush to get married and that he was dating a Spanish woman. The therapist asked him to role-play the conversation with the mediator, who, of course, translated the entire exchange as per usual. The therapist then asked the mediator to comment on his sensations, reactions and emotions with the objective of providing the patient with a corrective experience or with possible reactions of his father.

Returning to the example of the mediator who considered that a Muslim woman would be offended by a question about extramarital sexual relations, in the junior co-therapist model proposed, the mediator could overtly comment that such themes can be delicate or indeed offensive in Muslim cultures. In such a situation the mediator would give voice to both cultural perspectives, that is, that of the patient's culture and that of the 'mental health' culture, opening a space in which all three participants could give their perspective on the issue. In this way the issue is placed on the table such that all have a more or less clear sense of things. If the patient does indeed feel uncomfortable, this can be expressed, providing the clinician with the necessary information 'in the open' with which to adapt the intervention.

The manner in which the mediator is incorporated into the therapy session is limited only by the imagination of the therapist, always, of course, putting therapeutic integrity as the priority.

Transference and countertransference

Clinical psychiatry and psychology frequently involve strong affect, unusual ideation and difficult life situations which can be emotionally demanding, particularly for those who are not specifically trained in mental health. For the mediator, given the interethnic interplay which is frequently present, is exposed, then, to potentially complex transferential reactions. Given that there are three participants, there are exponentially more transferential relationships than in standard dyadic therapy. The mediator may also have reactions to the clinician, on the one hand, and on the other, have her or his fantasies about the relationship between the clinician and the patient. If this is combined with the respective transferential reactions of the patient and clinician, there is considerable transferential material present when a mediator participates. Because the mediator is the only one who has unmediated (as it were) contact with each participant, both the patient and the clinician may be prone to wondering – and perhaps fantasising – as to whether or not the mediator is *really* communicating what is being said. In addition, the clinician and patient, because they are not privy to the exact interchange between the mediator and the other, may have fantasies about the nature of the relationship.

In short, transference and countertransference can be a potential impediment to effective treatment. It is thus essential that the mediator be trained to manage her or his emotional responses to the patient situation at hand to avoid interventions or behaviours that are not in the interest of the patient. At the same time, the transferential relationship can be used therapeutically.

The patient may identify with the mediator, and as such may feel closer to the mediator than the clinician, which in turn can evoke reactions in the clinician, who is unaccustomed to having anything or anyone come between herself or himself and the patient. Further, Bot

(2005) makes the interesting point that the clinician can never be sure whether what he or she treats is the experience of the patient or that of the interpreter.

In the standard intercultural mediator role, the mediator is constantly negotiating between the pull and push between clinician and patient. Depending on a host of contextual and personal factors, the mediator may be more closely allied with one or the other. These alliances are in large part a function of transference and they can remain hidden, having an invisible impact on the therapeutic process.

Untreated transference can complicate the therapy process considerably, and this is all the more so when there are exponentially more transferential relationships to be dealt with in the triadic relationship. Treating transference, however, in the conduit model is in effect incoherent because the model denies the active presence of the mediator. What this suggests is that the presence of the mediator must be explicitly acknowledged for transference to be effectively treated.

The clinician, who is responsible for the therapeutic process, is the one who should direct any clinical exploration of transference. It goes without saying that transference between clinician and mediator is best attended to without the presence of the patient, to minimise the impact on the therapeutic relationship.

Mental health treatment and the culturally different

In the growing literature addressing psychological and psychiatric treatment of immigrant patients there is considerable variability as to what sort of adaptations, if any, are required (Comas-Diaz, 2003). Differences in the concept of self, of causality, of locus of control, among others, can have a profound impact on the way change and the treatment process are understood.

Cultural competence has been introduced as a means of managing such differences (Qureshi *et al.*, 2008); however, it does not necessarily follow that the work of the mediator would be reduced to 'mere translation' with a well trained clinician. The specific role of the mediator in the face of process-related differences is complex, because it is directly related to the very nature of mental health treatment with the culturally different. In large part the question revolves around the degree to which, and in what way, treatment should be modified. From an absolutist perspective, no interesting adjustment is required as it views all humans as made of the same stuff. From a universalist or derived etic perspective, although all humans are biological creatures, we are also cultural, and to that end the goals, tasks and perhaps even the process of therapy will have to take culture and difference into consideration and adapt accordingly. Finally, from a relativist perspective, culture is so central to human experience that only a culture-specific sort of treatment will be effective, to the extent that psychotherapy as we know it will not be appropriate for many non-western peoples.

Two issues come into play here, revolving around the respective vision of the clinician and mediator of. On the one hand, the mediator may opt for a more relativist perspective than the clinician; on the other, the mediator may be more culturally competent than the clinician. The two could overlap, most certainly; however, a mediator who adopts a relativist stance could in effect clash with a culturally competent clinician who adopts a derived etic approach. A possible situation is one in which the mediator feels that the clinician relies excessively on an absolutist perspective, well exemplified by Messent (2003, p. 136), who reports on an interpreter who did not feel that a Bangladeshi family would understand that they would be included in the treatment process for a son. The interpreter felt that he would have to explain, in detail, what the clinician meant by the phrase, 'we will work together until we find a way of helping him get better'. Key here is, in Messent's words, 'The interpreter knew that the parents' initial expectation of their consultation with the psychiatrist would be that she would make a diagnosis and then a medical intervention' (page 136). What is at issue here is who has responsibility for what. A competent clinician will be aware that many service users, immigrant or nationals, may have a minimal idea of what is involved in mental health treatment, and thus at the very outset the treatment process should be explained, and, as appropriate, negotiated. To what extent the example given by Messent represents good interpreter practice and to what extent it reveals clinical incompetence is debatable. Furthermore, the very notion that anyone 'knows' the initial expectations of a client, a priori, itself is dubious, as it veers closely towards cultural reductionism.

The junior co-therapist role of the mediator is advantageous here because, once again, rather than the mediator taking her or his own initiative in the face of what she or he feels is a potential source of cultural misunderstanding, the issue itself can be addressed by all participants. The mediator can say, to the patient, translating what the clinician has said 'we will work together until we find a way of helping him get better. Does this make sense?' He could then say to the clinician, 'because many Bangladeshis are not familiar with psychotherapy, I asked if the idea of working together makes sense'. This could easily give rise to a conversation about the expectations about the treatment process in which the next steps and roles of each participant could be negotiated.

The danger of leaving much unsaid is that, unless perspectives are made explicit, the mediator may feel a professional obligation to respond in the face of what they may perceive as cultural incompetence of the clinician, even if the clinician is 'competent' yet has a different perspective. Of course, much of this can be avoided by addressing strategies and the like during a briefing session prior to the visit; however, it is also the case that not everything can be anticipated. At a very minimum the therapeutic orientation should be addressed explicitly. This will also allow for the overall issue of adaptation to be overtly discussed. The junior co-therapist role allows the mediator to raise issues as deemed pertinent in the context of the authority of the clinician, rather than as something that needs to be inserted into the therapeutic space at whatever cost.

Working with an interintercultural mediator

Even when the interintercultural mediator is highly competent and well trained, to fully take advantage of her or his presence requires that the professionals adapt their working style. Although in this chapter we have suggested that the mediator be viewed as a junior co-therapist, this requires that the mediator is sufficiently trained in mental health, which is not always the case. Put differently, effective use of an intercultural mediator requires that the clinician have a solid understanding of what he or she can expect from the mediator, be disposed to set forth the parameters for the intervention, and then adapt the interview accordingly (see Tribe and Lane, 2009 for an overview of working with interpreters in mental health). To that end it is essential that the clinician and mediator meet prior to the interview with the patient. Ground rules and expectations should be outlined, the clinician should advise the mediator as to the objective of the interview and any potentially sensitive or difficult issues can be discussed. It provides the opportunity for both parties to clarify how they work and what can be expected from each other during the session. It is during the briefing that strategies can be identified, in which the therapist can alert the mediator to the sorts of interventions that he or she has in mind, such as role plays, and suppressive or expressive techniques. It also provides the mediator with the chance to advise the therapist as to the cultural appropriateness of the intervention in question.

As the mediator is conventionally understood to function as the voice of clinician and patient, the standard recommendation is that the mediator speak in the first person. In the junior co-therapist model, there is no pretence towards an absent presence, giving more leeway for the mediator to speak in her or his own voice. The switching from first person to second or third person can have clinical relevance. On the one hand, the mediator may switch to third person as a means of distanciation from overwhelming emotional material. On the other, it could be the case that the specific format used by the patient is itself therapeutically relevant, and, could get 'lost in translation' by strict adherence to first person usage.

The 'rule' that the clinician and patient should always direct themselves to each other becomes less rigid precisely because, in the suggested approach, the specific interactions in the room can be incorporated into the therapeutic dialogue. This is not to say that it is not recommended that the clinician and patient speak directly to each other since they do form the primary therapeutic relationship. It could be clinically relevant, and thus worth exploring, if, for example, the patient looks at the mediator when speaking of certain issues and at the clinician when speaking of others.

Given the nature of mental healthcare, the ethical principles of precision, neutrality and impartiality are key for an effective therapeutic approach. The clinician and mediator must work effectively together to create a comfortable and safe psychotherapeutic environment. This demands that the mediator provides a self-presentation as the therapeutic relationship develops in a system of three. The skills and attitudes of the mediator play a central role in the trust that the patient grants both professionals.

The participation of the mediator, who more than likely provides consecutive translation, means that shorter, more concise language should be used that avoids jargon and argot as much as possible. At first it may feel that the session is choppy and that there is a loss of flow and, given that extra time is needed for the translation, this is certainly true. By active incorporation of the mediator into the session as a junior co-therapist in the context of a three-person psychology, the inclusion of the mediator will be more comfortable and effective. This means that, rather than acting as though the mediator is not present, the mediator's participation is acknowledged and indeed used to advantage. Clearly, however, this requires that the mediator have the ability and know-how to respond, that he or she understands where the clinician is headed.

To facilitate neutrality in the mediator and precision in communication, a debriefing session between mediator and clinician is highly useful. In the post-session interview the two can review any doubts, suggestions or insights, as well as discuss how the clinical team managed the therapeutic exchange.

The professionalisation of intercultural mediation: training, trust and wellbeing

The junior co-therapist role is tenable if and only if both clinician and mediator are well prepared. This is because the shift is such that what is traditionally a much more limited mediator role transforms from an absent presence to a present presence.

For intercultural mediation to be effective, whatever the specific role, it is imperative that the clinician can trust that the mediator will not only faithfully reproduce the meanings and not function as a gatekeeper, but also that the presence and participation of the mediator will do no harm to the therapeutic process. Given the complexity of intercultural mediation, particularly the model proposed in this paper, in-depth training is essential.

Whereas in the USA the tendency has been towards medical interpretation, in European countries such as Belgium, France, Switzerland and Spain, the trend has been towards intercultural mediation. As may be evident from this article, the latter places greater focus on intercultural communication and healthcare than that present in medical interpretation. For example, in Catalonia, Spain, a training initiative funded by the foundation of the Bank la Caixa and organised by the Catalan Department of Health consists of some 200 hours of training in such diverse modules as medical anthropology, community health, cultural competence, ethics, intercultural mediation in distinct healthcare contexts, professional identity and intercultural communication. In addition, the students receive 40 hours of role playing and group supervision as well as individual supervision in their workplace. This training has been certified by the Catalan Health Studies Institute, representing an important step towards the professionalisation of this model.

As has been noted throughout this article, the mediator is exposed to considerable stress and emotional pressure. To that end, it is essential that individual and/or group supervision be made available (Tribe and Lane, 2009; Verrept, 2008). As part of the project referred to above, individual and group supervision is carried out throughout the year-long training programme, and subsequently group supervision is made available to all mediators. The objective of the supervision is to provide a forum in which to explore and attempt to resolve complications and difficulties at emotional, technical, conceptual and institutional levels related to intercultural mediation. The supervision follows the general format and spirit of psychotherapy supervision, and is generally valued as the most useful aspect of the clinical training. The question of boundaries and the difficulties of clarifying their role in the triadic relationship, as well as the management of emotions, are the issues most frequently addressed.

Conclusion

The notion that a 'two-person' model can be maintained with the presence of an interinter-cultural mediator is untenable for both practical and systemic reasons. On the one hand, despite the ideal of an absent presence in which the mediator in effect lends his or her voice to the clinician and patient, in actual practice the mediator adopts a 'co-diagnostician' role which is characterised by boundary violations, some of which can have deleterious effects on the clinical process. On the other hand, in the context of mental healthcare, the very notion that the addition of a third party to the clinical space will have no impact, particularly when the mediator controls the linguistic flow, is inconsistent with systems theory and contextu-alism. We have proposed shifting the view to a 'three-person' model in which the mediator is overtly recognised and incorporated into the clinical process, in which he or she adopts a sort of junior co-therapist role. The adoption of such a model clarifies role issues sufficiently to avoid transgressive boundary crossings, provides the mediator with clear guidelines from which to clarify messages and contextualise cultural issues, allows the clinician to control the therapeutic process more smoothly, and affords a variety of process interventions that could be clinically useful.

Intercultural mental healthcare can be very challenging, which requires that the clinician incorporate new information as well as methodological and attitudinal changes in their engagement with culturally different patients. Intercultural mediation is a solid proposal given that it facilitates not only communication, in the broadest sense of the word, but also the therapeutic relationship.

The model proposed here is particularly appropriate in mental healthcare because it is responsive to the needs of the field. Inasmuch as the participation of the mediator improves the quality of linguistic, contextual and cultural interpretation as well as the therapeutic relationship with the clinician, the entire process is highly beneficial if the clinician has a solid understanding of the role of the interintercultural mediator and how best to make use of him or her.

We understand that fluidity and transparency are essential in mental healthcare; however, in other medical fields in which more often than not there is not even the time to discuss the patient's symptoms, transparency is not crucial to diagnosis and treatment, and is thus expendable in the interest of speeding up the process. At the same time, the junior co-therapist role can indirectly facilitate the patient's trust in the healthcare system, treatment adherence and lead to a greater sense of satisfaction for all involved. Thus it is essential that not only are mediators provided with solid training but that clinicians themselves receive training in cultural competence and intercultural mediation.

References

Beltran, M. (2001). *The Role of the Health Care Interpreter: An Evolving Dialogue*: The National Council on Interpretation in Health Care. Working Paper Series, Chicago, 15.

Bhui, K., Warfa, N., Edonya, P., McKenzie, K., Bhugra, D. (2007). Cultural competence in mental health care: a review of model evaluations. *BMC Health Service Research*, 7, 15.

Blue, H. C., Gonzalez, C. A. (1992). The meaning of ethnocultural difference: its impact on and use in the psychotherapeutic process. In D. Greenfeld (ed.) *Treating Diverse Disorders with Psychotherapy. New Directions for Mental Health Services*, Vol. 55. New York: Jossey-Bass, 73–84.

Bolton, J. (2002). The third presence: a psychiatrist's experience of working with non-English speaking patients and interpreters. *Transcultural Psychiatry*, 39 (1), 97–114.

Bot, H. (2003). The myth of the uninvolved interpreter: interpreting in mental health and the development of a three person psychology. In L. Brunette, I. Bastin and H. Clarke (eds), *The Critical Link* 3.

Amsterdam/Philadelphia: John Benjamins, 27–35.

Bot, H. (2005). *Dialogue Interpreting in Mental Health*. Amsterdam: Rodopi.

Bot, H., Wadensjö, C. (2004). The presence of a third party: a dialogical view on interpreter-assisted treatment. In J. P. Wilson and B. Drozđek (eds) *Broken Spirits: The Treatment of Traumatized Asylum Seekers, Refugees, War and Torture Victims*. New York: Brunner Routledge.

Collazos, F., Qureshi, A., Casas, M. (2005). La mediación cultural en salud mental. *Monografías de Psiquiatría*, 4, 18–23.

Comas-Diaz, L. (2003). Culture and psychotherapy: a guide to clinical practice. *Journal of Nervous and Mental Disease*, 191 (8), 556.

Davidson, B. (2000). The interpreter as institutional gatekeeper: the social-linguistic role of interpreters in Spanish–English medical discourse. *Journal of Sociolinguistics*, 4/3, 379–405.

Drennan, G., Swartz, L. (2002). The paradoxical use of interpreting in psychiatry. *Social Science and Medicine*, 54, 1836–66.

Dysart-Gale, D. (2005). Communication Models, professionalization, and the work of medical interpreters. *Health Communication*, **17**(1), 91–103.

Hsieh, E. (2007). Interpreters as co-diagnosticians: overlapping roles and services between providers and interpreters. *Social Science and Medicine*, **64**, 924–37.

Hsieh, E. (2008). "I am not a robot!" Interpreters views of their roles in health care settings. *Qualitative Health Research*, **18**(10), 1367–1383.

Jacobs, L. (1992). Insights from psychoanalytic self psychology and intersubjectivity theory for gestalt therapists. *The Gestalt Journal*, **15** (2), 25–60.

Joe, G. W., Simpson, D. D., Dansereau, D. F., Rowan-Szal, G. F. (2001). Relationships between counseling rapport and drug abuse treatment outcomes. *Psychiatric Services*, **52**(9), 1223–9.

Martin, D. J., Garske, J. P., Davis, M. K. (2000). Relation of therapeutic alliance with outcome and other variables: a meta-analytic review. *Journal of Consulting and Clinical Psychology*, **68**(3), 438–50.

Messent, P. (2003). From postmen to makers of meaning: a model for collaborative work between clinicians and interpreters. In R. Tribe and H. Raval (eds) *Working with Interpreters in Mental Health*. Hove: Brunner-Routledge, 135–50.

Miller, K. E., Martell, Z. L., Pazdirek, L., Caruth, M., Lopez, D. (2005). The role of interpreters in psychotherapy with refugees: an exploratory study. *American Journal of Orthopsychiatry*, **75**(1), 27–39.

Norcross, J. C. (ed.) (2002). *Psychotherapy Relationships that Work: Therapist Contributions and Responsiveness to Patients*. Oxford: Oxford University Press.

Orange, D. M., Atwood, G. E., Stolorow, R. D. (2001). *Working Intersubjectively: Contextualism in Psychoanalytic Practice*. Hillsdale, NJ: The Analytic Press.

Paris, M. J., Añez, L. M., Bedregal, L. E., Andrés-Hyman, R. C., Davidson, L. (2005). Help seeking and satisfaction among Latinas: the roles of setting, ethnic identity, and therapeutic alliance. *Journal of Community Psychology*, **33**(3), 299–312.

Qureshi, A. (2005). Dialogical relationship and cultural imagination: a hermeneutic approach to intercultural psychotherapy. *American Journal of Psychotherapy*, **59**(2), 119–35.

Qureshi, A., Collazos, F., Ramos, M., Casas, M. (2008). Cultural competency training in psychiatry. *European Psychiatry*, **23**(Suppl. 1), 49–58.

Raval, H., Smith, J. A. (2003). Therapists' experiences of working with language interpreters. *International Journal of Mental Health*, **32**(2), 6–31.

Razban, M. (2003). An interpreter's perspective. In R. Tribe and H. Raval (eds) *Working with Interpreters in Mental Health*. Hove, UK: Brunner-Routledge.

Tribe, R., Lane, P. (2009). Working with interpreters across language and culture in mental health. *Journal of Mental Health*, **18**(3), 233–41.

Tribe, R., Morrisey, J. (2004). Good practice issues in working with interpreters in mental health. *Intervention*, **2**(2), 129–42.

Verrept, H. (2008). Intercultural mediation: an answer to healthcare disparities? In C. Valero Garces and A. Martin (eds) *Crossing Borders in Community Interpreting: Definitions and Dilemmas*. London: John Benjamins, 187–201.

von Bertalanffy, L. (1968). *General System Theory: Foundations, Developments, Applications*. New York: Braziller.

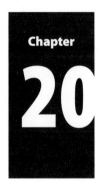

Chapter 20

Migrants and mental health: working across culture and language

Rachel Tribe

Editors' introduction

Mental health services have often been found inaccessible or inappropriate by members of migrant, black and minority ethnic (BME) and other minority communities, and usage has been reported to be poor compared to the white community. Requirements for mental health services are very varied. Using interpreters has both advantages and disadvantages, and clinicians must therefore be aware of how to use them effectively. Trained interpreters can be an important part of the therapeutic team and allow appropriate assessment and engagement with the patient.

Evidence has begun to emerge to suggest that services developed in conjunction with service users and the communities they serve lead to better usage, more appropriate and accessible services, and to an improved sense of inclusivity. Consultation and engagement with the communities' health trusts also allows services to develop in a dynamic way based on need, and in line with any changes in the population as well as the requirements of the complete community. This accords with a number of UK governmental directives. The issue of communication across language and culture appears to be key here, and this paper will draw attention to a range of practice issues and relevant guidelines.

Introduction

The term migrant can be understood to mean 'any person who lives temporarily or permanently in a country where he or she was not born, and has acquired some significant social ties to this country'. However, this may be a too-narrow definition when considering that, according to some states' policies, a person can be considered as a migrant even when he or she is born in the country (UNESCO, 2009).

The exact definition of a migrant is contested (Migrant Clinicians Network, 2006; Office for National Statistics, 2009; UNESCO, 2009), but migrants are normally identified as people who migrate across national or regional borders and have significant ties to the new country of residence and usually to the country from which they migrated as well. A more commonly used term is black and minority ethnic (BME), which appears to carry more inclusive connotations than the term 'migrant', while other terms used include black and Asian minority ethnic (BAMH) (National Black Carers and Carers Workers Network, 2008). Racism may play a role in the lives of many migrants, and there is a developing literature that shows that perceived discrimination may adversely affect psychological wellbeing

Migration and Mental Health, ed. Dinesh Bhugra & Susham Gupta. Published by Cambridge University Press. © Cambridge University Press 2011.

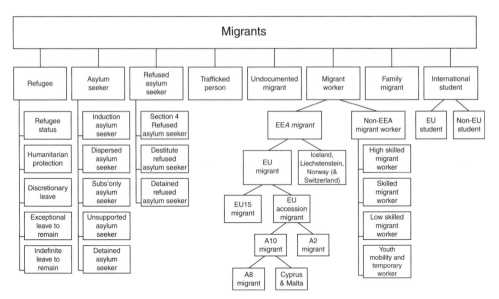

Figure 20.1 One classification system of migrants used within the UK. Reproduced with the kind permission of Yorkshire and Humber Regional Migration Partnership and partners.

(Fernando, 2007; Karlsen *et al.*, 2005; McKenzie, 2003). The term migrant should not be conflated with skin colour, as there has always been significant migration to the UK from a range of countries, including Europe both during and after World War 2. Figure 20.1 details how migrants may be classified within the UK.

Migration from Eastern Europe over the past few years has included large numbers of people moving across European borders. This underlines the fact that the composition of migrant communities changes over time, with some migrant groups having been in Britain for generations and some being more recent arrivals. For example, in 2004, after Poland joined the European Union, there was a large migration of Polish people to the UK (Drinkwater *et al.*, 2006). Subsequently, a number returned to Poland, and therefore the size of the Polish community in Britain decreased. While the Commission for Equality and Human Rights notes, in a practice briefing document, that it is important 'to focus on what new and existing communities have in common alongside a recognition of the value of diversity', health commissioners and providers may need to be mindful of the changing nature of migration and the need to monitor the accessibility and appropriateness of mental health services for all migrant communities. This has been emphasised in the National Institute for Health and Clinical Excellence (NICE, 2008) guidance on *Community Engagement to Improve Health*. However, while the guidance does recognise that many BME communities often have specific needs, it does not offer specific advice on how to consult these diverse communities. This may be done through a range of methods (for further details see Lane and Tribe, 2010).

If psychiatrists are to work effectively with issues of diversity, it is important to consider the individuality of patients, and not to make assumptions or stereotypes based upon ethnicity, gender, religion, age, sexual orientation or any other variable. The literature developed in the west has often stressed the importance of understanding other cultures, but has paid less attention to the need for practitioners in the west to consider the limitations or cultural relativism of their own position in their clinical practice. As Patel *et al.* (2000) says, 'An individual practitioner may strive admirably to understand the contribution of their client's culture to the conversation created between them in therapy, but will rarely give the same scrutiny to the role of their own culturally-determined belief system'.

Migrants are frequently divided into two distinct groups, although other categorisations are possible. Within any grouping, there will be a number of subgroups.

First, there will be people who migrated for family or economic reasons and are often referred to as voluntary migrants; these migrants were able to make a decision to migrate over time and make some of the necessary practical and psychological preparations for this move. Second, there are forced migrants (which include refugees and asylum seekers) who were forced to leave their country of origin often at short notice for reasons of war, human rights abuses, persecution on grounds of religion, gender or ethnicity and disasters (McColl *et al.*, 2008; Tribe, 2002); these migrants may have had little time to make the necessary psychological or practical preparations for this move.

There will also be temporary and permanent migrants. The former group will include, for example, people who have come to study in the UK intending to return to their country of origin, but who will reside in the UK for a number of years.

Definitions: refugees and asylum seekers[1,2]

The group listed above as forced migrants will include refugees and asylum seekers. The following definitions clarify the differences which, besides being legally distinct, will also affect entitlements to health and social care services, including mental health services.

An *asylum seeker* is someone who has left their country of origin and applied for refugee status and is awaiting a decision on their application.

The legal definition of a *refugee* is based on the United Nations High Commission for Refugees (UNHCR) convention of 1951 and is defined as a person who:

> owing to well-founded fear of being persecuted for reasons of race, religion, nationality, membership of a particular social group or political opinion, is outside the country of his or her nationality and is unable or, owing to such fear, is unwilling to avail him or herself of the protection of that country.
>
> The 1951 Convention Relating to the Status of Refugees Article 1 (A)(2)

In other words, a refugee is someone whose asylum claim has been granted, and who is thus protected by the Convention Relating to the Status of Refugees 1951 (UKTS 39 (1954) Cmd 9171), which came into force in 1954 and to which the UK is a party.

The difficulties experienced by asylum seekers are likely to be different to those experienced by refugees, as asylum seekers are living with uncertainty on a daily basis, waiting to hear whether they will be allowed to remain in the UK or whether they will be deported. This uncertainty does not bode well for psychological health (McColl *et al.*, 2008; Tribe, 2002).

---

[1] The Royal College of Psychiatrists (2007) consensus statement on *Improving Services for Refugees and Asylum Seekers: Position Statement* is available from www.rcp.ac.uk/docs/refugee%20asylum%20seeker%20consensus%20finaldoc.

[2] Details of services for refugees and asylum seekers can be located at www.refugeecouncil.org. In addition, they provide a range of downloadable information in numerous languages.

Humanitarian protection (granted after April 2003)

This may be granted when an individual does not qualify for refugee status but has been given humanitarian protection by a government. This will be granted for a number of years, after which it will be reviewed and may or may not be renewed.

Internally displaced persons

An internally displaced person (IDP) is usually someone who has been forced to flee their home and community through civil war or persecution, often on political or religious grounds, but has been displaced within their country of origin rather than to a different country. In addition, IDPs may find access to health provision severely curtailed. IDPs are frequently held in camps where conditions are not conducive to good mental health, and where only limited or emergency healthcare is available (UNHCR, 1996). Turner *et al.* (2009: p.9) notes: 'Internally displaced people living in transitional camps are a vulnerable population and specific interventions need to be targeted at this population to address the health inequalities that they report to be experiencing'.

A stateless person

Statelessness can occur when countries cease to exist or when people fail or are denied citizenship in the successor state/country. It may also arise on occasions as the result of countries failing to have gender-neutral policies and enforcing a patriarchal system where nationality can only be passed on via the male line. Without identification papers to prove citizenship, a stateless person cannot vote, obtain travel documents, work or access other government services (Goris *et al.*, 2009). The Council of Europe (2006) estimated that there were approximately 5.5 million irregular migrants residing in the EU. Estimates of the current number of stateless people worldwide ranges from 11 to 15 million. Strang (2009) has argued that the existing legal framework requires attention and that the EU needs to develop an EU-wide regularisation scheme for stateless people. Access to medical services and other provisions will be severely curtailed for this group, who consequently may have to live in the margins of society.

Mental health services have often been found to be inaccessible or inappropriate by members of BME and other minority communities, and usage has been reported to be poor compared to the white community (Patel *et al.*, 2000). The usage of services by migrants has shown that mental healthcare sometimes fails to meet migrants' needs (Fernando, 2007; Watters, 2002). This may be for a number of reasons. These may include a lack of awareness of availability or perceived appropriateness of services, different explanatory models, concerns about stigma associated with having mental health concerns and different help-seeking behaviours. There may be diagnostic difficulties across languages and cultures. Also, the categorisation of mental disorders across cultures can be problematic as epidemiological data is often generated from a particular classificatory perspective which may not always be appropriately applied across cultures (MacLachlan, 2005). In addition, some migrants will not be fluent in English and will require the services of an interpreter to enable them to access mental health services.

Working across language and culture

To know another language is the best and most exciting way of discovering the strengths – and limitations – of the one with which one has grown up . . . I have come to value my own translators as my wisest readers – they ask searching questions about precise meanings, they hear the rhythms of long stretches of interwoven writing, they send lists of alternative translations of particular words, all of which add a little meaning in the other language here, and take it away there, all of which are possible, none of which are perfect equivalents.

A. S. Byatt, *The Times*, 11 February 2006

Communicating across language and culture can be a rich and fascinating experience. It requires careful consideration when a mental health consultation is taking place as, without a common language, effective communication may be difficult. As language forms a major tool within psychiatry, this is a serious concern. In addition to language differences, the psychiatrist, patient and, on occasions, the interpreter may all hold different explanatory health models in relation to mental health. All of these may have been learned from within their own cultural paradigm and may be present in the consultation (Bhui and Bhugra, 2002; Fernando, 2007). Ivbijaro *et al.* (2005) argue that, in a richly diverse society, GPs can fail to recognise mental health problems or may offer inappropriate treatments if they are not aware of how different cultures describe mental distress, with the consequence that some patients may not be referred to secondary care and to the help they may require. This complex issue is discussed further elsewhere in this book.

The exact relationship between language and culture is complex and is still debated; it appears that language bears a close relationship to particular ways of construing meaning that may not be shared across cultures (Mudakiri, 2003). Social constructionists would argue that language acts as a defining structure in itself (Anderson and Goolishian, 1992; Burr, 1995). As such, languages may contain racist and sexist views, reflecting elements of the wider culture. For example, the words 'negro' and 'black' have very different connotations, as do a range of other words associated with race, culture, gender and age, in addition to those used as descriptors in mental health. Hoffman (1989), writing of her personal experience of living between two languages and the innate cultural constructions of words and meanings, writes:

All immigrants and exiles know the peculiar restlessness of an imagination that can never again have faith in its absoluteness . . . Because I have learned the relativity of cultural meanings on my skin, I can never take one set of meanings as final.

Eva Hoffman (1989: p.221)

The relationship between language and culture within the context of mental health is likewise complex. A colleague working in Sri Lanka during the civil war and conducting a mental health assessment, commenting on the relevance of western psychological models and language, stated:

When you ask them the classical . . . the whole thing, the PTSD criteria would be there, but these are all leading questions, this is the other problem. When you ask 'do you have intrusive memories?; one thing is that it is easier to say 'intrusive memory' in English, but trying to put it into Sinhala or Tamil, you see, is very difficult and by the time you have explained all that, they know that the patient has to answer in the positive. So these are the shortcomings.   Sivayogan, 1996, personal communication

Language is a dynamic medium which is constantly changing, with new words entering the language and usage subtly changing; for example, the word wicked is now used by some people as an adjective to mean 'very good, excellent, cool' or as an adverb to mean 'very, really, extremely' (online slang dictionary, 2009). Dictionaries are regularly updated as language usage changes. Neither is it a neutral medium (Holder, 2002). For example, the title used by a woman in England illustrates how language may interact with cultural values. In Victorian or earlier times, a title was ascribed to a woman on the basis of a marital relationship or lack of it with a man, and she was expected to take his name whereas men were automatically ascribed the title Mr, often in their teenage years or on reaching 18 years of age, and the title was not predicated on a marital relationship with a woman. In more sexist times, women were always known as Miss or Mrs. Use of the more recent title Ms gives a woman a title of her own and a choice which does not define her name or identity in relation to a marital relationship with a man, so reflecting changing times and the legal position and rights of women within most English-speaking cultures.

Language has also been used at various times in history to restrict access to due legal process; for example, in South Africa under apartheid all legal proceedings were conducted in English or Afrikaans. This apparently excluded more than half the population (Sacks, 2000). Not speaking the majority language may make patients feel vulnerable and exposed, having 'literally lost their voice' and on occasion becoming infantalised and ashamed by an inability to speak for themselves. Being reliant upon another person can replicate experiences of disempowerment and clinicians may need to be mindful of this. The need to rely on another person to represent our emotions and concerns is likely to be challenging (Tribe, 2007). The dilemmas associated with not speaking a dominant language can be exacerbated in a mental health, legal or welfare context, where the outcomes of the various meetings may be extremely significant for the patient. This is not to say that some people may choose not to learn the dominant language of the country of residence for a variety of reasons which may include but are not limited to gender politics and related issues.

As McNamee and Gergen (1992) write in relation to therapy as social construction, 'We not only bear languages that furnish the rationale for our looking, but also vocabularies of description and explanation for what is observed' (McNamee and Gergen, 1992 p.1). When issues of mental health are being discussed across languages and cultures, it is important to pay particular attention to the complexities involved, to ensure that an equitable, appropriate and accessible service is being delivered to all members of the community, including migrants. Most psychiatrists working in the west trained there, and this is highly likely to have influenced their world view and the models of mental health utilised. Everyone will develop explanatory health models based on the prevailing beliefs contained within their culture and training. It is easy to reify this knowledge and assume that it is immutable and fixed and applicable worldwide rather than one possible construction. Cultural differences are sometimes minimised and seen as additional or marginal factors rather than as constitutive of an individual and their experience of themselves (Patel and Newland, 2005). The whole issue of cultural relativism and applicability of ideas generated by western psychiatry and applied across cultures is contested by some authors. For example, Summerfield (2002, page 248) claims that many parts of western psychiatry have not adequately considered their own ethnocentricity and location within a western world view.

> DSM and ICD are not, as some imagine, atheoretical and purely descriptive nosologies with universal validity. They are western cultural documents, carrying ontological notions of what constitutes a real disorder, epistemological ideas about what counts as scientific evidence, and methodological ideas as to how research should be conducted.

Dilemmas associated with working with an interpreter

Clinicians often report feeling challenged when they are first asked to work with an interpreter. The reasons they give include feeling that they lack the requisite skills, assumptions about the difficulties of linguistic and cultural differences, concerns about splitting, issues of transference, and general concerns that it will change the dynamics of the meeting (Tribe and Thompson, 2009). Gerrish *et al.* (2004), noting the reluctance of health professionals to work with interpreters, argues that this ambivalence is something that may require attention by commissioners, managers, individual clinicians, training providers and professional associations. Wadensjo (2001) claims that within the medical literature, interpreting and interpreters are rarely mentioned, and that when they are, they are frequently viewed as a methodological problem within medical practice or research rather than as a helpful addition. Wiener and Rivera (2004) claim that it is imperative that healthcare providers are aware of the importance of interpretive services and become skilled in the use of interpreters; they noted that lack of language fluency was 'predictive of poor satisfaction with a medical encounter and a poor understanding and compliance with medical instructions' (p.93). Minas *et al.* (1994), after surveying psychiatrists in Australia, claimed that the crucial role language plays in all aspects of mental health provision had been largely ignored, and argued that it required immediate attention. Farooq and Fear (2003) described a similar situation in the UK. Several researchers have found that clinicians/participants reported that, after initial concerns, actually working with an interpreter enhanced their work, that their initial discomfort faded, and that they saw the experience as both helpful and informative (Miller *et al.*, 2005; Raval, 1996).

Benefits of working with an interpreter

If we are to provide a service to all members of the community, we need to work with interpreters to enable those not fluent in English to access services when they are needed. In addition to this, there is extensive evidence on the benefits of working with an interpreter. Once an interpreter is introduced, the way in which language is used, often without thinking, is thrown into sharp relief, often with very useful consequences (Raval, 1996). Farooq *et al.* (1997) found that the use of an *experienced* interpreter provided reliable data for psychiatric diagnosis. Hillier *et al.* (1994) and Kaufert and Koolage (1984) argue that interpreters can usefully assist in establishing rapport and negotiating complex terminology and different explanatory models of health, and clients have reported a host of benefits, including feeling better understood and heard (Hillier *et al.*, 1994; Kline *et al.*, 1980; Mudarikri; 2003). It was also noted that patients using an interpreter had a higher return rate following assessment, and believed they had received better professional attention (Faust and Drickey, 1986). An interpreter can also function as a safe attachment figure (Alexander *et al.*, 2004). A range of studies has reported positive experiences on the part of patients having an interpreter available, with benefits including improved access to and quality of care (Ziguras *et al.*, 2003). An increase in trust in the process and rapport with the health provider has also been noted, along with better compliance with treatment (Manson, 1988; Ramirez, 2003). Other studies of relationships between access to healthcare and quality of communication aided by interpreters have also reported improvement in appointment keeping, fewer emergency visits, greater patient satisfaction and improved compliance with health regimes (Lee *et al.*, 2002; Morales *et al.*, 1999; Riddick, 1998).

In summary, working with an interpreter brought many benefits for the patient and the clinician, enabling a better history to be taken and better rapport to be established, and allowed the clinician to be more reflective in offering services to patients who were not fluent in English. Guidelines on working with an interpreter in mental health can be located either in your trust, at Tribe and Raval (2003) or at www.bps.org.uk/publications/guidelines-for-practitioners/guidelines-for-practitioners.cfm. A short 10-minute training DVD funded by the Department of Health on working with an interpreter in mental health is downloadable with accompanying notes from www.dh.gov.uk.

Training requirements

The need for training for both interpreters and clinicians is increasingly recognised by mental health practitioners (Miller *et al.*, 2005; Tribe and Raval, 2003; Verrept and Louckx, 1997), as are the advantages for patients of a trained and experienced interpreter (Farooq and Fear, 2003). Bischoff *et al.* (2003), writing about primary care physicians claim that the quality of communication as perceived by service users who do not speak the local language can be improved with *specific training* for primary care physicians. Further research is necessary but the same may well be true for psychiatrists.

Given that a good therapeutic alliance is seen as central to much of the work of a psychiatric or therapeutic nature, working successfully in partnership with interpreters can be of key importance. It will also ensure that people not fluent in English are not denied access to services. In addition, the issue of whether or not interpreters should merely translate the spoken word or should also consider cultural issues is an important one. Tribe (1998) has suggested four modes of interpreting as presented below. Other writers, for example Mudarikiri (2003), offer slightly different accounts.

Models of interpretation

1. The linguistic mode, where the interpreter tries to interpret as far as possible word-for-word and adopts a neutral and distanced position (Cushing, 2003; Tribe, 1998).
2. The psychotherapeutic or constructionist mode, where the meaning/feeling of the words is most important, and the interpreter is primarily concerned with the meaning to be conveyed and contextual variables rather than word-for-word interpretation (Raval, 2003; Tribe, 1998, 1999).
3. The advocate or community interpreter, where the interpreter takes the role of advocate for the client (sometimes called a link worker or health advocate in the UK), either at the individual or wider group or community level, and represents their interests within a health setting beyond interpreting language for them (Baylav, 2003; Drennan and Swartz, 1999; Razban, 2003).
4. Cultural broker/bicultural worker, where the interpreter interprets not only the spoken word but also relevant cultural and contextual variables (Drennan and Swartz, 1999; Tribe, 1998). In some European countries, for example Belgium and Spain, this is known as an intercultural mediator (Qureshi *et al.*, 2010; Verrept and Louckx, 1997).

An experienced interpreter can move between the roles – all have their place depending on requirements and context.

Relationship between a mother tongue and emotion

Research shows that languages are not directly interchangeable; meanings may be coded, emotionally processed and internalised in one language and not always be directly accessible in another (Keefe, 2008). Also, the relationship between a mother tongue and emotion is very complicated although the literature is still developing. A number of writers, including Amati-Mehler *et al.* (1993), Antinucci-Mark (1990), Burck (2004), Greenson

(1950), Perez-Foster (1998), Tesone (1996) and others have studied therapy with multi-lingual patients. It is not possible to discuss all the complexities here, but it is clear that the relationship between a mother tongue, second language and emotions is complex, and clinicians need to consider how they work with this and the availability of emotions or clinical features in a first and second language. Further research needs to be conducted.

Recommendations on good practice when working with interpreters

The British Psychological Society guidelines for psychologists in health settings (2008) makes the following recommendations for practice, (adapted here with permission). They apply to all mental health professionals.

- Undertake a language-needs analysis for the population that your service covers, and consider how you will best meet this need.
- If you have not undertaken training in working with interpreters, do so. If this is really not feasible, e.g. if you will be working with an interpreter unexpectedly, read the guidelines and allow time to consider the issues or discuss them with a more experienced colleague in advance of your first session with an interpreter. Clinicians should consider attending deaf awareness training run by their NHS trust before working with a British sign language interpreter (BSLI).
- Check that the interpreter is qualified and appropriate for the consultation/meeting.
- Allow 10–15 minutes before the session to brief the interpreter about the purpose of the meeting and to enable them to brief you about any cultural issues which may be relevant to the session. For example, a mental state examination will take a rather different form to a family therapy session, with different objectives and ways of working.
- Be mindful of issues of confidentiality and trust when working with someone from a small language community (including the deaf community) as the client may be anxious about being identifiable and mistrustful of an interpreter's professionalism.
- State clearly in the consultation that you alone hold clinical responsibility for the meeting.
- Create a good atmosphere where each member of the triad feels able to ask for clarification if anything is unclear, and be respectful to your interpreter, who is an important member of the team who makes your work possible.
- Match when appropriate for gender and age. Do not use a relative, and never use a child.
- Be aware of the wellbeing of your interpreter and the possibility of your interpreter suffering from vicarious traumatisation. Consider what support they may be offered.
- At the end of the session allocate 10–15 minutes to debrief the interpreter about the session and offer support and supervision as appropriate.
- All written translations used should have been back-translated to ensure they are fit for purpose.
- Extreme caution should be exercised when considering the use of translated psychometric tests. See the International Test Commission Guidelines on Test Adaptation (2000) for a comprehensive review of these issues.
- Commissioners need to ensure that there are clear pathways to support members of their local community, including those who do not speak English.

In summary, to ensure that some groups are not denied access to psychological services, working effectively with interpreters should be a skill possessed by every clinician. To this end, all clinicians should receive training in working with interpreters as a core part of their professional training. If this is not available within your trust or professional association, it is recommended that it is undertaken as part of continuing professional development. Training courses are available in much of the country.

Acknowledgement

Apart from direct quotes, the case material presented in this chapter is based on a composite of patients, with all identifying material changed to ensure that patient confidentiality is maintained.

References

Alexander, C., Edwards, R., Temple, B. *et al*. (2004). *Access to Services with Interpreters, User Views*. York: Joseph Rowntree Foundation.

Amati-Mehler J., Argentieri, S., Canestri, J. (1993). *The Babel of the Unconscious, Mother Tongue and Foreign Languages in the Psychoanalytic Tradition*. Madison: International Universities Press.

Anderson, H., Goolishian, H. (1992). Client as expert. In S. Mcnamee and K. Gergen (eds). *Therapy as a Social Construction*. London: Sage.

Antinucci-Mark, G. (1990). Speaking in tongues in the consulting room or the dialectic of foreignness. *British Journal of Psychotherapy*, **6**(4), 375–83.

Baylav, A. (2003). Issues of language provision in health care services. In R. Tribe and H. Raval *Undertaking Mental Health Work Using Interpreters*. London: Routledge.

Bhui, K., Bhugra, D. (2002). Explanatory models for mental distress: implications for clinical practice and research. *British Journal of Psychiatry*, **181**, 6–7.

Bischoff, A., Perneger, T. V., Bovier, P. A., Louton, L., Stalder, H. (2003). Improving communication between physicians and patients who speak a foreign language. *British Journal of General Practice*, **53**, 541–6.

British Psychological Society Guidelines on Working with an Interpreter (2008). www. bps.org.uk/publications/guidelines-for-practitioners/guidelines-for-practitioners.

cfm (scroll down to the bottom of the page) (accessed 24 September 2009).

Burck, C. (2004). Living in several languages: implications for therapy. *Journal of Family Therapy*, **26**(4), 314–39.

Burr, V. (1995). *An Introduction to Social Constructionism*. London: Routledge.

Council of Europe(2006). Convention on the Avoidance of Statelessness http:// conventions.coe.int/Treaty/EN/treaties/ Html/200.htm (accessed 24 September 2009).

Cushing, A. (2003). Interpreters in medical consultations. In R. Tribe and H. Raval (eds) *Working with Interpreters in Mental Health*. London & New York: Routledge.

Delivering Race Equality (DRE) in mental health care: an action plan for reform inside and outside services. www.dh.gov.uk/en/ Publicationsandstatistics/Publications/ PublicationsPolicyAndGuidance/ DH_4100773%20 (accessed 24 September 2009).

Drennan, G., Swartz, L. (1999). A concept overburdened: institutional roles for psychiatric interpreters in post-apartheid South Africa. *Interpreting*, **4**(2), 169–98.

Drinkwater, S., Eade, J., Garapich, M. (2006). *Poles Apart? EU Enlargement and the Labour Market Outcomes of Immigrants in the UK IZA Discussion Paper No. 2410*. Available at SSRN: http://ssrn.com/ abstract=944475 (accessed 24 September 2009).

Farooq, S., Fear, C. (2003). Working through interpreters. *Advances in Psychiatric Treatment*, **9**, 104–9.

Farooq, S., Fear, C., Oyebode, F. (1997). An investigation of the adequacy of psychiatric interviews conducted through an interpreter. *Psychiatric Bulletin*, **21**, 209–13.

Fernando, S. (2007). Race and culture conference. British Psychological Society Conference. London.

Faust, S., Drickey, R. (1986). Working with interpreters. *Journal of Family Practice*, **22** (2), 134–8.

Gerrish, K., Chua, R., Sobowale, A., Birks, E. (2004). Bridging the language barrier: the use of interpreters in primary care nursing. *Health, Social Care in the Community*, **12**, 407–13.

Goris, I., Harrington, J., Köhn, S. (2009). Statelessness: what it is and why it matters. *Forced Migration Review*, **32**, 4–7.

Greenson, R. (1950). The mother tongue and the mother. *International Journal of Psychoanalysis*, **31**, 18–23.

Hillier, S., Huq, A., Loshak, R., Marks, F., Rahman, S. (1994). An evaluation of child psychiatric services for Bangladeshi parents. *Journal of Mental Health*, **3**, 332–7.

Hoffman, E. (1989). *Lost in Translation*. London: Minerva.

Holder, R. (2002). *The Impact of Mediated Communication on Psychological Therapy with Refugees and Asylum Seekers: Practitioners' Experiences*. Unpublished MSc dissertation, London: City University.

International Test Commission Guidelines on Test Adaptation (2000). www.intestcom. org/Guidelines/test+adaptation.php (accessed 24 September 2009).

Ivbijaro, G. O., Kolkiewicz, L. A., Palazidou, E. (2005). Mental health in primary care: ways of working: the impact of culture. *Primary Care Mental Health*, **3**, 45.

Karlsen, S., Nazroo, J. Y., McKenzie, K. *et al.* (2005). Racism, psychosis and common mental disorder among ethnic minority groups in England. *Psychological Medicine*, **35**, 1795–803.

Kaufart, J. M., Koolage, W. W. (1984). Role conflict among 'cultural brokers', the experience of native Canadian medical interpreters. *Social Science & Medicine*, **18**, 283–6.

Keefe, A. (2008). *Absent Language: Mother–Child Communication in the Absence of a Common Mother-Tongue*. Westminster Postoral Foundation: Unpublished MA thesis.

Kline, F., Acosta, F. X., Austin, W., Johnson, R. G. (1980). The misunderstood Spanish-speaking patient. *American Journal of Psychiatry*, **137**(12), 1530–3.

Lane, P., Tribe, R. (2010). Following NICE 2008: a practical guide for health professionals: community engagement with local black and minority ethnic (BME) community groups. *Diversity, Health & Social Care*, **7** (2), 105–14.

Lee L. J., Batal, H. A., Masselli, J. H., Kutner, J. S. (2002). Effect of Spanish interpretation method on patient satisfaction in an urban walk-in clinic. *Journal of General Internal Medicine*, **17**, 641–6.

MacLachlan, M. (2005). *Culture and Health*, 2nd edn. Chichester: Wiley.

Manson, A. (1988). Language concordance as a determinant of patient compliance and emergency room use in patients with asthma. *Medical Care*, **26**, 1119–28.

McColl, H., McKenzie, K., Bhui, K. (2008). Mental healthcare of asylum-seekers and refugees. *Advances in Psychiatric Treatment*, **14**, 452–4.

McKenzie, K. (2003). Racism and health. *British Medical Journal*, **326**, 65–6.

McNamee S., Gergen, K. (1992). (eds) *Therapy as Social Construction*. London: Sage.

Migrant Clinicians Network (2006). www. migrantclinician.org/toolsource/resource/ discussion-current-definition-migrant-used-migrant-and-community-health-centers (accessed 14 August 2009).

Miller, K., Martell, Z., Pazdinek, L., Carruth, M., Lopez, F. (2005). The role of interpreters in psychotherapy with refugees: an exploratory study. *American Journal of Orthopsychiatry*, **75**(1), 27–39.

Minas, I. H., Stuart, G. W., Klimidis, S. (1994). Language, culture and psychiatric services: a survey of Victorian clinical staff. *Australian and New Zealand Journal of Psychiatry*, **32**, 424–33.

Morales, L., Cunningham, W., Brown, J., Liu, H., Hays, R. (1999). Are Latinos less satisfied with communication by health care providers? *Journal of General Internal Medicine*, **14**, 409–17.

Mudakiri, M. M. (2003). Working with interpreters in adult mental health. In R. Tribe and H. Raval (eds) *Undertaking Mental Health Work Using Interpreters*. London: Routledge.

National Black Carers and Carers Workers Network (2008). Beyond We Care Too: Putting Black Carers in the Picture. www. www.afiya-trust.org (accessed 13 August 2009).

NICE (2008). *Community Engagement to Improve Health National Institute for Clinical Excellence*. http://www.nice.org.uk/nicemedia/pdf/PH009Guidance.pdf (accessed March 2009).

Office for National Statistics (ONS) (2009). www. statistics.gov.uk/hub/index.html (accessed 24 September 2009).

Perez-Foster, R. (1998). *The Power of Language in the Clinical Process: Assessing and Treating the Bilingual Person*. New Jersey: Aronson.

Patel, N., Bennett, E., Dennis, M. *et al.* (2000). *Clinical Psychology, 'Race' and Culture: A Training Manual*. Leicester: BPS Books.

Patel, N., Newland, J. (2005). Professional and ethical practice in multicultural and multiethnic society. In R. Tribe and J. Morrissey (eds) *The Handbook of Professional and Ethical Practice for Psychologists, Psychotherapists & Counsellors*. London: Brunner-Routledge.

Qureshi, A., Revollo, H-W., Collazos, F. *et al.* (2010) Intercultural mediation: reconstructing Hermes: the messenger gets a Voice. In D. Bhugra and S. Gupta (eds) *Migrants and Mental Health*. Cambridge: Cambridge University Press.

Ramirez, A. G. (2003). Consumer–provider communication research with special populations. *Patient Education Counsel*, **50**, 51–4.

Raval, H. (1996). A systemic perspective on working with interpreters. *Clinical Child Psychology & Psychiatry*, **1**(1), 29–43.

Raval, H. (2003). An overview of the issues in the work with interpreters. In R. Tribe and H. Raval (eds) *Undertaking Mental Health Work Using Interpreters*. London: Routledge.

Razban, M. (2003). An interpreter's perspective. In R. Tribe and H. Raval (eds) *Undertaking Mental Health Work Using Interpreters*. London: Routledge.

Riddick, S. (1998). Improving access for limited English-speaking consumers: a review of strategies in health care settings. *Journal of Health Care for the Poor and Underserved*, **9** (Suppl.), S40–S61.

Sacks, V. (2000). Can law protect language? Law, language and human rights in the South African constitution. *International Journal of Discrimination and the Law*, **4**, 343–68.

Strang, A. (2009). Towards an EU-wide regularisation scheme. Statelessness: what it is and why it matters. *Forced Migration Review*, **32**, 63–5.

Summerfield, D. (2002). Commentary on Tribe, R: mental health of refugees and asylum-seekers. *Advances in Psychiatric Treatment*, **8**, 247.

Tesone, J-E. (1996). Multi-lingualism, word-presentations, thing-presentations and psychic reality. *International Journal of Psychoanalysis*, 77, 871–81.

Tribe, R. (1998). A critical analysis of a support and clinical supervision group for interpreters working with refugees located in Britain. *Group Work Journal*, **10**(3), 196–214.

Tribe, R. (1999). Bridging the gap or damming the flow? Bicultural workers; some observations on using interpreters when working with refugee clients, many of whom have been tortured. *British Journal of Medical Psychology*, 72, 567–76.

Tribe, R. (2002). Mental health and refugees. *Advances In Psychiatric Treatment*, **8**(4), 240–8.

Tribe, R. (2007). Working with interpreters. *The Psychologist*, **20**(3), 159–61.

Tribe, R., Raval, H. (2003). (eds) *Working with Interpreters in Mental Health*. London & New York: Brunner-Routledge.

Tribe, R., Thompson, K. (2009). Exploring the three way relationship in therapeutic work with interpreters. *International Journal of Migration, Health and Social Care*, **5**(2), 35–43.

Turner, A., Pathirana, S., Daley, A., Gill, P. S. (2009). Sri Lankan tsunami refugees: a cross sectional study of the relationships between housing conditions and self-reported health. *BMC International Health and Human Rights*, **9**, 16.

UNESCO (2009). http://portal.unesco.org/shs/en/ev.php-URL_ID=3020&URL_DO=DO_TOPIC&URL_SECTION=201.html (accessed 17 August 2009).

UNHCR (1951). *The 1951 Refugee Convention.* Geneva: UNHCR.

UNHCR (1996). *Refugee Emergencies. A Community-Based Approach.* Geneva: UNHCR.

Verrept, H., Louckx, F. (1997). Health advocates in Belgian health care. In A. Uggalle and G. Cardenas (eds) *Health and Social Services Among International Labor.* Austin: University of Texas Press, 67–87.

Wadensjo, C. (2001). Interpreting in crisis; the interpreter's position in therapeutic encounters. In L. Mason (ed.) *Triadic Exchanges: Studies in Dialogue Interpreting.* Manchester: St. Jerome, 71–85.

Watters, C. (2002). Migration and mental health care in Europe: report of a preliminary mapping exercise. *Journal of Ethnic and Migration Studies*, **28**, 153–72.

Who are Migrants? www.nysp.org.uk/downloads/RIM_who_are_migrantsNov08v2.pdf?PHPSESSID=3831481a34af52ea3998ece954faa67f (accessed 12 September 2009).

Wiener, E. S., Rivera, M. I. (2004). Bridging language barriers: how to work with an interpreter. *Clinical Pediatric Emergency Medicine*, **5**(2), 93–101.

Ziguras, S., Klimidis, S., Lewis, J., Stuart, G. (2003). Ethnic matching of clients and clinicians and use of mental health services by ethnic minority clients. *Psychiatric Service*, **54**, 535–41.

Psychological therapies for immigrant communities

Stephen Turner and Dinesh Bhugra

Editors' introduction

Migrants may have experienced losses and may be suffering from common mental disorders. As far as psychological therapies are concerned, one size does not fit all. Depending upon cultures of origin, education, socio-economic status and religious values, the world view of the migrant will be formed. Their acceptance or rejection of the psychological interventions will be influenced by the models of therapy on offer. It is possible that ethnic matching of the therapist may facilitate initial engagement. However, unless there is considerable agreement on respective world views, it is unlikely that therapy can progress effectively and successfully. In this chapter the authors raise general principles of psychotherapy as applied across cultures. It is likely that refugees and asylum seekers may be more traumatised and may require specific strategies. However, ego-based psychotherapies may not be easily accepted across other cultures. Although some types of behavioural therapy have been used successfully across some cultures, due attention must be paid to ensure that cognitive behavioural therapy is modified according to underlying cognitive schema. In working with couples or families it is possible that individuals may have reached different levels of acculturation, thereby making the task more difficult.

Introduction

Immigrants face particular challenges when seeking assistance from psychotherapy services, not least their belief that such services may not apply to them, or be useful for them. Arriving in the west from a very different cultural milieu, and perhaps not having English as a first language, may be perceived by both therapists and patients themselves as being insurmountable barriers. However, this is not the case, and migrants can benefit immensely from psychotherapy for mental distress. It is necessary, however, for therapists to be sensitive to cultural differences, and to recognise that the psychotherapeutic approaches taken with patients from immigrant communities may require modification from those used with patients from the ethnic and cultural majority.

We begin by considering the cultural specificity of a particular psychotherapeutic approach. We discuss whether an approach which is acceptable in western society can reasonably be applied to other, very different, cultures. It may be the case that the theoretical underpinnings of the approach may seem reasonable and acceptable, but the presentation of the approach requires modification. We give some examples of where the approach is theoretically sound, but requires 'translation' into a style which can be effectively applied to another culture. We consider cultural influences on the expected role of the therapist and

Migration and Mental Health, ed. Dinesh Bhugra & Susham Gupta. Published by Cambridge University Press. © Cambridge University Press 2011.

how the therapist can best present himself to members of an ethnic minority to develop rapport and promote a useful therapeutic alliance. We go on to consider how cultural, racial and ethnic differences between therapist and patient can affect therapy with both individuals and couples. We conclude with a discussion of special issues, concentrating in particular on the specific problems that can arise when dealing with gay and lesbian immigrants, and with traumatised populations such as refugees and asylum seekers.

Psychotherapy in non-western cultures

When westerners talk about psychotherapy, they are usually referring to an approach which is a confiding and emotional professional relationship between two people, with the ultimate purpose of relieving mental distress. However, this definition implicitly assumes that therapy is a private matter, and that discussions which take place within the setting of the therapeutic encounter can be translated by the patient and applied to their relationship with the world as they see fit. People come to therapy for many reasons, but a frequent and general motivation is a sense of internal and external *dissociation*, a sense of feeling *alienated*. Reintegration of the self – which Jung referred to as *individuation* – is, from the psychoanalytical perspective, approached as an internal and personal process involving discussion, imagination and fantasy. An implicit assumption in this style of psychotherapy is that, as the patient becomes more *integrated* with the self through therapy, then their interaction with external reality will naturally also become more functional, fluid and adaptive. Through this process, the sense of dissociation which created the patient's difficulties can be overcome, and mental distress relieved.

This simplistic description of the processes involved in psychotherapy apply mainly to a society in which personal identification with the ego – being an *individual*; being *my own man*; being *independent* – are considered positive qualities to be aspired towards. In other words, they apply to western, capitalist societies where one's sense of personal contentedness is assumed, in the main, to be a personal matter.

An alternative definition of the psychotherapeutic encounter is provided by Frank (1993), who defined psychotherapy as 'a procedure to counter demoralisation which makes use of: an emotionally charged confiding relationship with a helpful person; a healing setting; a rationale, conceptual scheme, or myth; a ritual'. This definition is more encompassing, and more useful as we try to understand how best to modify psychotherapeutic approaches to assist patients who may come from a non-egocentric cultural background. Bhugra and Tantam (1998) refer to 'mind healing' as being more than just talking therapy: it can involve the entirety of a person's experience, including their family and social relationships as well as their religious beliefs and awareness as an integral part of the healing process. Hence, an accurate understanding of a person's cultural background is an essential prerequisite to effecting a helpful therapeutic relationship.

For a psychotherapeutic encounter to be helpful, the philosophical basis of the approach must be acceptable to the patient. As Varma and Gupta (2008) point out, 'Psychoanalysis became popular in the USA because of the emphasis on individualism, rational thinking, free expression, and tolerance of dissent.' They go on to explain that politically motivated forms of social control (such as 'work-therapy' in the Soviet Union) became popular as they resonated with the political fashion of that time. Western psychoanalysis has assumed, throughout its evolution, that the philosophical basis of its insights are universal. It assumed that the underpinnings of the psychoanalytical model can be usefully applied to a patient irrespective of whether the patient hails from downtown Manhattan or the backstreets of

Delhi – the only differences being concerned with superficial matters such as presentation and language. Berne (1960) takes this viewpoint to an extreme when he states that 'Psychotherapeutic manoeuvres can be readily transferred from one culture to another. The principles learned in the treatment of young women in Connecticut or California are just as effective in the South Pacific.' However, this extreme belief neglects completely the reality, which is that people in traditional societies often view psychological problems – and, indeed, the changing circumstances of all of one's life experience – from a strong magico-religious perspective. Adopting a paternalistic and rational attitude to such belief systems risks disengaging the patient. In addition, when the concepts of self vary across cultures and to ignore these realities is a major shortfall in any therapeutic armamentarium. As Hofstede (2001) has very cogently described, cultures can be divided into collectivist and individualistic or sociocentric and egocentric, masculine or feminine and what the power distance in the cultureis.

These characteristics thus raise very pertinent questions about differences across cultures and differing world views which any therapist has to bear in mind if they are to succeed in engaging people for therapeutic benefits. These challenges are worth bearing in mind when the therapist sees any patient no matter whether they belong to the majority or the minority culture. Neki *et al.* (1985), in their review of the applicability of western therapies, state the obvious when they note, 'After all, the therapist must attract and keep the patient before he can expect anything from him.' A more helpful approach would be for the therapist to allow his technique to be modulated by the belief systems of the patients (and their families or carers, who may have a significant effect on the patient) rather than the other way around. To do otherwise would be to discard a lifetime's immersion in a particular belief system, and that is, of course, too much to ask, or even to wish for. More adaptive and useful is to tailor the approach to therapy with an individual patient by taking the most relevant components of western psychotherapy and the patient's own belief systems to effect the most useful therapeutic encounter. Jung (1961) summarises this approach by stating 'We need a different language for each patient.' Although principles of therapy may remain the same, the approach has to be tailor-made for each patient. Koss (1987) compared the expectation of improvement and the perceived improvement between the users of a community mental health centre psychotherapy service and those attending a spiritually focused centre in Puerto Rico. He found that there was a significant difference in the *expectation* of improvement between the two groups (with the attendees of the spiritualist centre having *higher* expectations), whereas the actual *perceived* improvement following the differing interventions was the same. This outcome suggests that the cultural acceptability of the approach is of at least equal importance to the philosophical underpinnings – rational or otherwise – of the therapeutic approach itself. It is cultural acceptability that will improve therapeutic adherence and alliance.

Accepting that the style of therapy needs to be adjusted to take into account the patient's cultural background is not to assume that the western psychoanalytical approach does not have, at least some, universal applicability. Moacanin (2003) draws a direct comparison between the techniques of Jungian psychoanalysis and the meditative practices of Tibetan Buddhism. In so doing she demonstrates that the similarities between these approaches are greater than their differences, despite the vast differences between the cultures which gave rise to each. In particular, the role of a 'guru' or 'spiritual teacher' (analogous to the therapist) is central; however, the manner in which he or she presents himself to the disciple (or patient) is completely different. The process and ultimate aim of the therapeutic encounter is similar and arguably universal; but the actual style of the process is culturally specific. In India, Bose (1999) developed psychoanalytical strategies independent of Freud and communicated these with Freud and used a different model of oedipal complex. It is worth noting that in joint or extended families the notions of a classical oedipal complex may be difficult to sustain as the parenting may well be spread across different individuals and ages.

Psychoanalytical psychotherapy is, of course, only one approach. It is long term and requires a great deal of investment in terms of time and energy, and aims to address the causes and origins of mental distress at a fundamental level. Most patients who come to therapy – migrants or not – may have different goals to those who select other forms of therapy. More short-term interventions can be effective in assisting patients to address specific problems which they bring to therapy. However, once again, to be effective, these approaches need also to be sensitive to cultural difference.

We consider two of these: cognitive behavioural therapy (CBT) and group psychotherapy.

Cognitive behavioural therapy

CBT aims to assist patients in examining the characteristic way in which they think and act, to produce more healthy and adaptive styles of cognition. Unlike psychoanalysis, it is less concerned with why these patterns of thinking developed in an individual and more concerned with how they can be modified. Hence, it is symptom-focused, less concerned with a patient's personal narrative and history, and aimed at addressing a patient's present and future concerns.

In keeping with this short-term, issue-specific emphasis, CBT traditionally does not focus on the developmental history of the individual after the initial assessment. However, in migrant communities it may be necessary to revise this approach to assist in establishing initial rapport. Many of the issues that migrant patients bring to therapy may derive from their experience of racism, of trauma and an experience of war, economic hardship or enforced relocation. To brush these concerns aside after the initial assessment may leave a patient feeling that their problems were not being taken seriously, or that they were not being listened to. Such a belief on the part of a patient, particularly at an early stage in therapy, would be disastrous for any possibility of therapeutic success. Although spending significant time allowing a patient to vent his negative experiences and personal narrative would be unusual for a CBT approach, it is likely to be time well spent in allowing rapport to develop. Rathod *et al.* (2009) refer to work done with African-Caribbean patients in which it was necessary to allow the discussion of issues of slavery, racism and discrimination to be raised in CBT to allow progress to occur.

The degree of acculturation of a patient is also relevant. The length of time spent by the patient in the majority culture – in other words, the number of years since the patient first arrived – needs to be taken into account. In addition, the level of acculturation between generations will be different. Those who stay at home will acculturate more slowly than those who go out to work or school. Rathod *et al.* (2009) comment: 'With successive generations, individuals' values adapt to their country of residence. The initial task for the CBT therapist for these patients in multicultural settings is the assessment of the degree of acculturation, and whereabouts their cultural beliefs lie on the spectrum between the different cultures'.

A more general point (to which we shall return in the section on Individual therapy) is concerned with cultural influences affecting the approach of the therapist to his patients, and the expectations of the patient of their therapist. Asian and Chinese patients, for example, tend to regard professionals as authority figures, and expect their therapeutic encounter to be a process of being told what is wrong with them and what needs to be done. At an early stage in the therapeutic process with these patients, it may be necessary for the therapist to go against their predisposition and adopt a didactic style to be considered competent by the patient so that progress can begin. Another note of caution for the therapist is to ensure that they are familiar with the cognitive styles within a given culture. It may not be possible for every individual to carry the same concepts of guilt as compared with shame or 'I-ness' and concepts of the self alluded to above; therefore, individual assessments in the context of their culture become very important.

Group psychotherapy

Group psychotherapy presents significant challenges to patients from different cultural groups, and the fact that first generation immigrants are even less well represented in group psychotherapy than in other schools of therapy is evidence of this (Salvendy, 1999). Language differences present particular problems in group psychotherapy, since a patient who is able to follow a conversation in individual therapy may struggle with a fast-flowing group dialogue. In addition, an ethnically diverse group may leave group members splitting into racial factions – a process with which the therapist facilitating such a group would need to be cognisant. Ethnic or racial stereotypes may be promoted by members feeling that they are 'representing' their ethnic group rather than speaking from their own perspective, which can, in turn, lead to power imbalances between majority and minority group members. Active participation in the group process requires a certain level of self-disclosure, and cultural prohibitions on disclosure to strangers may inhibit participation.

The question of whether it is more therapeutically useful for a group to be multicultural or composed mainly or specifically of members from one ethnic group is context-dependent. If an individual is struggling with issues concerning acculturation, then a multicultural group setting is likely to be more effective. Monocultural group psychotherapy has the potential to reinforce ethnic stereotypes and promote subcultural norms. However, an exception to this may be in addressing religious fundamentalist groups or political fanaticism in a group setting. Silverstein (1995) states 'adherents of fundamentalist religious populations and politically or nationalistically fanatic groups and sects will be more effectively treated in homogeneous groups'.

Despite these potential difficulties, evidence suggests that group psychotherapy can be effective in assisting migrants with mental distress. Jenkins (1990) states 'interracial and/or interethnic group therapy can be effective if the minority members satisfy themselves that the therapist is sensitive to their socio-cultural and personal situation'. Hence, in a group setting with an ethnically diverse population, the responsibility lies with the therapist to ensure that these difficulties do not inhibit the success of group therapy.

Individual therapy

In the therapeutic encounter, both patient and therapist bring to the interaction their own racial and ethnic background. An important question is whether cultural and ethnic resonance or dissonance has a significant impact on the likely success of therapy. The development of a *therapeutic alliance* between patient and therapist is essential to doing fruitful work. An understanding of the influence of cultural difference between therapist and patient on the development of such an alliance is essential to avoid pitfalls which may block the potential to do useful work.

It has been a misconception that immigrant communities lacked the 'psychological sophistication' and capacity for introspection to engage usefully with psychotherapy, as it is understood in the west. Varma and Gupta (2008) define psychological sophistication as 'The ability to understand one's emotions and actions, conflicts and difficulties in intra-psychic rather than emotional terms'. However, this capacity for understanding needs to be translated into verbal expression for a therapeutic alliance to develop, and for therapy to progress. This involves the use of language, and the role of language difficulties in therapy have been overplayed: for example, Kline *et al.* (1980) found that Spanish-speaking patients who used an interpreter to speak to their therapists reported a more positive engagement than bilingual Mexican–Americans who spoke to their therapists in English. Further work (Ghassemzadeh, 2007; Hays, 1995) has indicated that the use of interpreters has little influence on the likely success of therapy (also see Chapter 20). Language barriers have been used as a justification for ethnic minorities being under-represented in the patient group for psychotherapy services, but research indicates that this explanation is inadequate.

When a patient is approaching psychotherapy for the first time, they are likely to have in mind a personal fantasy of their therapist, and what to expect from them. This fantasy will be culturally moulded, at least to some extent, and the level to which the therapist fulfils the expected role will influence the development of initial rapport. Patients from traditional societies are more likely to adopt a subservient role in their interaction with the therapist, and a therapist who fails to address this dependency need and does not react assertively with such a patient at the start of therapy is less likely to be able to establish initial rapport and the beginnings of a positive therapeutic alliance. Varma and Gupta (2008) state 'Indian patients have been observed to feel more free in terms of being dependent', an experience which is likely to seem alien to western therapists and patients. Hence, the approach of a therapist to a patient or patient group from a traditional society may require the engage-ment of a stylistic approach – at least initially – which goes against the grain of western psychotherapy.

Patients from a traditional background in eastern culture may perceive the role of the therapist to be analogous to the role of the *guru* or 'spiritual teacher'. This is not simply a doctor or healer in the western sense, but someone who has 'devoted themselves to under-standing and helping people in their totality' (Varma and Gupta, 2008; also see Neki, 1973 for the guru–chela paradigm). Within Tibetan Buddhist society, it is assumed that the Lama, or guru, possesses special powers to understand and determine the problems of the patient without recourse to verbal enquiry (Clifford, 1991). Similarly, in traditional African culture – specifically in some parts of Nigeria – 'the belief prevails that the most powerful healers know what the person's problem is before the person says anything. Taking a history is, according to this view, a symptom of therapeutic weakness' (Bhugra and Tantam, 1998). In this case it is likely that the therapist would need to give the patient a realistic explanation of the patient's capabilities prior to starting therapy, while still being aware that the therapist will be expected to adopt an assertive and didactic role in the therapeutic encounter.

The cultural acceptance of medical psychotherapy in the west has led to western patients recognising and expressing mental distress in psychological terms. Seeking out a therapist and receiving therapy is now a subject of dinner party chat in some sectors of western society, and the social stigma previously associated with mental distress is evaporating. However, patients from more traditional cultures are less likely to express such distress in the same terms. In these patients, physical somatisation, or the opinion that mental health problems are associated with spirit possession or the influence of climate factors, is more common.

Paradoxically, such opinions can be helpful in the healing process if they are properly understood, as they can be expressions of a sense of disconnectedness from their family or culture. As we mentioned previously, patients often come to therapy because of a sense of 'dissociation', either from themselves or the people around them. A traditional healer, therefore, may involve the patient's family and social contacts in the healing ritual, and in so doing assist the patient in reconnecting with those around them through their involvement in the ritual. Conversely, in the west, a therapist who is unable to translate the expression of symptoms in magico-religious or somatic terms is at risk of missing the expression of important psychological distress in their patients. Devereux (1980) has identified patterns of symptom expression in culturally diverse patients that are related to impoverishment, dedifferentiation, and disindividualisation. Bhugra and Tantam (1998) refer to this work when they state 'The clinician or therapist who understands the culture can predict the pattern, and therefore understand the patient's distress in a cultural framework and plan appropriate interventions'.

Couple therapy across cultures

Psychotherapy with couples in a multicultural society can involve both therapists and each member of the couple coming from widely differing cultural backgrounds. This can lead to a variety of potential pitfalls which can compound the already complex area of couple therapy. If we define a 'majority' culture and multiple 'minority' cultures, there are four possible scenarios (Bhugra and DeSilva, 2000):

1. Therapist comes from majority culture; couple from a minority culture
2. Therapist from minority culture; couple from majority culture
3. Therapist and couple both from the same minority culture
4. Therapist from one minority culture; couple from a different minority culture.

Each of these possible scenarios is becoming increasingly common in western psychotherapy, and each requires an awareness of the specific issues which may come up in therapy as a result.

The interaction between therapist and patient is influenced by both external and internal factors. External factors include race, class, educational level, gender and language; whereas internal factors include self-concept and identity, which can have multiple meanings, and values and religious beliefs which will be influenced by culture. In addition, the therapist's experience in general, and in working with ethnic minorities in particular, will have an influence, as will the patient's prior experience (if any) of being in therapy, as well as expectations from the therapeutic encounter.

No matter how 'objective' the therapist may attempt to be, the dynamic of the therapeutic interaction will be influenced depending on which of the above four scenarios pertains in a particular situation. The specific ethnicity of the three people involved will play a part, as will any imbalances of power related to communication and language, and the participants' prior experience of racial discrimination. The level of dissonance between the cultural backgrounds of those involved and the mainstream culture will play a part, as will the level of acculturation of the couple, both individually and as a unit. It is likely to be the case that the therapist, by virtue of their position, may be more likely to identify with the host culture to a greater extent than their patients. D'Ardenne (1991) reflects on this and suggests to the therapists, 'All therapists have some power over their patients, but the situation between patients from a minority culture and a therapist from the majority culture compounds this power imbalance further. The patients' perception of your age, social class, professional background and cultural skills will also affect your status, and how your patients see it.' To some extent this has been discussed in the previous section, where we raised the issue of 'what patients expect' from their therapist, and the role they are expected to play.

The situation in which the two people in a couple come from different cultural backgrounds (i.e. mixed race or inter-cultural couples) raises specific issues. In this case, the acceptance (or lack of it) on the part of one or both of the extended families involved may be a significant factor in causing the couple to come to therapy, and in the potential success of the therapeutic process. Non-acceptance of the relationship by one or both of the families is likely to be a significant cause of mental distress, with the level of distress being related to the level of rejection experienced. In extreme cases, the lives of one or both of the patients can be in danger if the union of the couple occurred against the wishes of the extended family. In the UK, the phenomenon of 'honour killings' of women by male family members has received a media profile in the recent past (Bingham, 2009). In the case of an inter-cultural couple, it would be easy and attractive to hope that the fact that the couple are together despite family opposition is an indication of the relationship's robustness. However, it could be the case that the union occurred during a period of passionate idealism, and the reality of the situation, and the ensuing distress, evolved later. It is reasonable to assume, however, that a significant level of mental distress will be caused by familial or racial rejection of one or both partners, or of the entire union itself.

Conflict between the host culture's expectations regarding the roles of men and women in a relationship, and the expectations of the two partners, can also give rise to friction. In several countries, women are expected to have a subservient role in the relationship, and not to associate with anyone outside of the family home without the permission of the husband. A man who has grown up in such a society, and who then emigrates to the west, may have expectations about the role and behaviour of his wife – and women in general – that do not resonate well with mainstream western culture. Conversely, a woman who has married within such a culture, then comes to the west with her husband, may experience a desire to explore her newfound freedoms. This is likely to cause friction within the relationship, and with the extended families involved. In therapy with such intercultural couples, the gender and cultural background of the therapist (two of the 'external factors' described above) is likely to be of critical importance, and the therapist must be highly sensitive to the possibility of being seen to collude with one or other of the two partners for these 'external' reasons. The manner in which such a couple approaches therapy may not, at first, indicate that cultural difference between the two partners is the causative factor for the symptomatology: such a couple may complain in general terms of 'incompatibility' or 'unreasonableness'. In such a situation the therapist must probe a little more deeply, while being cognisant of the role of cultural difference in the relationship.

An intercultural relationship may contain factors that are stabilising for the relationship, despite the problems mentioned above. Bhugra and DeSilva (2000) summarise the main issues concerning the pros and cons associated with an intercultural relationship, and on the plus side they note that mixed race relationships can be characterised by the points in Table 21.1.

In conducting therapy with ethnic minority couples, the therapist must be aware of issues of race and culture. A potential pitfall is the issue of 'colour blindness', where the therapist

Table 21.1 Intercultural relationships: some advantages (from Bhugra and De Silva, 2000)

1. More thorough preparation for marriage
2. A greater degree of commitment
3. Broader opportunities for learning and growth
4. Greater opportunities for children
5. More accepting of differences
6. Greater degree of self–other:
a. Differentiation
b. Tolerance
c. Respect
d. Acceptance

Table 21.2 Common pitfalls in therapy with ethnic minorities (from Bhugra and De Silva, 2000)

Colour consciousness: all problems result from minority status
Cultural transference: patient's feelings result from therapist's race
Cultural countertransference: therapist's feelings towards patient result from their race
Cultural ambivalence: therapist wishes to help but needs to control to maintain power
Over-identification: minority therapist over-identifies everything in terms of racism and defines problems as racially based (same as colour consciousness)
Identification with oppressor: minority therapist denies his/her status by virtue of power and because it is painful

overlooks the cultural differences between therapist and patient. Other issues are illustrated in Table 21.2. It is important for therapists to be aware of these issues, since such an awareness will reduce the likelihood of these issues becoming problematic within therapy.

Special issues

In the preceding discussion, we have concentrated implicitly on issues concerning heterosexual individuals and couples from ethnic minority groups, and the influence of culture and family on the therapeutic process. However, there are special groups which require a different and specific approach. Of these, we concentrate here on two in particular: gay and lesbian migrants; and refugees and asylum seekers who have special issues that clinicians must take into account in both their assessment and management.

Gay and lesbian migrants

In the world at present, there are 93 countries in which homosexual relationships are illegal, and seven in which they carry the death penalty (Iran, Saudi Arabia, Yemen, United Arab Emirates, Sudan, Nigeria and Mauritania). The UK government now recognises being gay as a possible reason to give an individual asylum in Britain. This immigration reform recognises the level of threat which can be faced by gay and lesbian people in their own countries (also see Chapter 17).

In the twenty-first century, the clerical authorities of the three main monotheistic religions (Christianity, Islam and Judaism) agree on little; however, condemnation of homosexuality and the refusal to accept equal civil rights for homosexual people is perhaps the only issue on which they all speak with the same voice. Even in western countries, where legal reform has recognised the value and validity of homosexual relationships, there remains a deeply ingrained homophobia in society. Gay people face bullying in school and college, rejection by their family and religion, and discrimination in the workplace. Physical attacks on gay people are common, and deaths as a result continue to occur and these incidents will precipitate migration if possible.

Gay people have much higher rates of psychological morbidity than the national average, and rates of suicide are also higher (see Chapter 17). Given the level and intensity of the rejection that gay people routinely experience, it is understandable that they often come to the therapist for assistance. When the patient comes from an ethnic minority, their problems are compounded: in addition to all of the other issues discussed above, in the eyes of their ethnic community they may be considered to have committed the ultimate transgression. They may be isolated, fearful and suffering from severe mental distress.

Gay patients who have come to the UK to escape homophobia at home face different challenges from their heterosexual counterparts. Specifically, the social supports which may normally be afforded a new immigrant in a foreign country through their ethnic minority community may not be available due to rejection. They may have to face the issues of being a member of an ethnic minority group in a foreign country alone and unsupported. The level of integration of the person into the gay subculture in the UK can be a stabilising or a spoiling factor, depending on the component of the subculture with which the person becomes involved. For young immigrants facing economic hardship, the attraction of becoming a sex worker could be irresistible – although this is a risk for all young, new immigrants, gay or straight.

The development of a therapeutic relationship with gay people from ethnic minority groups is likely to represent a challenge to the therapist. The question of whether it is therapeutically useful for the therapist to be gay himself or herself relates very closely to the issues described in Table 21.2 and in the section on Couple therapy, with 'gay' replacing cultural/ethnic/racial difference. It need not be significant that the therapists are gay themselves, although it may be the case that a patient would prefer to see a therapist with the same sexuality as their own. This may provide a sense of security in that there is a feeling that they are more likely to be understood and accepted. Gay ethnic minority patients' experience of rejection may make it more difficult to win trust and develop rapport, irrespective of the sexuality or ethnicity of the therapist. Patients may approach therapy with an expectation that they will be rejected, since that may have been their predominant experience of relationships during their lives. The therapist needs to be sensitive to these issues during the initial stages of therapy.

Refugees and asylum seekers

In addressing the issues surrounding refugees and asylum seekers, we are effectively addressing the question of how best to manage traumatised patients. In the twenty-first century there are ongoing conflicts around the globe, with civil unrest, political violence and war continuing to cause mass migration of very distressed people. With international air travel, these patients can find themselves in the UK, and it is becoming increasingly common for therapists to be involved with their care.

The uncertainty surrounding a patient's immigration status is likely to be a source of considerable anxiety, since this will impact on the individual's ability to settle and plan for their future. Currently in the UK there are many hundreds of individuals and families in immigration detention centres awaiting a decision on their applications. These locations regularly experience unrest, children's education is disrupted and considerable strain is placed on family relationships. Many of these individuals will have experienced severe trauma, and symptoms of post-traumatic stress disorder may be present (see Chapter 8).

The approach of these patients to the therapist may be to regard the therapist as an authority figure who, they may hope, can assist the patient with an attempt to remain in the country. Hence, the initial approach in therapy may be to explain to the patient the purpose of the therapeutic encounter, and set realistic expectations concerning what can reasonably be achieved. It is necessary for the therapist to be aware that the therapy may be terminated with little warning if the patient's asylum application is unsuccessful. In working with these patients, the therapist needs to be aware of the patient's cultural background and the trauma which they may have experienced. The role of the therapist, at least initially, may simply be to listen and allow the patient to vent their feelings and their experience. Patients who have experienced political violence or who have been in a war zone may be mistrustful of individuals perceived to be authority figures, given their possible past experiences with armed forces or the police in their own countries. In the initial therapeutic encounter, the therapist is likely to adopt a passive role, allowing the patients to express themselves in the best way they can, and state what they consider their problems to be, and what they hope to achieve through therapy. It may well be helpful if the therapist and the patient agree on the priorities and the expected outcomes of therapy. This will enable both sides to be absolutely clear of expectations so the chances of hopes/expectations being dashed will be minimised.

The manner in which ethnic minority patients express mental distress may be less obvious than with those from the west. In some cultures, mental distress is expressed through somatisation or through the attribution of symptoms to magico-religious phenomena such as spirit possession, or even to the weather. It may require some subtlety and sensitivity for the therapist to elucidate symptoms and translate them into a psychiatric diagnosis. Patients who attribute external causes to their mental distress may be resistant to such a diagnosis, and the therapist should be aware that the expression of an explicit diagnosis to the patient, at least initially, may negatively impact on the therapeutic relationship. However, it is possible to engage patients with different beliefs and explanatory models as long as their views are not denigrated.

Conclusions

Ethnic minorities are often under-represented in psychotherapy services. The reasons for this are related to inaccurate and possibly prejudiced ideas concerning the influence of 'psychological sophistication' and communication on the ability of ethnic minority patients to participate effectively in the therapeutic encounter. We have explained how a particular patient's cultural background may have an influence on their approach both to therapy and to the therapist. By understanding and developing a sensitivity to such cultural differences, therapists may be more likely to present themselves in a manner that is likely to improve the development of rapport and the possibility of promoting helpful therapy. Differences in the ethnic and cultural background of both therapist and patient can influence the therapeutic alliance in subtle ways, and therapists need to be aware of these effects. We live in an increasingly multicultural society, and training programmes for psychotherapists need to be improved in order to take into account the specific issues that arise in working with ethnic minority patients.

References

Berne, E. (1960). The cultural problem: psychotherapy in Tahiti. *American Journal of Psychiatry*, **116**, 1076.

Bhugra, D., De Silva, P. (2000). Couple therapy across cultures. *Sexual and Relationship Therapy*, 15(2), 184–92.

Bhugra, D., Tantam, D. (1998). Psychotherapy, culture and ethnicity. In D. Tantan (ed.) *Clinical Topics in Psychotherapy*. London: Gaskell.

Bingham, J. (2009). Honour killing: father convicted of murder of Tulay Goren. *Daily Telegraph*, 17 Dec 2009.

Bose, G. (1999). The Genesis and adjustment of the Oedipus wish. In T.G. Vaidyanathan & J. J. Kripal: *Vishnu on Freud's desk*. New Delhi: OUP pp 21–38.

Clifford, T. (1991). *Tibetan Buddhist Medicine and Psychiatry*. York Beach: Simon Weiser.

D'Ardenne, P. (1991). Transcultural issues in couple therapy. In D. Hooper and W. Dryden (eds) *Couple Therapy: A Handbook*. Milton Keynes: Open University Press.

Devereux, G. (1980). Normal and abnormal. In B. Gulati and G. Devereux (eds) *Basic Problems of Ethnopsychiatry*. Chicago: University of Chicago Press, 1–34.

Frank, J. D. (1993). The views of a therapist. In M. Shepherd and N. Sartorius (eds) *Non-specific Aspects of Treatment*. Bern: Huber.

Ghassemzadeh, H. (2007). The practice of cognitive-behaviour therapy in Roozbeh hospital: some cultural and clinical implications of psychological treatment in Iran. *American Journal of Psychotherapy*, 61(1), 53–69.

Hays, A. (1995). Multicultural applications of cognitive behaviour therapy. *Professional Psychology*, **26**, 309–15.

Hofstede, G. (2001). *Culture's Consequences: Comparing Values, Behaviors, Institutions and Organizations Across Nations*, 2nd edn. Thousand Oaks, CA: Sage.

Jenkins, A. (1990). Dynamics of the relationship in clinical work with African-American clients. *Group*, **14**(1), 36–43.

Jung, C. J. (1961). *Memories, Dreams, Reflections*. New York: Vintage Books.

Kline, F., Acosta, F., Austin, W. *et al.* (1980). The misunderstood Spanish-speaking patient. *American Journal of Psychiatry*, **137**, 1530–3.

Koss, J. D. (1987). Expectation and outcome for patients given mental health care or spiritist healing in Puerto Rico. *American Journal of Psychiatry*, **144**, 56–61.

Moacanin, R. (2003). *The Essence of Jung's Psychology and Tibetan Buddhism*. USA: Wisdom Books.

Neki, J. S. (1973). Guru–chela relationship: the possibility of a therapeutic paradigm. *American Journal of Orthopsychiatry*, **43**, 755–66.

Neki, J. S., Joinet, B., Hogan, M. *et al.* (1985). The cultural perspective of therapeutic relationship – a viewpoint from Africa. *Acta Psychiatrica Scandinavica*, **71**, 543–50.

Rathod, S., Kingdon, D., Phiri, P., Gobbi, M. (2009). Developing culturally sensitive cognitive-behaviour therapy for psychosis for ethnic minority patients by exploration and incorporation of service users' and health professionals' views and opinions. Report to Department of Health Delivering Race Equality Project Group.

Salvendy, J. (1999). Ethnocultural considerations in group psychotherapy. *International Journal of Group Psychotherapy*, **49**(4), 429–64.

Silverstein, R. (1995). Bending the conventional rules when treating the ultra-orthodox in group setting. *International Journal of Group Psychotherapy*, **45**(2), 237–49.

Varma, V. K., Gupta, N. (2008). *Psychotherapy in a Traditional Society: Context, Concept and Practice*. New Delhi: Jaypee.

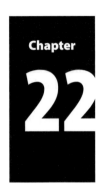

Ethno-psychopharmacology

Norman Poole

Editors' introduction

In any given therapeutic encounter, both medication and psychological interventions take place. The acceptance and adherence to any treatment modality will depend upon the patient's explanatory models and the differences between the patient's and clinician's models. It is possible that the culture will affect these models and also the expectations of any given treatment. There is considerable evidence in the literature that some ethnic and cultural groups are prescribed higher doses of medication and develop higher levels of side effects on smaller doses. These responses depend upon a number of factors, including pharmacological factors such as pharmacodynamics and pharmacokinetics, and non-pharmacological factors such as the use of complementary and alternative medicines, diet, smoking, placebo effect and religious taboos. In this chapter, Poole reviews the literature on pharmacokinetics and pharmacodynamics of antipsychotic and antidepressant drugs. He suggests that ethnic differences related to pharmacokinetics and pharmacodynamics are related to side effects, but equally important are the influences of cultural and religious factors, including diet. He points out that, as ever, at the core of this interaction is the doctor–patient relationship, where the style of the doctor, whether collaborative or authoritarian, works well. Clinicians must therefore be aware of the cultural expectations of their patients prior to pharmacotherapeutic interventions.

Introduction

There can be few areas of psychiatry where science and practice are at such odds as in ethno-psychopharmacology. There is now a large and growing body of evidence showing that drug metabolism and response differs markedly between ethnic groups, yet those known to metabolise psychotropic drugs poorly are frequently prescribed higher doses and polypharmacy.

A central tenet of racism is that each 'race' has distinct biological characteristics that can be considered more or less valuable. The inglorious history of the science of race and the policies advocated by its adherents stimulated a post-World War 2 consensus that all differences between ethnic groups can be explained by culture rather than biology (Tooby and Cosmides, 1992). This has, at times, had a stifling effect upon an emerging ethno-psychopharmacology. Self-defined ethnicity has, however, been shown to correlate with genetic variability (Sinha *et al.*, 2006), although it should be borne in mind that variation occurs in only around 0.02% of nucleotides and no single genetic marker of ethnicity has ever

Migration and Mental Health, ed. Dinesh Bhugra & Susham Gupta. Published by Cambridge University Press. © Cambridge University Press 2011.

variability in the rates of PMs and UMs. Those who are CYP2D6 PMs have a three-fold increased risk of adverse events on a standard dose regimen compared with EMs, and are six times more likely to discontinue their treatment (de Leon *et al.*, 2005b). The high proportion of Asians who are IMs explains why lower doses of risperidone are effective (mean dose 1.5 mg in first episode psychosis) (Luo, 2004) and are recommended to prevent EPSE.

Pharmacokinetics of antidepressant drugs

The major tricyclic antidepressants (TCAs) – amitriptyline, clomipramine, desipramine, imipramine and nortriptyline – are all substrates of CYP2D6 so should be prone to wide ethnic variation in metabolism (Poolsup *et al.*, 2000). Given the TCAs have a narrow therapeutic window, these differences may result in side effects, intolerance, toxicity or, in UMs, lack of efficacy. Indeed, a number of studies have demonstrated that serum concentrations of a TCA after a single dose are higher in Asians than in white subjects (Allen *et al.*, 1977; Pi *et al.*, 1989), who have far lower prevalence rates of the intermediate metaboliser (IM) CYP2D6*10. African-American patients have also been shown to have higher plasma levels of amitriptyline and nortriptyline than an, admittedly, unmatched white group (Ziegler and Biggs, 1977). Intriguingly, Asians may respond equally well to a lower serum concentration of desipramine and imipramine, though this effect may be mediated by pharmacodynamic ethnic variation, which is further discussed in the relevant section below.

A recent paper reports that Dutch PMs of CYP2D6 are at five-fold risk of switching from a TCA to another antidepressant during the first 6 weeks of treatment (to exclude those switched for poor response) compared with EMs (Bijl *et al.*, 2008). The PMs on an SSRI were not more likely to switch, perhaps because they have a wider therapeutic window. The newer antidepressants are not immune from the effects of CYP2D6 polymorphisms. Japanese homozygous for the CYP2D6*10 allele had a peak concentration of venlafaxine nearly 300% higher than those with the 'wild' version of the enzyme (Fukuda *et al.*, 2000).

The SSRIs fluoxetine, sertraline and paroxetine are mainly metabolised by CYP2D6 and 2C19. The effectiveness of sertraline, which is also a substrate for CYP3A4, has been studied in three ethnic groups: Australian whites, Australian Chinese and Malaysian Chinese (Hong Ng *et al.*, 2006). Comparing Australian Chinese with Malaysian Chinese enabled the investigators to assess the influence of environmental factors that could confound the results. Higher doses were required by the white group for the same clinical efficacy, despite plasma concentration being lower in the Asian groups. More Asians dropped out of treatment, possibly indicating increased sensitivity to side effects.

Pharmacokinetics of anxiolytics and mood stabilisers

The benzodiazepines, carbamazepine and lamotrigine are all metabolised by CYP3A4 and so the same considerations apply as with quetiapine, detailed above. Ethnic variations in the plasma concentration after a single dose of alprazolam have been shown, with Asians seeming to metabolise more slowly than whites (Lin *et al.*, 1988). Diazepam is also metabolised by CYP2C19 so is likely to be affected by PM polymorphisms. Asians, who have a higher prevalence of such polymorphisms, have been shown to require lower doses for the same clinical effect, although this may be explained by differences in body fat, which is greater in whites (Poolsup *et al.*, 2000).

Pharmacodynamics and ethnicity

It has been suggested that the capacity for inter-individual variation in the CYP will be selected for because so many substrates of this system are exogenous. The variability increases the likelihood that a novel exogenous toxin can be metabolised by at least some members of the species. Differences in neuroreceptor structure and function are, on the other hand, predicted to be low for they are evolutionarily ancient and required to respond stably to their ligand. However, Asians have been found to respond to lower serum concentrations of sertraline (Hong Ng *et al.*, 2006) and the TCAs desipramine and imipramine (Hu *et al.*, 1983), which suggests an increased sensitivity to these drugs' therapeutic effects.

A number of antidepressants block the serotonin transporter 5-HTTLPR, which increases the 5-HT concentration in the somatodendritic area to cause a downregulation of presynaptic and postsynaptic receptors (Stahl, 2008). The gene for 5-HTTLPR can be either a long allele (*l*) or a short allele (*s*), and the *l* form has been associated with a 50% reduction in transcriptional activity and serotonin uptake (Heils *et al.*, 1996). Those homozygous for the long allele (*l/l*) show less fear and attenuated amygdala responses to fearful stimuli than do heterozygotes or those with the *s/s* form (Hariri *et al.*, 2002). Numerous studies have demonstrated superior response to antidepressants in depressed patients with *l/l* and *l/s* (Kirchheiner *et al.*, 2004) and the *s* allele has been associated with the occurrence of side effects. Of relevance for ethno-psychopharmacology is the wide variability in frequency of the alleles in different ethnic groups. The *l* allele occurs in 14% of Koreans, 57% of whites (Lesch *et al.*, 1996) and up to 70% of those from sub-Saharan Africa. The relevance of this awaits clarification. Some studies have shown improved antidepressant response in Asians with the *s/s* form (Kim *et al.*, 2006), although a recent cross-cultural study found higher rates of *l/l* in whites, and more *s/l* and *s/s* in the Asian group but no differences in symptom level, response or adverse effects between the genotype groups (Ng *et al.*, 2006).

A genetic association study conducted on those entering the Sequenced Treatment Alternatives for Depression (STAR*D) study found a link between response to citalopram, the first treatment step, and a polymorphism of the gene coding for the 5-HT$_{2A}$ receptor (McMahon *et al.*, 2006). Those homozygous for the variant HTR$_{2A}$ allele had an 18% decreased absolute risk of not responding compared to those homozygous for the other allele. In addition, the allele associated with better response occurred six times more frequently in white subjects than in African Americans. This corresponds with previous studies that show lower response rates for SSRI treatment of depressive disorder in African Americans (Brown *et al.*, 1999). An association between two polymorphisms of the 5-HT$_{2A}$ receptor (10-T/C and His452Tyr) and poor response to clozapine has also been identified by meta-analysis (Arranz *et al.*, 1998). It is not yet clear, though, if these polymorphs vary in prevalence between ethnic groups.

Early studies of lithium response in Asians with bipolar affective disorder indicated that smaller doses and lower blood lithium levels were needed in Japanese (Takahashi, 1979) and Taiwanese (Yang, 1985) patients. These findings were confirmed in a cross-cultural study that demonstrated that white Caucasians require higher blood levels than a matched group of Taiwanese and Chinese Asians (0.98 versus 0.71–0.73 mEq/l). John Cade, credited with the discovery of lithium's effect on bipolar disorder, apparently noticed this differential response, so on the basis of this astute clinical observation he may be said to have pioneered ethno-psychopharmacology shortly after founding psychopharmacology (Schweitzer, 2008). As no inter-ethnic pharmacokinetic differences could be discerned after receiving a single lithium dose, the explanation for this is instead likely to be pharmacodynamic. A recent pharmaco-genetic study of lithium prophylaxis in Greeks with bipolar affective disorder found significantly fewer relapses in those heterozygous for the short and long alleles of 5-HTTLPR and a trend towards poor response in the *l/l* group (Serretti *et al.*, 2004). Perhaps the greater frequency of the *s* form in Asians explains the lower mean dosages required, though this awaits elucidation.

Adverse effects and ethnicity

Unless inter-ethnic differences in CYP metabolism are considered when prescribing psychotropics, dose-dependent side effects and treatment discontinuation will be higher than expected. As clinicians gain knowledge about a drug's range of effective doses based on treatment of the majority ethnic group they may inadvertently over-prescribe to the ethnic minorities they serve. Consequent adverse effects may exacerbate the feelings of alienation and incomprehensibility the patient already feels towards psychiatry. A number of studies have already demonstrated that some ethnic groups have an increased vulnerability to side effects. For example, with a fixed dose regimen of haloperidol, Asians experienced significantly more EPSEs than whites, but when the dose was titrated against clinical effect they received a lower dose and EPSE rates reduced to a level found in the white patients (Lin *et al.*, 1989). Similarly, Hispanics are reported to require half the dose of a tricyclic antidepressant to achieve therapeutic benefit but are also more sensitive to side effects (Marcos and Cancro, 1982). It is not known whether this finding reflects pharmacokinetic or pharmacodynamic differences.

Not all increases in side effect rates can be explained by metabolic factors, however. African Americans are at greater risk of developing lithium toxicity because the lithium–sodium counter-transport pathway, a genetically determined mechanism that exchanges intracellular lithium for extracellular sodium, is less effective (Strickland *et al.*, 1995). The intracellular lithium concentration in red blood cells was 60% higher in black patients with bipolar disorder and they also experienced more fatigue, dizziness, loss of initiative and urinary frequency. Red blood cell lithium concentration might then be a better correlate of intracerebral and intraneuronal lithium than the traditionally used serum concentration.

The infrequent but serious clozapine-induced agranulocytosis (CIA) is thought to be an immune response that is associated with particular human leukocyte antigens (HLAs) (Dettling *et al.*, 2007). As with the CYP system, large genetic variability in HLAs is to be expected to maximise survival against a novel threat, and the frequency of particular alleles differs by ethnicity. The B38, DR4 and DQw3 HLA haplotypes are found in 10–12% of Jewish people, but only 0.4–0.8% of whites carry them. Lieberman *et al.* (1990) noted that 20% of their Jewish patients on clozapine developed agranulocytosis, far higher than the usual 1%. All five of their Jewish patients who developed agranulocytosis carried the B38, DR4, DQw3 combination, so it was hugely over-represented in the CIA group. A large scale study of those in clozapine monitoring in Ireland and the UK identified a hazard ratio of 2.4 for Asians compared with other ethnicities (Munro *et al.*, 1999). The authors suggested the increased risk might reflect differences in metabolite toxicity as a result of CYP ethnic variability. Such findings raise the hope that genotyping will enable prediction of serious side effects. In the meantime, ethnicity should be a factor in considerations on drug choice.

Ethnicity and prescribing practices

The clinical use of psychotropic medications should conform to principles of evidence-based medicine and rational prescribing. The practice of prescribing is often, however, at variance with much of the pharmacokinetic and dynamic science outlined above. Although African-Americans are known to be at twice the risk of developing tardive dyskinesia (Morgenstern and Glazer, 1993), young black men with schizophrenia are half as likely to receive an atypical antipsychotic, which is believed to mitigate this risk, as white Americans (Herbeck *et al.*, 2004). It may be the prescribing practices to which black patients are exposed that cause the higher incidence of tardive dyskinesia rather than any genetically determined vulnerability. Studies in the USA have repeatedly shown that African-Americans receive higher doses of antipsychotics in the community and in emergency settings, are at increased risk of polypharmacy, and are prescribed antipsychotics as a depot in greater numbers (Chaudhry *et al.*, 2008). It will be recalled that many of those from black ethnic groups have less efficient CYP2D6 isoenzymes. Yet typical antipsychotics have a greater affinity for the 2D6 enzyme family than the second generation drugs (except risperidone), so it is sadly ironic that these are being withheld. This state of affairs is also true for clozapine (Kuno and Rothbard, 2002), the antipsychotic least likely to cause tardive dyskinesia, and is recommended as a rational treatment response when it develops. Perhaps clinicians are wary of prescribing clozapine to blacks because they are concerned about benign ethnic neutropenia, which is commonly present, or they balk at the risk of inducing metabolic syndrome.

Ethnic disparity in prescribing is not restricted to the antipsychotics though. The schizophrenia patient outcomes research team (PORT) client survey found minorities are more likely to be prescribed drugs at higher than recommended doses and are less likely to receive an antidepressant when depressed (Lehman and Steinwachs, 1998). Half as many African-Americans as white Americans who completed suicide were given an antidepressant in the year leading up to the act (Ray *et al.*, 2007). Prescribing inequality is not universal and a recent UK study that controlled for relevant factors revealed no relationship between prescribing practice and ethnicity, except in one centre that they diplomatically did not identify where polypharmacy was more prevalent in black patients (Connolly and Taylor, 2008).

Culture and psychopharmacology

The explanation for these discrepancies is a complex story involving more than just inadequate cultural competence on the part of the prescriber, though this undoubtedly plays a part. An ethnic group may have developed a set of health and illness beliefs quite at odds with those inculcated in the west. On the one hand, psychiatry is sometimes viewed as pathologising of normal or spiritual experiences and on the other, particular cultures are inordinately stigmatising of mental illness. Cultural beliefs will therefore influence a patient's conception of the problem and its solution, which the family and social system either confirms or contests. Ethnic groups with a strong tradition of herbal remedies hold beliefs antithetical to the advanced practice of psychopharmacology: the patient engages in home preparation of the herbs; dosages are fixed; rapid relief is anticipated; side effects minimal; and switching to a new regimen is straightforward (Westermeyer, 1989). If a medication fails to meet these ideals it will be discontinued and the corresponding illness model disparaged.

A sizeable proportion of improvement to psychotropics is attributable to the placebo response, a major explanatory model for which is expectancy theory: a placebo treatment produces an expectation of a certain effect that the expectation itself produces

(Stewart-Williams and Podd, 2004). It may achieve this by ameliorating anxiety, reducing negative cognitions while strengthening coping cognitions that cause salutary modifications in behaviour and arousal, or by directly affecting physiological pathways specific to the particular expectation. Expectancies are influenced by the information given about the placebo, hence a placebo can cause sedation or stimulation depending on the alleged effect. Although little studied, there is some evidence that placebo response is greater in non-western ethnic groups (Ng and Klimidis, 2008), perhaps because they expect western medicines to be stronger or more potent. A similar heightening of expectations might explain the intriguing discovery that in clinical trials of antidepressants both placebo and treatment response rates are positively correlated with year of publication (Walsh et al., 2002), though to date the role of ethnicity has not been investigated.

Cultural attitudes also affect the interpretation of side effects, even where no ethnically founded pharmacokinetic or pharmacodynamic difference exists. The side effect profile of lithium use is thought to be universal but certain effects convey a culturally salient meaning (Lee, 1993). Chinese patients on long-term lithium were unperturbed by polydipsia and polyuria because these are compatible with the removal of toxins from the body, but the fatigue was regarded with trepidation, perhaps because fatigue signifies loss of vital energy in Asian cultures (Sumathipala et al., 2004).

Adherence, it is known, is greatly influenced by the quality of the doctor–patient relationship. However, the physician as expert in collaboratively managing chronic conditions currently favoured by professional bodies and patient groups in the west might not conform to the 'good' doctor in other cultures where a more authoritative style wins respect. The doctor's own cultural heritage cannot be ignored. Where the patient and clinician's cultural groups have been in recent or traditional conflict, a cultural transference and counter-transference develops that can foster non-adherence (Comas-Díaz and Jacobsen, 1991). Indeed, the reduced compliance with psychiatric treatment found in African Americans (Herbeck et al., 2004) may have its origins here.

Cultural practices will also directly impact upon the pharmacokinetics of a drug. For example, CYP3A4 is inhibited by grapefruit juice while CYP1A2 is inhibited by caffeine but induced by cruciferous vegetables (cabbage, broccoli and brussels sprouts) and smoking. The induction of CYP1A2 by polycyclic aromatic hydrocarbons (PAH) found in cigarette smoke is a major reason for reduced plasma dose of commonly used antidepressants and anti-psychotics, particularly in those with the *1C and *1D alleles (Arranz and Kapur, 2008). Smoking rates vary significantly across ethnic groups and even more between genders within ethnic groups. For example, in the UK over 40% of Bangladeshi men smoke though only a tiny minority of Bangladeshi women do so (Health Survey for England 1999, 2001). Grilling meat over a dry heat also produces PAH so CYP1A2 induction will occur in places where this is common, such as Turkey, USA and many Asian countries.

Complementary medicines, often assumed to be benign so not declared to the doctor, can have significant pharmacological interactions. In combination with an SSRI, St John's Wort can precipitate the serotonin syndrome. It also induces CYP1A2, 2C9 and 3A4 and is known to decrease the bioavailability of many commonly used western medications (Mills et al., 2004). Liquorice, which is commonly used in traditional Chinese medicine, can increase the plasma level of active metabolites of tricyclics, thereby causing higher rates of side effects (Yu, 2008). Herbal medicines may act by similar mechanisms to standard psychiatric drugs. An extract from the Japanese stephania root demonstrates partial dopamine D1 agonism and D2 antagonism, and has been shown to have a similar efficacy to perphenazine in the treatment of inpatients with schizophrenia (Yu, 2008). Unani medicine, which is related to Ayurveda and likewise has its roots in ancient Greek and Arabic practice, is popular in the Indian subcontinent. Based on Galen's concept of the four humours, medications are employed to restore balance, many of which contain large quantities of heavy metals that can cause toxicity such as gold, silver, tin, copper, barium, lead, mercury, zinc, antimony and iron. A complementary physician may recommend a period of dietary restriction and increased fluid intake that can alter the pharmacokinetics of absorption and distribution of concomitant psychotropics. Likewise, religious taboos, such as not consuming anything, including medications, during daylight hours over the period of Ramadan, can similarly alter the efficacy and tolerability of a prescribed drug. During an episode of illness, spiritual and religious beliefs and practices assume even greater significance for the sufferer, though will often not be divulged to their doctor.

In practice, it is important to enquire about the use of complementary medicines, religious observances and taboos, diet and use of tobacco and alcohol. If it is agreed that a psychopharmacological agent is indicated for a patient who uses complementary medicine, then start at a low dose, monitor for interactions and side effects, and ensure the patient is as fully informed as the available evidence allows.

Conclusions

Ethno-psychopharmacology is a subdiscipline that, in an increasingly globalised world, cannot be ignored by psychiatrists. The practice of ethno-psychopharmacology should come readily to psychiatrists, being biopsychosocial in orientation. Beliefs about medications, concurrent use of complementary remedies, the meaning of symptoms and nature of support structures should be elicited and used to inform the formulation and treatment plan. The major CYP pathway for commonly used psychotropics and frequency of IM, PM and UMs in the ethnic minorities one serves should be readily to hand and used to guide treatment decisions. If side effects develop or there is no response, then choose another medication metabolised by a different route. The science is progressing rapidly so keeping up to date is imperative if psychiatric patients are to receive the highest quality treatment. Iniquitous prescribing highlights the need for some ethno-psychopharmacological insights to be rapidly converted into practice, while yet others provide an intriguing glimpse of an emergent psychopharmacogenetics.

References

Allen, J. J., Rack, P. H., Vaddadi, K. S. (1977). Differences in the effects of clomipramine on English and Asian volunteers. Preliminary report on a pilot study. *Postgraduate Medical Journal*, **53**(4), 79–86.

Arranz, M. J., Kapur, S. (2008). Pharmacogenetics in psychiatry: are we ready for widespread clinical use? *Schizophrenia Bulletin*, **34**(6), 1130–44.

Arranz, M. J., Munro, J., Sham, P. *et al.* (1998). Meta-analysis of studies on genetic variation in 5-HT$_{2A}$ receptors and clozapine response. *Schizophrenia Research*, **32**, 93–9.

Bijl, M. J., Visser, L. E., Hofman, A. *et al.* (2008). Influence of the CYP2D6*4 polymorphism on dose, switching and discontinuation of antidepressants. *British Journal of Clinical Pharmacology*, **65**(4), 558–64.

Brown, C., Schulberg, H. C., Sacco, D., Perel, J. M., Houck, P. R. (1999). Effectiveness of treatments for major depression in primary medical care practice: a post hoc analysis of outcomes for African American and white patients. *Journal of Affective Disorders*, **53**, 185–92.

Chaudhry, I. B., Neelam, K., Duddu, V., Husain, N. (2008). Ethnicity and psychopharmacology. *Journal of Psychopharmacology*, **22**, 673–80.

Comas-Díaz, L., Jacobsen, F. M. (1991). Ethnocultural transference and countertransference in the therapeutic dyad. *American Journal of Orthopsychiatry*, **61**(3), 392–402.

Connolly, A., Taylor, D. (2008). Ethnicity and quality of prescribing among in-patients in south London. *British Journal of Psychiatry*, **193**, 161–2.

de Leon, J., Armstrong, S. C., Cozza, K. L. (2005a). The dosing of atypical antipsychotics. *Psychosomatics*, **46**, 262–73.

de Leon, J., Susce, M. T., Pan, R. M. *et al.* (2005b). The CYP2D6 poor metabolizer phenotype may be associated with risperidone adverse drug reactions and discontinuation. *Journal of Clinical Psychiatry*, **66**, 15–27.

Dettling, M., Cascorbi, I., Opgen-Rhein, C., Schaub, R. (2007). Clozapine-induced agranulocytosis in schizophrenic Caucasians: confirming clues for associations with human leukocyte class I and II antigens. *The Pharmacogenomics Journal*, **7**, 325–32.

Fukuda, T., Nishida, Y., Zhou, Q. *et al.* (2000). The impact of the CYP2D6 and CYP2C19 genotypes on venlafaxine pharmacokinetics in a Japanese population. *European Journal of Clinical Pharmacology*, **56**(2), 175–80.

Hariri, A. R., Mattay, V. S., Tessitore, A. *et al.* (2002). Serotonin transporter genetic variations and the response of the human amygdala. *Science*, **297**(5580), 400–3.

Health Survey for England 1999 (2001). *The Health of Minority Ethnic Groups*, London: The Stationery Office.

Heils, A., Teufel, A., Petri, S. *et al.* (1996). Allelic variation of human serotonin transporter gene expression. *Journal of Neurochemistry*, **66**, 2621–4.

Herbeck, D. M., West, J. C., Ruditis, I. *et al.* (2004). Variations in use of second-generation antipsychotic medication by race among adult psychiatric patients. *Psychiatric Services*, **55**, 677–84.

Hong Ng, C., Norman, T. R., Naing, K. O. *et al.* (2006). A comparative study of sertraline dosages, plasma concentrations, efficacy and adverse reactions in Chinese versus Caucasian patients. *International Clinical Psychopharmacology*, **21**, 87–92.

Hu, W. H., Lee, C. F., Yang, Y. Y., Tseng, Y. T. (1983). Imipramine plasma levels and clinical response. *Bulletin of Chinese Social Neuroscience and Psychiatry*, **9**, 40–9.

Israili, Z. H., Dayton, P. G. (2001). Human alpha-1-glycoprotein and its interaction with drugs. *Drug Metabolism Reviews*, **33**(2), 161–235.

Jones, D. S., Perlis, R. H. (2006). Pharmacogenetics, race and psychiatry: prospects and challenges. *Harvard Review of Psychiatry*, **14**, 92–108.

Kim, H., Lim, S. W., Kim, S. *et al.* (2006). Monoamine transporter gene polymorphisms and antidepressant response in Koreans with late-life depression. *Journal of the American Medical Association*, **296**, 1609–18.

Kirchheiner, J., Nickchen, K., Bauer, M. *et al.* (2004). Pharmacogenetics of antidepressants and antipsychotics: the contribution of allelic variations to the phenotype of drug response. *Molecular Psychiatry*, **9**, 442–73.

Kuno, E., Rothbard, A. B. (2002). Racial disparities in antipsychotic prescribing prescription patterns for patients with schizophrenia. *American Journal of Psychiatry*, **159**, 567–72.

Lambert, T., Norman, T. R. (2008). Ethnic differences in psychotropic drug response and pharmacokinetics. In C. H. Ng, K-M. Lin, B. S. Singh and E. Chiu (eds) *Ethno-Psychopharmacology: Advances in Current Practice*. Cambridge: Cambridge University Press, 38–61.

Lee, S. (1993). Side effects of chronic lithium therapy in Hong Kong Chinese: an ethnopsychiatric perspective. *Culture Medicine and Psychiatry*, **17**(3), 301–20.

Lehman, A. F., Steinwachs, D. M. (1998). Patterns of usual care for schizophrenia: initial results from the schizophrenia patient outcomes research team (PORT) client survey. *Schizophrenia Bulletin*, **24**(1), 11–20.

Lesch, K. P., Bengel, D., Heils, A. *et al.* (1996). Association of anxiety-related traits with a polymorphism in the serotonin transporter gene regulatory region. *Science*, **274**, 1527–31.

Lieberman, J. A., Yunis, J., Egea, E. *et al.* (1990). Agranulocytosis in Jewish patients with schizophrenia. *Archives of General Psychiatry*, **47**, 945–8.

Lin, K. M., Finder, E. (1983). Neuroleptic dosages for Asians. *American Journal of Psychiatry*, **140**(4), 490–1.

Lin, K. M., Lau, J. K., Smith, R. *et al.* (1988). Comparison of alprazolam plasma levels in normal Asian and Caucasian male volunteers. *Psychopharmacology*, **96**, 365–9.

Lin, K. M., Poland, R. E., Nuccio, I. *et al.* (1989). A longitudinal assessment of haloperidol doses and serum concentrations in Asian and Caucasian schizophrenic patients. *American Journal of Psychiatry*, **146**(10), 1307–11.

Lin, K. M., Chen, C. H., Yu, S. H., Wang, S. C. (2008). Culture and ethnicity in psychopharmacotherapy. In C. H. Ng, K-M. Lin, B. S. Singh and E. Chiu (eds) *Ethno-Psychopharmacology: Advances in Current Practice*. Cambridge: Cambridge University Press, 27–37.

Luo, N. (2004). Drug utilization review of risperidone for outpatients in a tertiary referral hospital in Singapore. *Human Psychopharmacology*, **19**, 259–64.

Marcos, L. R., Cancro, R. C. (1982). Pharmacotherapy of Hispanic depressed patients: clinical observations. *American Journal of Psychotherapy*, **36**, 505–13.

McMahon, F. J., Buervenich, S., Charney, D. *et al.* (2006). Variation in the gene encoding the serotonin 2A receptor is associated with outcome of antidepressant treatment. *American Journal of Human Genetics*, **78**(5), 804–14.

Melkersson, K. I., Scordo, M, G., Gunes, A., Dahl, M. L. (2007). Impact of CYP1A2 and CYP2D6 polymorphisms on drug metabolism and on insulin and lipid elevations and insulin resistance in

clozapine-treated patients. *Journal of Clinical Psychiatry*, **68**, 697–704.

Mills, E., Montori, V. M., Wu, P. *et al.* (2004). Interaction of St John's wort with conventional drugs: a systematic review of clinical trials. *British Medical Journal*, **329** (7456), 27–30.

Morgenstern, H., Glazer, W. M. (1993). Identifying risk factors for tardive dyskinesia among long-term outpatients maintained with neuroleptic medications. *Archives of General Psychiatry*, **50**(9), 723–33.

Mori, A., Maruo, Y., Iwai, M., Sato H., Takeuchi, Y. (2005). UDP-glucuronosyltransferase 1A4 polymorphisms in a Japanese population and kinetics of clozapine glucuronidation. *Drug Metabolism and Disposition*, **33**, 672–5.

Munro, J., O'Sullivan, D., Andrews, C. *et al.* (1999). Active monitoring of 12760 clozapine recipients in the UK and Ireland: beyond pharmacovigilance. *British Journal of Psychiatry*, **175**, 576–80.

Ng, C. H., Klimidis, S. (2008). Cultural factors and the use of psychotropic medications. In C. H. Ng, K.-M. Lin, B. S. Singh and E. Chiu (eds) *Ethno-Psychopharmacology: Advances in Current Practice*. Cambridge: Cambridge University Press, Chapter 10.

Ng, C. H., Schweitzer, I., Norman, T., Easteal, S. (2004). The emerging role of pharmacogenetics: implications for clinical psychiatry. *Australian and New Zealand Journal of Psychiatry*, **38**(7), 483–9.

Ng, C. H., Chong, S. A., Lambert, T. *et al.* (2005). An inter-ethnic comparision study of clozapine dosage, clinical response and plasma levels. *International Clinical Psychopharmacology*, **20**(3), 163–8.

Ng, C. H., Easteal, S., Tan, S. *et al.* (2006). Serotonin transporter polymorphisms and clinical response to sertraline across ethnicities. *Progress in Neuro-Psychopharmacology and Biological Psychiatry*, **30**(5), 953–7.

Pi, E. H., Tran-Johnson, T. K., Walker, N. R. *et al.* (1989). Pharmacokinetics of desipramine in Asian and Caucasian volunteers. *Psychopharmacology Bulletin*, **25**, 483–7.

Poolsup, N., Li Wan Po, A., Knight, T. L. (2000). Pharmacogenetics and psychopharmacotherapy. *Journal of Clinical Pharmacy and Therapeutics*, 25(3), 197–220.

Ray, W. A., Hall, K., Meador, K. G. (2007). Racial differences in antidepressant treatment preceding suicide in a Medicaid population. *Psychiatric Services*, 58(10), 1317–23.

Schweitzer, I. (2008). Introduction. In C. H. Ng, K-M. Lin, B. S. Singh and E. Chiu (eds) *Ethno-Psychopharmacology: Advances in Current Practice*. Cambridge: Cambridge University Press, 1–4.

Serretti, A., Malitas, P. N. Mandelli, *et al.* (2004). Further evidence for a possible association between serotonin transporter gene and lithium prophylaxis for mood disorders. *The Pharmacogenomics Journal*, 4, 267–73.

Sinha, M., Larkin, E. K., Elston, R. C., Redline, S. (2006). Self-reported race and genetic admixture. *New England Journal of Medicine*, 354, 421–2.

Stahl, S. M. (2008). *Stahl's Essential Psychopharmacology: Neuroscientific Basis and Practical Applications*. Cambridge: Cambridge University Press.

Stewart-Williams, S., Podd, J. (2004). The placebo effect: dissolving the expectancy versus conditioning debate. *Psychological Bulletin*, 130(2), 324–40.

Strickland, T., Lin, K., Fu, P., Anderson, D., Zheng, Y. (1995). Comparison of lithium ratio between African-American and Caucasian bipolar patients. *Biological Psychiatry*, 37(5), 325–30.

Sumathipala, A., Siribaddana, S. H., Bhugra, D. (2004). Culture-bound syndromes: the story of dhat syndrome. *British Journal of Psychiatry*, 184, 200–9.

Takahashi, R. (1979). Lithium treatment in affective disorders: therapeutic plasma level. *Psychopharmacology Bulletin*, 15, 32–5.

Tooby, J., Cosmides, L. (1992). The psychological foundations of culture. In: J. H. Barkow, L. Cosmides and J. Tooby (eds) *The Adapted Mind: Evolutionary Psychology and the Generation of Culture*. Oxford: Oxford University Press. Chapter 1.

Walsh, B. T., Seidman, S. N., Sysko, R., Gould, M. (2002). Placebo response in studies of major depression: variable, substantial, and growing. *Journal of the American Medical Association*, 287(14), 1840–7.

Wang, S. L., Huang, J. D., Lai, M. D., Liu, B. H., Lai. M. L. (1993). Molecular basis of genetic variation in debrisoquin hydroxylation in Chinese subjects: polymorphism in RFLP and DNA sequence of CYP2D6. *Clinical Pharmacology & Therapeutics*, 53, 410–18.

Westermeyer, J. (1989). Somatotherapies. In J. H. Gold (ed.) *Psychiatric Care of Migrants: A Clinical Guide*. Washington DC: American Psychiatric Press, 139–68.

Yang, Y. Y. (1985). Prophylactic efficacy of lithium and its effective plasma levels in Chinese bipolar patients. *Acta Psychiatrica Scandinavia*, 71, 171–5.

Yu, X. (2008). Complementary medicines in mental disorders. In C. H. Ng, K-M. Lin, B. S. Singh and E. Chiu (eds) *Ethno-Psychopharmacology: Advances in Current Practice*. Cambridge: Cambridge University Press, Chapter 9.

Zhou, H. H., Adedoyin, A., Wilkinson G. R. (1990). Differences in plasma binding of drugs between Caucasians and Chinese subjects. *Clinical Pharmacology and Therapeutics*, 48(1), 10–17.

Zhou, S. F., Liu, J. P., Chowbay, B. (2009). Polymorphism of human cytochrome P450 enzymes and its clinical impact. *Drug Metabolism Reviews*, 41(2), 89–295.

Ziegler, V. E., Biggs, J. T. (1977). Tricyclic plasma levels: effects of age, race, sex and smoking. *Journal of American Medical Association*, 238, 2167–9.

Chapter 23

Migration and physical illnesses

Gurvinder Kalra, Priyadarshini Natarajan and Dinesh Bhugra

Editors' introduction

Physical health and mental health are inextricably linked, and mind–body dualism may not be accepted by certain cultures. There are differences in the prevalence of physical diseases related to ethnicity and cultures. However, transition across cultures can expose individuals to previously unknown aetiological agents such as viruses and harmful emissions. These exposures can affect the immunity of the migrant and, with rapid travel times, the chances of spreading infection across a wide area can be extremely high. Clinicians must recognise that physical illnesses will affect the mental health of migrants and vice versa, and therefore they must be cognisant of physical factors. Migrant physical and mental health issues can be complex, and informed by infections and organic factors. As the authors highlight in this chapter, it is important to be aware of the potential impact both of migration as a stressor and also leading to long-term physical changes related to changes in diet and lifestyle. Their health beliefs and models of illness will be affected by culture and idioms of distress and use of metaphors may not be easily picked up by clinicians. As there is evidence to suggest that migrants may be more prone to infections and to industrial accidents, education and prevention gain prime importance. Medically unexplained symptoms may add further to the burden of care. With awareness of variation in physical illness, the clinician can avoid mistakes and provide more suitable and appropriate treatments. Addressing these issues can bring benefit to the new society.

Introduction

The interaction between physical and mental health is a complex one. Physical ill-health will affect mental health, and emotional distress in turn influences physical health. However, a key to understanding help-seeking is the way in which individuals and their families and cultures see mind–body dualism. In western cultures, even now people who 'somatise' their symptoms are seen as psychologically inferior and are often treated with disdain. However, if cultures do not make a clear distinction between mind and body, it is logical that poor functioning of one will lead to poor functioning of the other, as they are inter-related. Furthermore, individuals may use somatic or physical metaphors to describe their distress. For example, 'I feel gutted' or 'my heart is sinking' are both expressions of feeling low or anxious. Thus, clinicians must be aware of specific terms and idioms of distress used in specific cultures.

Migration and Mental Health, ed. Dinesh Bhugra & Susham Gupta. Published by Cambridge University Press. © Cambridge University Press 2011.

The other key point to be aware of in relation to other cultures is the role of the life cycle and associated rituals and taboos, so that clinicians do not confuse normal variants with pathology. The life cycle course allows an intimate understanding of the core values of a culture, with social transitions linked with physiological transitions. These allow cultures to celebrate transitional states. The key stages in a life course are pregnancy and childbirth, infancy, childhood, puberty (menstruation), adulthood, transition into old age (retirement, reaching 60, menopause) and end of life. Pregnancy and childbirth are heavily influenced by culture. Diet and proscription of foods and rituals in pregnancy will affect the size and growth of the fetus as well as complications in pregnancy and outcome of birth. The role of medicine and untrained or partly trained midwives in childbirth will vary across cultures. Antenatal care and access to such care will also depend upon a number of factors. Transition to motherhood is celebrated in different ways, with varying amounts of rest recommended after parturition. Socio-economic factors will affect when the mother goes back to work. Postnatal psychosis and depression will occur across cultures, but different modalities of treatment will be used and be acceptable. With child mortality being high in low- and middle-income (LAMI) countries, it is possible that specific rituals are carried out to celebrate 'social birth' and acceptance into the society, occurring a few days, few weeks or months after physical birth. Feeding of infants will be heavily influenced by cultural norms, where specific rituals will need to be carried out in celebration of the introduction of the baby to semi-solid food. Cultural notions of weaning foods are significant to new mothers and families. Childcare may be handed over to older siblings or other members of the joint or extended family at an early stage. Similarly, attitudes to and mores of bringing up children will vary across cultures. Notions of physical or corporal punishment acceptable in one culture may be totally unacceptable and, indeed, illegal in another, and this may produce an element of conflict in migrants. Expectations of educating girls and somewhat different gender role expectations will add another layer of complexity to the interaction between migrants and the new culture. Social transition from puberty to adulthood brings with it additional responsibilities, both for the individual and their families, and clinicians in the new culture may not be aware of this. For girls in particular, the onset of menstruation (and resulting perceived impurity) may be a significant step in some cultures. Transition after menopause brings cultural issues of their own when menopause is medicalised as a matter of routine, thus creating further tensions.

Death and resulting bereavement raise management issues for clinicians. In some cultures, the official period of bereavement and grief may be up to a year, thereby making the clinical diagnosis of abnormal grief reaction erroneous if using western periods as the norm. Death in itself may be medicalised and construed as a failure of modern medicine, whereas in many cultures it is a fact of life and a step towards reincarnation or *nirvana*. The care and disposal of the dead body has different connotations and procedures which vary cross-culturally.

Physical health of migrants can be seen in different stages, including acute phase, transition, chronic or long-term care. New migrants may present with acute conditions, infections and traumatic injuries. In the transition phase, 3–6 years after arrival, Kurdish refugees in the USA in 1991–1992 believed that they would go back and their focus was on their children's health as they were expected to grow up to be the next generation of freedom fighters and adults' care was second in preference. After initial infectious diseases, chronic diseases like diabetes and hypertension started to emerge (Kemp and Rasbridge, 2004, page 29). Ten or more years later, following a period of settlement, chronic physical and psychological problems may emerge. Chronic poor health may be further complicated by the breakdown of family structures, social isolation, alienation and accumulation of unrecognised or untreated conditions and being unaware of the new healthcare systems or pathways. The health risks across the globe include malnutrition, intestinal parasites, hepatitis B, tuberculosis, low rates of immunisation, malaria, dental caries, STIs (including HIV), diarrhoeal illness, rheumatic heart disease, epilepsy, etc. Kemp and Rasbridge (2004, page 34) go on to note that global screening recommendations include tuberculosis (TB), intestinal parasites, hepatitis, HIV, VDRL (syphilis), Hansen's disease, other STIs, full blood count, malaria, immunisation and nutritional status. Religious influences on health and taboos must not be overlooked.

Migrant health

Migrants' health is important at all levels, including the community of origin, transit and destination, and also includes periodical migration as well as permanent migration. As the presence of immigrants increases, it becomes ever more important to assess their health needs and utilisation of health services, so that adequate programmes and policies can be promoted, bearing in mind how the migrants may have different health risks and health behaviour. Reeske et al. (2009) have hypothesised that these differences might diminish with time passed since migration, thus referring to migration as a 'health transition'. Mobile people interact with and potentially affect and adopt the health profile of all communities along their migration route.

Mobility implies not only the physical displacement of a person or population, but also the mobility of culture, health beliefs and epidemiological factors that occur along with the individual. The legal status of the migrant in the host country is one of the most important factors that determine access to health and social services. Irregular migration that does not follow the laws, policies and regulations of the land, including human trafficking, can result in migrants hiding in host countries, carrying with them various infectious or newer lifestyle diseases in their prodromal phases. During the migration-exile, the cultural barrier, social degradation, guilt, social passivity and ideological alienation cause a changed identity and low control, which increase the vulnerability to psychological distress and physical disease (Sundquist et al., 1995). This trauma, resulting from migration, stress and prolonged affect-laden situations, may precipitate a physical illness (Gonzalez et al., 1999). Other factors responsible may be: limited access to regular medical services, lack of insurance coverage, high cost of healthcare and inflexible work schedules, resulting in use of unsupervised self-treatment or substandard care (Hong et al., 2006). Times have changed from earlier day's when rural-to-urban migration of people in search of seasonal jobs led to the spread of acutely infectious illnesses like cholera (especially in India). Now lifestyle diseases also spread with the developing-to-developed nation migration.

An additional issue that needs to be explored is the role of culture and ethnicity. Ethnicity is an important factor in understanding the origin of some physical illnesses. Race is a biological construct and ethnicity is self-ascription by the individuals. However, racial and ethnic differences do matter in some physical conditions. Among the Ashkenazi Jews from Eastern Europe there is a high incidence of Tay–Sachs syndrome which presents with learning disability and apathy in adults. We also know that sickle cell anaemia may offer some protection from malaria, and the genetic variant for sickle cell trait is common among the sub-Saharan population in Africa and among the African-Caribbean population.

Hospitalisation and migrants

Access to medical care may include access to primary care services, in secondary care from simple outpatient access to full inpatient admissions, both of which may be different in the migrant individuals. Studies have found lower hospitalisation rates in adult immigrants except for some specific causes (injuries, particularly for men, infectious diseases, deliveries and induced abortions), which were higher in the immigrants than for the resident population (Cacciani *et al.*, 2006). The migrants may thus make contact with the healthcare system purely following emergencies or accidents (owing to poor living and working conditions) or only when the illness becomes unbearable for them. In fact, there are surveys of injuries at work conducted in Italy that have suggested a higher risk for immigrants (Capacci *et al.*, 2005; INAIL Report, 2002). Similarly, reports suggest that migrant workers have higher rates of occupational accidents and consequent disability than native workers (Egger *et al.*, 1990). A Danish study showed that the duration of hospital stay is longer for foreigners than for residents for some diagnoses but shorter for others (Krasnik *et al.*, 2002), while earlier researchers had suggested that immigrants have an epidemiological profile similar to the disadvantaged Dutch (Uniken Venema *et al.*, 1995). Another study from the Netherlands reported a lower use of specialised healthcare among immigrants, possibly because of difficulties of access (Stronks *et al.*, 2001).

Looking at health status and hospital utilisation by recent immigrants to New York City, Muennig and Fans (2002) concluded that foreign-born people living there appeared to be healthier and consumed fewer hospital resources than US-born populations. Thus, the lower utilisation of healthcare services may be either because of the healthcare barriers or better health in the migrants. A meta-analysis (Gagnon *et al.*, 2009) showed that results for preterm birth, low birth weight and health-promoting behaviour in migrants were as good or better as those for receiving-country women in ≥50% of all studies that were included in the review. The latter can be interpreted in the light of 'the healthy and young migrate' scenario, though this may not always be true. When considered disease-wise, Cacciani *et al.* (2006) found that immigrants are more frequently hospitalised for infectious diseases, particularly HIV and TB, in their study. Healthy migrants' effect, as described by Parkin (1992), suggests that the healthiest and youngest people choose to go abroad in search of better living conditions. However, this effect may slowly decline as a consequence of both forced migration and displacement, and family reunions. One study conducted in Rome reported deliveries and injuries as the most frequent cause of hospitalisation (Arista and Marceca, 1998). Also in Italy, Lemma *et al.* (1993) found that migrants had higher rates of TB, trauma and pregnancy, although other analyses report a lower percentage of hospitalisations for immigrants compared with Italians (Barro *et al.*, 1993; Pennazza *et al.*, 2000).

Mortality risk among babies born to migrants is not consistently higher, but appears to be greatest among refugees, non-European migrants to Europe, and foreign-born blacks in the USA (Gissler *et al.*, 2009). These differences may be related to physical problems, stress or other factors which need to be explored further.

Infectious diseases and migrants

Travel time between destinations is often shorter than the incubation period of an infectious agent. This was particularly illustrated by the severe acute respiratory syndrome (SARS) and swine flu epidemics. The relationship between population migration and the emergence of previously unknown diseases such as HIV or SARS, as well as the re-emergence of known diseases such as tuberculosis and malaria, is increasingly being recognised as a major health problem. Reduced time of travel between countries helps in the quick spread of an infection before it can come to the attention of the health inspectors, giving rise to pandemics. The migrant population may be at risk for various infectious diseases in their newly acquired countries. Again, a number of factors are responsible for the same. Some of these individuals may already be harbouring the infectious agents or may acquire them afresh after migrating or during the process of migration. Migrants may carry a higher risk of infectious diseases, for example TB, owing to higher disease prevalence in a country/region they travelled from or through. TB has re-emerged in the industrialised world and this is largely associated with the increased arrival of people coming from geographical areas of high TB prevalence. Worldwide TB control and surveillance systems have failed to appreciate the scope and patterns of migration and this has contributed to the emerging field of migration health among the many factors. The former is an important point to consider in infections like TB, which has moved from the isoniazid (INH)-sensitive to the multidrug-resistant (MDR) cases and now to the ever-growing cases of extensively drug-resistant (XDR) TB. Many of the XDR patients may never have been treated for TB, implying that they had a primary infection with the XDR strain of *Mycobacterium tuberculosis*. XDR tuberculosis has now become a global threat and is of great significance in the field of public health. Migrants with either MDR or XDR TB in the incubation period pose a high threat to the native population. Whereas infections like yellow fever are easy to control with vaccinations at the immigration counters, TB does not provide the health providers with such opportunities. TB is an example of a disease that can be easily screened and treated at the outset with drugs that are available at a low cost worldwide, leading to socio-economic benefits to the host countries.

XDR tuberculosis or even simple TB has major implications for patients with HIV–AIDS. HIV–AIDS has become the biggest 'pandemic' to sweep scores of people globally. With people migrating from rural to urban areas and from developing to developed countries or vice versa, the chances of sexually transmitted HIV have increased, thanks to the anonymity factor in the immigrants and the sexual 'highs' that they may sometimes go on in their newly found independence.

SARS is a recent example of a regional outbreak in one country that spread within weeks along the routes of international air travel to over 25 countries and five continents. The affected migrants spread quickly through the new countries before the health inspectors had time to quarantine them at the entry points, infecting more people.

Persons trafficked for sexual exploitation face significant risks to their mental and reproductive health, such as sexual violence, unwanted and unsafe pregnancy, STIs (including HIV), substance abuse and risk of infectious diseases such as hepatitis and TB. With the involvement of younger boys and girls for sexual trafficking, the risk that these individuals face regarding STIs is great. Cacciani *et al.* (2006) reported a higher proportion of infectious and parasitic diseases in migrant youths in Italy, and Uniken Venema *et al.* (1995) in the Netherlands also noted that rates of infectious diseases and child mortality were higher among Turkish and Moroccan immigrants.

Depression may well accompany many infectious diseases and may not be diagnosed if the diagnosis focuses only on infectious diseases. Clinicians therefore need to be aware of not only different symptoms of depression across cultures but also idioms of distress that migrants may use.

Lifestyle diseases and migrants

Not only are infectious diseases important as far as the issue of migration is concerned but, with the westernisation of many countries, lifestyle diseases have evolved as an important group of illnesses in these population groups. The prevalence of diabetes, other cardiovascular risk factors and cardiovascular morbidity and mortality varies between immigrant groups in western societies.

Some of the best documented examples of health effects attributed to migration are studies of the acculturation of people of Japanese descent to the westernised way of life in the USA. The difference in health outcomes can be observed in the differences between people of Japanese ancestry who have acculturated to the American lifestyle compared to those who maintain a traditional lifestyle in their country of origin. The latter subjects, who maintained a less acculturated lifestyle, including a more traditional diet of lower fat, animal protein and overall caloric intake, placed themselves at lower risk for non-insulin-dependent diabetes mellitus (NIDDM) (Huang *et al.*, 1996; Leonetti *et al.*, 1989; Tsunehara *et al.*, 1990). NIDDM, on the other hand, was found to be higher in those who had acculturated themselves to the US lifestyle, which formed the basis to the claim of obesity resulting from excessive caloric intake, a high percentage of calories from fat and animal protein, increased risk directly proportional to ageing, and a sedentary western lifestyle leading to decreased physical activity (Huang *et al.*, 1996; Tsunehara *et al.*, 1990).

In one study, diabetes mellitus was more prevalent in Turkish and Moroccan immigrants, and smoking was more prevalent in Turkish males and very rare in Moroccan females, which could be explained on grounds of religious values (Uitewaal *et al.*, 2004).

In the wake of rapid globalisation and the rapid transition of lifestyle, the change in the epidemiology of cardiovascular diseases (CVD), another important group of lifestyle disorders, cannot be forgotten. The overall burden of CVD continues to grow in low-, middle- and high-income countries. The expected rate of increase in CVD in LAMI countries may soon be almost twice that in developed countries (Gaziano, 2005). Indians tend to have premature coronary heart disease (CHD), at least a decade earlier than their counterparts in the developed countries (Prabhakaran *et al.*, 2005), indicating that there may be different factors at play. McKeigue *et al.* (1993), in a study on early onset of CHD in South Asian men, suggested that higher insulin resistance among South Asians could provide a causal link. Rapid demographic transitions currently taking place in India may contribute to the change in the epidemiology of these diseases in both the native population of the country plus the people who are affected by the brain drain phenomenon. In a longitudinal follow-up study on rural-to-urban migration and CVD risk factors in young Guatemalan adults, Torun *et al.* (2002) showed migration-induced differences in undesirable eating habits, physical inactivity, higher body fat percentage and adverse lipid profiles among rural-to-urban migrants compared to non-migrants. A study on the influence of country of birth on mortality from CVDs in Sweden revealed a significantly higher CHD mortality rate among women born in Finland or Eastern Europe compared to the native Swedish population (Sundquist and Johansson, 1997). Although Indian Asians are more likely than Europeans to seek medical advice for symptoms suggestive of angina, Chaturvedi *et al.* (1997) demonstrated that they may be less likely to be referred for exercise testing, wait longer to be seen by a cardiologist, wait longer for angiography, and are less likely to receive thrombolysis for ST segment elevated myocardial infarction. South Asians also have a high risk of stroke that is raised 1.5-fold compared to Europeans in the UK (Wild and McKeigue, 1997). Prevalence studies using country of birth as the ethnic identifier also reported higher CHD prevalence rate among South Asians compared to Europeans (Hughes *et al.*, 1990; McKeigue *et al.*, 1993; Palaniappan *et al.*, 2004; Wild *et al.*, 2007). With respect to the within country situation, a higher prevalence rate of CHD in Indians living in highly urban areas compared with rural Indians has been documented (Ahmad and Bhopal, 2005; Gupta and Gupta, 1996).

In the case of multiple sclerosis, it has been seen that migrants who move from an area where the disease is common to an area where it is rarer show a decrease in the rate of the disease, while people who migrate in the opposite direction tend to retain the low risk of their country of origin. Although migrants from low-risk countries to high-risk countries retain their low risk, their children have a risk of multiple sclerosis that approaches that of the host country. Migrant studies add little to our understanding of the genetics of multiple sclerosis but they emphasise the importance of environmental factors (Gale and Martyn, 1995). An Australian study suggested that the risk from environmental factors in multiple sclerosis may operate over a period of many years and not only in childhood and early adult life as was previously thought (Hammond *et al.*, 2000). Patel *et al.* (2006) compared Gujaratis (Indians) in Britain and their contemporaries in villages of origin in India and concluded that exposure to increased fat intake and obesity induced by migration is likely to explain the disproportionate combination of established risk factors (higher mean body mass index, greater dietary energy intake, fat intake, blood pressure and fasting serum total cholesterol) and emerging risk factors (higher apolipoprotein B, triglycerides, non-esterified fatty acids and C-reactive protein) prevalent in Gujaratis in Britain.

A factor that may be considered important in the difference in lifestyle disorders in migrants is diet (Landman and Cruickshank, 2001). Darmon and Khlat (2001) hypothesised that the diet of Mediterranean adults living in France may partly explain the low rates of chronic diseases and high adult life expectancy observed in migrant men from northern Africa. A French study (Méjean *et al.*, 2007) found that Tunisian immigrants presently residing in the south of France enjoyed better health than their French counterparts. The migrant Tunisians were less affected by nutrition-related non-communicable diseases (NR-NCD) than the non-migrant Tunisians. This study also found that, compared to the French, migrants had a more balanced and varied diet owing to a higher consumption of nuts and beans. A previous French national survey (Wanner *et al.*, 1995) showed that North African migrants in France consumed more vegetables than local-born French but similar quantities of fruit. The healthy diet habits included a higher consumption of olive oil in the Tunisian migrants than the French, which has a high monounsaturated fat: saturated fat ratio.

Medically unexplained symptoms and migrants

Medically unexplained symptoms (MUS) are one of the most commonly presenting quagmires in medical practice. These are symptoms for which no specific medical cause can be found or delineated by the treating physicians and hence no proper scientific consensus can be reached. Such patients comprise 15–30% of all primary care consultations (Fink *et al.*, 1999; Kirmayer and Robbins, 1991). Physicians may often assume a psychiatric causation for these symptoms, with the patients ending up with psychiatric referrals. Some patients may reject these referrals outright because of the stigma that it may carry. Even physicians may find these patients frustrating and controlling (Page and Wessely, 2003). The patients may provide the physician with all sorts of explanations, who might offer them reassurance, or may normalise their symptoms, or just offer no explanation at all (Dowrick *et al.*, 2004).

In case of immigrants, psychosocial distress may lead to MUS, but this is not the only factor responsible. This may be the predominant reason that patients with common mental disorders such as depression or anxiety present in primary care. Rates of mental and physical dysfunction may be high. Also, it may become difficult for the physician to understand the terminologies used by these individuals to refer to their symptoms. MUS such as 'low blood pressure' are often given by Indian female patients, which is viewed to be caused by underlying weakness. However, it is not possible to verify such a diagnosis (Robbins *et al.*, 1982). Other MUS include unexplained chronic pain, chronic unexplainable headache, irritable bowel syndrome (IBS), chronic fatigue syndrome, etc. IBS is one of the most commonly presenting MUS (Page and Wessely, 2003). A cross-sectional study revealed a high prevalence of chronic headache as well as a very low utilisation of adequate medical care in first generation Turkish immigrants in Germany (Kavuk *et al.*, 2006). Page and Wessely (2003) discuss how labelling the MUS of a patient may afford the sufferer legitimacy, ensuring that the dysfunction is not seen by others as 'in the patient's head' along with reducing the stigma of a psychiatric illness. These illness labels may be associated with a specific set of beliefs and attitudes.

The treating physician should understand that the problem of the MUS is real and somatic, and not unnecessarily prescribe testing or surgery. Stress, depression and anxiety are a key part of such symptoms and medications may help (Smith *et al.*, 2003). This association with depression and anxiety disorders may increase with the number of unexplained symptoms reported by the patient (Kroenke, 2003; Kroenke and Rosmalen, 2006).

Cancer and migrants

Migrant populations have undergone a change in their sociocultural and physical environment, which has led to a corresponding change in risk for different cancers (Parkin and Khlat, 1996). Rapid changes in cancer risk following migration imply that lifestyle or environmental factors are of over-riding importance in aetiology of these cancers (McCredie, 1998). Studies of first and second generation Japanese migrants to the USA have demonstrated considerable variations in the extent of post-migration change in the risk of different cancers (Haenszel, 1961; Haenszel *et al.*, 1973). Similarly, cervical cancer shows an important international variation in its incidence (Parkin *et al.*, 1992). Several risk factors have been related to this cancer, including the human papilloma virus (Bosch *et al.*, 1992). In one study, for instance, cases of cervical cancer were diagnosed at a more advanced stage and had a poorer prognosis in migrants from different parts within Spain (Borràs *et al.*, 1995). US Hispanics had consistently lower rates of breast, lung, prostate and colon cancers than non-Hispanics (Trapido *et al.*, 1995).

In France, the migrants originating from Morocco, and in Australia, the migrants originating from the Near East, have a lower mortality from all cancers than their host countries. Moroccans in France have a much lower risk than the local-born for lung cancer. They tend to have a relatively high risk for some cancers which are likely to have a viral aetiology, e.g. nasopharynx (Italians and Near Easterners), liver (Near Eastern males) and possibly cervix (Moroccans) (Khlat, 1995).

New Zealand migrants to England and Wales had a risk of cancer of the colon and prostate that was similar to or above New Zealand levels. In English and Welsh migrants to

New Zealand, risks of bladder cancer in each sex, and of scrotal and penile and pleural cancer in males, approximated to the risks in England and Wales; cervical cancer risk approximated to the New Zealand risk; and stomach, lung and ovarian cancers showed intermediate risks (Swerdlow *et al.*, 1995).

Key issues

Health requires a state of physical, mental and social wellbeing, and not only the absence of disease or infirmity. The ability of a migrant to integrate into a host society is based on combined mental, physical, cultural and social wellbeing. Integration into a host society is an important condition for a successful migration outcome and this notion has led to a comprehensive interpretation of 'migrant health' in line with the WHO definition of health.

With an increasing awareness of mental health in the migrant population, the underpinnings of the relation it shares with the physical illness cannot be underscored. As migration increases and the number of immigrants continue to increase, it has become all the more important to evaluate the impact they have on the health system of the new country or region, apart from the psychosocio-economic–cultural arena. It is thus important to study their epidemiological profile, understand their mental and physical healthcare needs, and improve their access to healthcare services, removing all the barriers to healthcare. Migrants bring with them social conditions, rituals, epidemiological risk factors and medical background of their country of origin, and these may be different from, and unknown to, that of the host community. Globalisation has created a new risk group which requires specific health policy interventions. A substantial number of immigrants do not hold a legal resident's permit; this group probably comprises individuals with different health needs (Caritas Roma, 2003), thus giving rise to a new subset of risk group within the migrant population, apart from the socio-economic subset. Even people who have legal status may not use the available health services if they do not know about them, if they do not understand them, or if the services offered are 'foreign' to their cultural and/or religious beliefs. Being an immigrant may have an influence on health through complex mechanisms, encompassing genetic, social, economic and cultural elements (Bollini and Siem, 1995). Being 'undocumented' means that migrants with irregular status such as trafficked persons, smuggled persons, economic migrants and certain subgroups of migrant workers, labour migrants and asylum seekers are more exposed to various health risks. These 'undocumented' or 'irregular' groups are a clandestine lot and make collection of health-related data difficult. Consequently, infectious diseases with long incubation periods and non-infectious conditions of public health interest are unlikely to be detected.

Physical illnesses thus form an important part of the overall health of the immigrants, with injuries for males and induced abortions for females being some of the critical areas for their health, in which public health interventions may be promoted (Baglio *et al.*, 2010).

Conclusions

Addressing migrant health provides certain benefits to the host societies. Inclusion of migrants into health programmes will facilitate the integration of migrants within communities, which can spare financial, social and political costs in the future. The healthy migrants may be contributing more to the new societies and may form an important workforce. Poor migrant health can lead to increased discrimination because new societies perceive migrants as carriers of infectious disease and as unproductive members of the community. The stress that results from all of the physical diseases in the migrants and the inability to reach out for the available or not really available health services for them, may lead to various mental problems in them. The mental health professionals need to be aware of these.

Pre-departure migration health assessment is one way of addressing population mobility and public health concerns. Such assessments detect and treat communicable diseases as well as non-communicable diseases that may be carried by migrants. Such assessments may reduce the need for quarantine in international travel and immigration. Health conditions that are of public health concern (for example, TB) are screened and treated before departure. The migrant may be allowed to migrate to the new country once his or her health condition is assessed as no longer posing a threat to public health, but ethical questions remain. Health assessment focuses on infectious or communicable diseases, including TB, parasitic diseases and sexually transmitted diseases. The international health regulations of the WHO and various national health regulations governing different countries in terms of managing infectious diseases are important aspects.

References

Ahmad, N., Bhopal, R. (2005). Is coronary heart disease rising in India? A systematic review based on ECG defined coronary heart disease. *Heart*, **91**, 719–25.

Arista, A. A., Marceca, M. (1998). [Request of health services by foreign patients in a Roman hospital: a 6 years survey (1990–1995)]. *Annali di Igiene*, **10**, 181–8 (Italian).

Baglio, G., Saunders, C., Spinelli, A., Osborn, J. (2010). Utilisation of hospital services in Italy: a comparative analysis of immigrant and Italian citizens. *Journal of Immigrant and Minority Health*, Feb 6 [Epub ahead of print].

Barro, G., Cislaghi, C., Costa, G., Lemma, P., Bandera, L. (1993). [Health problems of foreigners immigrated to Italy: the answer of institutions]. *Epidemiologica E Prevenzione*, **17**, 239–43 (Italian).

Bollini, P., Siem, H. (1995). No real progress towards equity: health of migrants and ethnic minorities on the eve of the year 2000. *Social Science and Medicine*, **41**, 819–28.

Borràs, J. M., Sánchez, V., Moreno, V., Izquierdo, A., Viladiu, P. (1995). Cervical cancer: incidence and survival in migrants within Spain. *Journal of Epidemiology & Community Health*, **49**(2), 153–7.

Bosch, F. X., Munoz, N., Shah, K. V., Meheus, A. (1992). Second international workshop on the epidemiology of cervical cancer and human papilloma virus. *International Journal of Cancer*, **52**, 171–3.

Cacciani, L., Baglio, G., Rossi, L. *et al.* (2006). Hospitalization among immigrants in Italy. *Emerging Themes in Epidemiology*, **3**, 4.

Capacci, F., Carnevale, F., Gazzano, N. (2005). The health of foreign workers in Italy. *International Journal of Occupational & Environmental Health*, **11**(1), 64–9.

Caritas Roma (2003). Contemporary immigration in Italy. *Current Trends and Future Prospects*. Roma: Nuova Anterem.

Chaturvedi, N., Rai, H., Ben-Shlomo, Y. (1997). Lay diagnosis and health-care-seeking behaviour for chest pain in South Asians and Europeans. *Lancet*, **350**, 1578–83.

Darmon, N., Khlat, M. (2001). An overview of the health status of migrants in France, in relation to their dietary practices. *Public Health Nutrition*, **4**(2), 163–72.

Dowrick, C. F., Ring, A., Humphris, G. M., Salmon, P. (2004). Normalisation of unexplained symptoms by general practitioners: a functional typology. *British Journal of General Practice*, **54**, 165–70.

Egger, M., Minder, C. E., Smith, G. D. (1990). Health inequalities and migrant workers in Switzerland. *Lancet*, **336**, 816.

Fink, P., Sorensen, L., Engberg, M., Holm, M., Munk-Jorgensen, P. (1999). Somatization in primary care: prevalence, health care utilization, and general practitioner recognition. *Psychosomatics*, **40**, 330–8.

Gagnon, A. J., Zimbeck, M., Zeitlin, J. *et al.* (2009). Migration to western industrialised countries and perinatal health: a systematic review. *Social Science and Medicine*, **69**(6), 934–46.

Gale, C. R., Martyn, C. N. (1995). Migrant studies in multiple sclerosis. *Progress in Neurobiology*, **47**(4–5), 425–48.

Gaziano, T. A. (2005). Cardiovascular disease in the developing world and its cost-effective management. *Circulation*, **112**, 3547–53.

Gissler, M., Alexander, S., MacFarlane, A. *et al.* (2009). Stillbirths and infant deaths among migrants in industrialized countries. *Acta Obstetricia et Gynecologica Scandinavica*, **88**(2), 134–48.

Gonzalez, E. A., Natale, R. A., Pimentel, C., Lane, R. C. (1999). The narcissistic injury and psychopathology of migration: the case of a Nicaraguan man. *Journal of Contemporary Psychotherapy*, **29**(3), 185–94.

Gupta, R., Gupta, V. P. (1996). Meta-analysis of coronary heart disease prevalence in India. *Indian Heart Journal*, **48**, 241–5.

Haenszel, W. (1961). Cancer mortality among the foreign born in the United States. *Journal of the National Cancer Institute*, **26**, 37–132.

Haenszel, W., Berg, J. W., Segi, M. *et al.* (1973). Large bowel cancer in Hawaiian Japanese. *Journal of the National Cancer Institute*, **51**, 1765–79.

Hammond, S. R., English, D. R., McLeod, J. G. (2000). The age-range of risk of developing multiple sclerosis: evidence from a migrant population in Australia. *Brain*, **123**(Pt5), 968–74.

Hong, Y., Li, X., Stanton, B. *et al.* (2006). Too costly to be ill: healthcare access and health-seeking behaviours among rural-to-urban migrants in China. *World Health Population*, **8**(2), 22–34.

Huang, B., Rodriguez, B. L., Burchfiel, C. M. *et al.* (1996). Acculturation and prevalence of diabetes among Japanese-American men. *American Journal of Epidemiology*, **144**, 674–81.

Hughes, K., Lun, K. C., Yeo, P. P. B. (1990). Cardiovascular disease in Chinese, Malays, and Indians in Singapore. Differences in mortality. *Journal of Epidemiology & Community Health*, **44**, 24–8.

Istituto Nazionale per l'Assicurazione degli Infortuni sul Lavoro (INAIL): Rapporto INAIL (2002). Rome 2003.

Kavuk, I., Weimar, C., Kim, B. T. *et al.* (2006). One-year prevalence and socio-cultural aspects of chronic headache in Turkish immigrants and German natives. *Cephalalgia*, **26**(10), 1177–81.

Kemp, C., Rasbridge, L. (2004). *Refugee and Immigrant Health*. Cambridge: Cambridge University Press.

Khlat, M. (1995). Cancer in Mediterranean migrants-based on studies in France and Australia. *Cancer Causes Control*, **6**(6), 525–31.

Kirmayer, L. J., Robbins, J. M. (1991). Three forms of somatization in primary care: prevalence, co-occurrence and sociodemographic characteristics. *Journal of Nervous & Mental Disease*, **179**, 647–55.

Krasnik, A., Norredam, M., Sorensen, T. M. *et al.* (2002). Effect of ethnic background on Danish hospital utilization patterns. *Social Science and Medicine*, **55**, 1207–11.

Kroenke, K. (2003). Patients presenting with somatic complaints: epidemiology, psychiatric co-morbidity and management. *International Journal of Methods in Psychiatric Research*, **12**(1), 34–43.

Kroenke, K., Rosmalen, J. G. (2006). Symptoms, syndromes, and the value of psychiatric diagnostics in patients who have functional somatic disorders. *Medical Clinics of North America*, **90**(4), 603–26.

Landman, J., Cruickshank, J. K. (2001). A review of ethnicity, health and nutrition-related diseases in relation to migration in the United Kingdom. *Public Health Nutrition*, **4**(2B), 647–57.

Lemma, P., Gogliani, F., Rossignoli, F., Triassi, M., Costa, G. (1993). [The health of the foreigners immigrated to Turin in the current informative system]. *Epidemiologia E Prevenzione*, **17**, 259–66 (Italian).

Leonetti, D. L., Fujimoto, W. Y., Wahl, P. W. (1989). Early-life background and the development of non-insulin dependent diabetes mellitus. *American Journal of Physical Anthropology*, **79**, 345–55.

McCredie, M. (1998). Cancer epidemiology in migrant populations. *Recent Results Cancer Research*, **154**, 298–305.

McKeigue, P. M., Ferrie, J. E., Pierpoint, T., Marmot, M. G. (1993). Association of early-onset coronary heart disease in South Asian men with glucose intolerance and hyperinsulinemia. *Circulation*, **87**, 152–61.

Méjean, C., Traissac, P., Eymard-Duvernay, S. *et al.* (2007). Diet quality of North African migrants in France partly explains their lower prevalence of diet-related chronic conditions relative to their native French peers. *Journal of Nutrition*, **137**(9), 2106–13.

Muennig, P., Fans, M. C. (2002). Health status and hospital utilization of recent immigrants to New York City. *Preventive Medicine*, **35**, 225–231.

Page, L. A., Wessely, S. (2003). Medically unexplained symptoms: exacerbating factors in the doctor-patient encounter. *Journal of the Royal Society of Medicine*, **96**(5), 223–7.

Palaniappan, L., Wang, Y., Fortmann, S. P. (2004). Coronary heart disease mortality for six ethnic groups in California, 1990–2000. *Annals of Epidemiology*, **14**, 499–506.

Parkin, D. M. (1992). Studies of cancer in migrant populations: methods and interpretation. *Revue d'Epidemiologie et de Sante Publique*, **40**, 410–24.

Parkin, D. M., Khlat, M. (1996). Studies of cancer in migrants: rationale and methodology. *European Journal of Cancer*, **32**A(5), 761–71.

Parkin, D. M., Muir, C., Whelan, S. *et al.* (eds) (1992). *Cancer Incidence in Five Continents*, vol. VI. Lyon: International Agency for Research on Cancer.

Patel, J. V., Vyas, A., Cruickshank, J. K. *et al.* (2006). Impact of migration on coronary heart disease risk factors: Comparison of Gujaratis in Britain and their contemporaries in villages of origins in India. *Atherosclerosis*, **185**, 297–306.

Pennazza, F., Boldrini, R., Fortino, A. (2000). *Rapporto Statistico il Ricovero Ospedaliero Degli Stranieri in Italia Nell'anno 2000*. Roma: Ministero della Salute, D.G. Sistema Informativo e Statistico e degli Investimenti Strutturali e Tecnologici Ufficio di Statistica.

Prabhakaran, D., Yusuf, S., Mehta, S. *et al.* (2005). Two-year outcomes in patients admitted with non-ST elevation acute coronary syndrome: results of the OASIS registry 1 and 2. *Indian Heart Journal*, **57**(3), 217–25.

Reeske, A., Spallek, J., Razum, O. (2009). Changes in smoking prevalence among first- and second-generation Turkish migrants in Germany – an analysis of the 2005 microcensus. *International Journal for Equity in Health*, **20**(8), 26.

Robbins, J. M., Korda, H., Shapiro, M. F. (1982). Treatment for a nondisease: the case of low blood pressure. *Social Science and Medicine*, **16**, 27–33.

Smith, R. C., Lein, C., Collins, C. *et al.* (2003). Treating patients with medically unexplained symptoms in primary care. *Journal of General Internal Medicine*, **18**(6), 478–89.

Stronks, K., Ravelli, A. C. J., Reijneveld, S. A. (2001). Immigrants in the Netherlands: equal access for equal needs? *Journal of Epidemiology and Community Health*, **55**, 701–7.

Sundquist, J., Johansson, S. E. (1997). The influence of country of birth on mortality from all causes and cardiovascular disease in Sweden 1979–1993. *International Journal of Epidemiology*, **26**, 279–87.

Sundquist, J., Iglesias, E., Isacsson, A. (1995). Migration and health: a study of Latin American refugees, their exile in Sweden and repatriation. *Scandinavian Journal of Primary Health Care*, **13**(2), 135–40.

Swerdlow, A. J., Cooke, K. R., Skegg, D. C., Wilkinson, J. (1995). Cancer incidence in England and Wales and New Zealand and in migrants between the two countries. *British Journal of Cancer*, **72**(1), 236–43.

Torun, B., Stein, A. D., Schcoeder, D. *et al.* (2002). Rural-to-urban migration and cardiovascular disease risk factors in young Guatemalan adults. *International Journal of Epidemiology*, **31**(1), 218–26.

Trapido, E. J., Burciaga Valdez, R., Obeso, J. L. *et al.* (1995). Epidemiology of cancer among Hispanics in the United States. *Journal of the National Cancer Institute Monographs*, **18**, 17–28.

Tsunehara, C. H., Leonetti, D. L., Fujimoto, W. Y. (1990). Diet of second-generation Japanese-American men with and without non-insulin-dependent diabetes. *American Journal of Clinical Nutrition*, **52**, 731S8.

Uitewaal, P. J., Manna, D. R., Bruijnzeels, M. A., Hoes, A. W., Thomas, S. (2004). Prevalence of type 2 diabetes mellitus, other cardiovascular risk factors, and cardiovascular disease in Turkish and Moroccan immigrants in North West Europe: a systematic review. *Preventive Medicine*, **39**(6), 1068–76.

Uniken Venema, H. P., Garretsen, H. F., van der Maas, P. J. (1995). Health of migrants and migrant health policy, The Netherlands as an example. *Social Science and Medicine*, **41**(6), 809–18.

Wanner, P., Khlat, M., Bouchardy, C. (1995). Life style and health behavior of southern European and North African immigrants in France. *Revue d'Epidemiol et de Sante Publique*, **43**, 548–59.

Wild, S., McKeigue, P. (1997). Cross sectional analysis of mortality by country of birth in England and Wales, 1970–92. *British Medical Journal*, **314**, 705–10.

Wild, S. H., Fischbacher, C., Brock, A., Griffiths, C., Bhopal, R. (2007). Mortality from all causes and circulatory disease by country of birth in England and Wales 2001–2003. *Journal of Public Health*, **29**, 191–8.

Mental health of migrants in China – is it a No Man's Land?

Roger Man Kin Ng

Editors' introduction

Internal migration within the same country may occur from rural areas to sprawling urban conurbations or in reverse, from urban areas to rural societies. Each of these types of movement has problems associated with migration. Changes in family structure and associated social support may produce further alienation and increased substance abuse or mental health problems. Using Hong Kong and China as examples, Ng illustrates the impact of migratory stress on migrants. Migrations from Vietnam to Hong Kong and of Filipina maids and subsequently from mainland China produced varying patterns of adjustment. Following migration, nearly one-third of new migrants were noted to have depression. However, children of migrants more likely to have higher self-esteem and used fewer withdrawal coping styles. Migration within mainland China has led to increased levels of alienation and frustration owing to poor housing, long working hours in poor working conditions and low economic means. These factors, combined with poor social support and factionalism, have led to further isolation. Ng concludes that the negative impact of migration may create further ripple effects towards other members of the family and the younger generation.

Introduction

China accounts for one-fifth of the total world population and has a diverse ethnic composition. Since the adoption of the Open Door Policy in the 1980s, there is marked economic progress in China. With the economic boom in coastal cities, there is a massive influx of migrants from rural areas to coastal cities. The economy has also thrived in Hong Kong in the past 30 years, attracting tens of thousands of foreign domestic workers from developing countries coming to work in Hong Kong. Since the handover of sovereignty of Hong Kong back to China in 1997, increased cross-border economic and social activities have also allowed many immigrants from mainland China to settle in Hong Kong by reasons of marriage and blood relations. The segregation of Hong Kong from mainland China in the past 100 years has led to unique migration patterns and sociocultural disparities that warrant separate discussions in this chapter.

Hong Kong, a special administrative region in China: 'One country, two systems'

Hong Kong has always been a land of refuge for immigrants. Hong Kong was a small fishing village when it was put under British colonial rule in 1842. Ever since Hong Kong became a

Migration and Mental Health, ed. Dinesh Bhugra & Susham Gupta. Published by Cambridge University Press. © Cambridge University Press 2011.

crown colony, it has witnessed the influx of refugees from mainland China during different periods of civil war and political turmoil in the mainland. The major influx of immigrants from the mainland occurred in 1949–1950, when many refugees left China after liberation by the Chinese communist regime. Since then, there have been several large waves of immigration from mainland China, mainly related to the various political movements in the 1950s and 1960s. It can be safely concluded that most citizens in Hong Kong are either immigrants themselves or descendants of immigrants over the past 100 years.

Hong Kong as a port of refuge: influx of Vietnamese refugees into Hong Kong in the 1970s–1980s

During the 1970s, the outbreak of the Vietnamese War led to a massive exodus of political refugees from Vietnam to nearby Asian countries. Under international pressure, the colonial government declared Hong Kong as one of the 'countries of first asylum' to these political refugees. Because of the slow screening process of the western governments in granting political asylum to these refugees, there was a gradual accumulation of Vietnamese refugees in Hong Kong. The situation worsened when many Vietnamese began to leave Vietnam to seek better economic opportunities in western countries. As they were not considered to be 'refugees' escaping from political persecution, they were then classified as 'Vietnamese Boat People' by the colonial government until proven otherwise, and they were faced with even more difficulties in seeking political asylum in western countries. As of 1 August 1984, 12 806 Vietnamese 'boat people' were housed in refugee camps in Hong Kong (Security Branch of Hong Kong Government Secretariat, 1984). Of these, 6309 were accommodated in two open centres (Kai Tak Centre and Jubilee Transit Centre), where refugees were allowed virtually unrestricted movement in and out, as well as being able to take up open employment. The remainder were detained in closed centres where they were not allowed to engage in outside work and were under strict surveillance by the correctional services department staff. The opening of these closed centres in the early 1980s was an attempt by the colonial government to discourage the refugees from choosing Hong Kong as a place of asylum (Chan and Loveridge, 1987). The Vietnamese in these closed centres were not allowed freedom of movement within the Hong Kong territory and were detained until they were granted political asylum in a western country. There are surprisingly few studies that looked into the psychological adjustment among these Vietnamese detainees in Hong Kong (Chan and Loveridge, 1987; Knudsen, 1983). In addition, these studies are mainly qualitative studies that provided in-depth investigations of the sense of learned helplessness and entrapment in these transit camps in Hong Kong, as well as the sense of alienation and paranoia towards refugees from the rival factions (North Vietnamese who were predominantly Chinese in ethnic origin versus South Vietnamese who were predominantly Vietnamese) and towards the detaining authority. Indeed, there were sporadic reports of outbreaks of protests and violence between various factions of Vietnamese in the camps and between the detainees and the correctional staff. Yet there was no systematic epidemiological study that investigated the prevalence of psychiatric disorders among this socially isolated ethnic minority group in Hong Kong in the era of 1980s, possibly because of lack of research resources and barriers to accessing this group of disadvantaged people for study. Studies conducted in the UK and Australia on Asian refugees settling in these countries have indirectly shed light on the high prevalence of psychiatric disorders, as well as the relation of psychiatric morbidity with pre-migration trauma and detention experiences in mother countries and in transit camps (Mollica et al., 1998; Steel et al., 2002).

Before the handover of sovereignty of Hong Kong back to China, there were still a substantial number of Vietnamese boat people who did not obtain the status of political refugees and could not be resettled in western countries. To resolve this impasse before the handover, the remaining boat people were eventually granted legal residence status in Hong Kong by the government. Owing to cultural and language barriers and prolonged periods of residence in institutions, these 'migrants' probably face major problems of adjustment in this predominantly Chinese society. However, no systematic cohort studies can be identified that specifically studied the psychological adjustment of this unique group of 'new migrants' in Hong Kong.

Economic boom in Hong Kong in the 1980s–1990s: recruitment of foreign domestic workers as a major workforce

During the influx of Vietnamese refugees into Hong Kong, there was also a parallel increase in arrival of foreign domestic workers in Hong Kong. With increasing economic prosperity in Hong Kong since the 1970s, females have become an increasingly important workforce in Hong Kong. To free up the female workforce from household chores, the Hong Kong government began the policy of introducing foreign domestic workers (FDWs) from neighbouring Asian countries (AMC, 2004; Gibson et al., 2001). FDWs are permitted to work as domestic workers for families. By the 2000s, there were more than 200 000 FDWs, mainly from the Philippines, Indonesia and Sri Lanka (Census and Statistics Department, 2008), reflecting the poor socio-economic conditions of these countries relative to their Asian neighbours. They are predominantly female workers, though there are a few males working as drivers for affluent families. Although they are often hailed as heroes in their mother countries as significant contributors to economies at home, they have to give up their own families and social network, as well as their relatively more sophisticated original jobs in the mother countries for domestic jobs in Hong Kong (Gibson et al., 2001). As their mother countries have cultures, religions and languages that are very different from Chinese society, it is perhaps not surprising that FDWs experienced acculturation problems (Gibson et al., 2001), not to mention the culture shock encountered upon living with their employers of very different culture. In addition, many domestic workers left their own families to work in Hong Kong, leading to marital and family problems in their homeland (Lau et al., 2009). A few studies conducted in Hong Kong have specifically investigated the mental health of this unique and yet significant population in Hong Kong (Chen et al., 2008; French and Lam, 1988; Holroyd et al., 2001; Lau et al., 2009). In general, the studies do confirm the general impression that FDWs experienced problems in communication, social relations, living conditions and psychological adjustment. In a retrospective chart review of all first psychiatric admissions to three regional hospitals in Hong Kong, Lau et al. (2009) found that there was a high incidence of stress-related acute psychosis (60% of all first psychiatric admissions for FDWs), an incidence not different from a similar study conducted in Kuwait (90% as caused by stress-related psychiatric disorders, including reactions to severe stress and acute transient psychosis) (Zahid et al., 2004). As fear of termination of contract upon revealing their mental health problems might reduce their willingness to seek early intervention, such hospital-based studies probably underestimated the extent of psychiatric morbidity in the whole population of FDWs. Furthermore, community-based studies conducted so far are usually restricted to samples recruited by convenient sampling, so the generalisability of these findings is again not clear. However, in view of the substantial proportion of the total

Hong Kong population made up by the FDW (3% of the total population and 6% of the total workforce in Hong Kong), a territory-wide epidemiological survey on the prevalence of psychiatric disorders among FDWs is urgently needed to assess the extent of the healthcare burden and the need for extra healthcare resources.

Post-1997: relaxation of border control

Since the handover of sovereignty of Hong Kong back to China in 1997, together with an increased level of economic prosperity in China, there is frequent bilateral trade and labour movement between Hong Kong and China. While many people in Hong Kong have settled in coastal cities in China to seek possible work opportunities, there are also many mainlanders from nearby cities who married Hong Kong citizens. Because of the 'one country, two systems' policy adopted by the central government to preserve prosperity and confidence in Hong Kong, residents of mainland China are required to apply for one-way permits to reside permanently in Hong Kong. In the past two decades, new arrivals from the mainland admitted under the one-way permit scheme contributed to 54.9% of Hong Kong's population growth, equivalent to 11.7% of the population of 6.92 million in 2004 (Chou, 2009). Owing to increased cross-border marriage, as mentioned previously, the main purpose of the one-way permit scheme is to facilitate family reunion for spouses and children in mainland China whose relatives are permanent residents in Hong Kong. Not surprisingly, most of these new immigrants are children (30% of the scheme applicants) and wives of Hong Kong residents (another 30% of the scheme applicants). Although these immigrants are also ethnic Han Chinese people with similar Chinese culture, many had poor psychological adjustment upon arrival in Hong Kong. In a fairly representative survey on new immigrants of less than 6 months, Chou (2009) found that around 30% of respondents were depressed. Furthermore, depression was predicted by poor pre-migration planning and moderated by better post-migration social support and optimism towards life. Almost 20% of the respondents reported not having prepared for their migration to Hong Kong (like pre-arranging their accommodation in Hong Kong), which Chou (2009) attributed to the long waiting time taken for the release of the one-way permits to applicants by the Hong Kong government. However, it is not clear if depression resolves spontaneously after further stay in Hong Kong, which can only be answered by further cohort studies on this group of immigrants from mainland China. Yet another intriguing study conducted in a convenient sample of secondary school students in Hong Kong found that the newly arrived migrant children had higher self-esteem and used fewer withdrawal coping styles compared to local-born schoolchildren (Tam and Lam, 2005). What is more alarming is that the children that migrated to Hong Kong at an earlier age and were presumably more acculturated were found to resemble local-born children in having lower self-esteem and more delinquent behaviours in comparison with the newly arrived immigrants. It again awaits further cohort studies to confirm or refute the hypothesis that disillusion and frustration with lack of opportunities for new young immigrants explain the above phenomenon. Nevertheless, crowded living environment and rapid pace of lifestyle in Hong Kong may still create a lot of stress for new immigrants after arrival in Hong Kong. The extent of personal optimism and positive support therefore appear to be important buffers against such stress (Bhugra, 2003). Although Hong Kong has provided funding to support programmes in facilitating the adjustment of new young immigrants (Rao and Yuen, 2001), the exact ingredients important for effective programmes await delineation by high-quality local research. With the extremely low birth rate in Hong

Kong in the past 10 years, these new arrivals from the mainland will remain the single most important source of population growth in Hong Kong. This is an important area of research, both from the point of view of healthcare planning for this emerging population group and from the research perspective of dismantling various risk factors of migration on mental health of migrants (language and lifestyle differences in the face of similarities in ethnicity and culture).

Mainland China

Migrant workers from rural to city regions: a curse or a blessing for the migrants?

With the adoption of the open door policy in China in the past 30 years, booming economies in cities have attracted billions of migrants seeking opportunities in the cities. It is estimated that 120–150 million migrant workers have moved to major cities in China over the past 20 years, and the number will reach 300 million in 2010 (Lague, 2003). Most of these migrant workers come from the relatively impoverished western and central inland regions and moved to the east and coastal cities to seek better jobs and economic opportunities. They are known as 'peasant workers' in Chinese literature ('nonminngong'). Because of the policies of the central government in stemming the massive flow of migrants from rural regions into cities in the 1950s, rural migrants into cities were not entitled to the housing and medical benefits enjoyed by city residents (Bai, 2007). The introduction of this household registration system ('*Hukou*' system) effectively leads to a disparity of the benefits received between migrant workers and local residents (in a survey of workers in Shanghai, among migrant workers, only 14% had health insurance plans and only 10% had pension schemes, while 79% and 91% of their city counterparts enjoyed these benefits, respectively) (Feng *et al.*, 2002). As such policies still remain in force in many cities in mainland China, expensive costs for private healthcare pose major barriers of accessibility to physical and mental health services for many migrant workers in the cities. Furthermore, partly due to exploitation by the employers and to the driving forces of cutting costs of production, migrant workers are usually paid less than city resident counterparts (Wong *et al.*, 2007). With their relatively low level of education, the migrants fail to compete with city residents for better jobs and have often been labelled negatively as 'local buns' ('tobaozi'). Many migrants take up manual jobs with long working hours and poor working environments that are disdained by the city residents (Tan, 2000). Poor living and work environments, low economic means and long working hours lead to much frustration among the migrant workers (Bai, 2007). An in-depth qualitative study using representative samples recruited from an epidemiological study found that migrant workers complained about being discriminated against by city residents (Jia and Wu, 2008). The respondents felt marginalised and alienated in the city environment. The reasons cited in the study for such marginalisation include a clash between rural and city cultures, lack of leisure time to socialise with city residents and to regulate their negative emotions, as well as discriminating attitudes from the city residents. Many migrant workers considered themselves as 'guests' in their cities ('guoke'), saying that they would return to their rural homeland once they had saved enough money from work (Bai, 2007). Several large-scale well-conducted epidemiological studies in different provinces (North Eastern provinces, Henan Province, Guangdong Province and Zhejiang Province), using similar instruments (symptom checklist-90), found that migrant workers, when compared with their city counterparts, were more depressed, anxious and paranoid (Jia and Wu, 2008; Luo *et al.*, 2006; Qian *et al.*, 2008; Sun, 2007). The prevalence of psychological maladjustment among migrant workers ranged from 5.4% (Luo *et al.*, 2006) to around 39% (Sun, 2007), with male respondents being psychologically more maladjusted than female respondents in some studies (Jia and Wu, 2008; Luo *et al.*, 2006; Wong *et al.*, 2007) and female respondents being more neurotic (Qian *et al.*, 2008; Sun, 2007). A similar result of poor psychological adjustment was found in another study in Weihai city of Shandong Province using the Kessler K-10 rating scale, with a prevalence rate of psychological distress at 19% (He *et al.*, 2008). Another study conducted in Shanghai using the Brief Symptom Inventory independently corroborated other studies in finding a high prevalence of psychological problems in the migrant workers (25% in male workers and 9% in female workers). The higher prevalence of psychological distress in male workers was postulated to be related to greater societal and cultural pressure on male workers to excel in work and to support the family, as well as different meanings ascribed by male and female workers to migration (Wong *et al.*, 2007). Female workers might view migration as an opportunity to escape from restrictive roles as housewives in their rural villages while male workers might shoulder a great burden in generating wealth for their rural families and in preserving 'face' for their families (Tan, 2000).

Migrant workers were also found to have poorer levels of objective and subjective social support, and were less willing to seek social support from others (Qian *et al.*, 2008). This lack of social support is understandable given that the migrant workers usually left behind their families in rural areas and came to look for job opportunities in the city (Qian *et al.*, 2008; Wong *et al.*, 2007). Their fear of rejection by city residents, combined with their actual experiences of discrimination, lead to understandable paranoia towards city dwellers and reluctance in seeking help and support from their city counterparts (Jia and Wu, 2008). Such feelings of marginalisation and alienation also lead to formation of gangs in construction sites and factories, where migrants from similar provinces and with similar dialects coalesce for self-protection and fighting for their rights (Bai, 2007). Fights among different rival factions in factories and construction sites are frequently reported in the newspapers. Apart from lack of social support, studies have also reported poor skills of regulating negative emotions, including limited utilisation of recreational resources in the city areas, and restricted access to appropriate psychological support (Bai, 2007; Qian *et al.*, 2008). Indeed, studies have reported increased prevalences of alcohol and substance misuse in migrant workers, especially among depressed females working in the commercial sex industry (Chen *et al.*, 2008). Substance misuse is regarded as a maladaptive coping of depressive symptoms, precipitated and maintained by stress and low self-esteem associated with jobs in sex-related industries like massage parlours and night clubs. It is also worth noting that the 30-day smoking rate, 30-day alcohol intoxication rate and lifetime prevalence rates of substance and alcohol abuse are all elevated in comparison with national data in all rural-to-city migrant workers in all work types, suggesting that substance and alcohol misuses are important public health problems among all migrant workers.

Ripple effect of migration stress on children of migrant families

The negative impact of migration from rural to city regions extends beyond the migrant workers to their children, as increasing numbers of migrant workers bring their families to the cities. The Beijing Migrant Census of 1997 found that 32% of migrants had relocated with their families (*China Daily*, 2003). Owing to the household registration system ('Hukou' system), children of migrant children are not entitled to receive 9 years of free education provided by the provincial government for the city residents. Inexpensive private education institutions were usually poor in teaching facilities and low in teacher quality. Furthermore, the discrimination faced by these children from schoolmates and teachers because of their heavy accents and out-of-date clothing leads to social isolation and marginalisation in school (Xie and Pan, 2007). It has been found in a recent epidemiological study in Shanghai that children of migrant families, compared to their counterparts of urban families, are more depressed and anxious (Wong *et al.*, 2009). Possible predictors of poor mental health identified include parent–child conflicts, discipline from teachers and discrimination in school. However, owing to the cross-sectional nature of this survey, it would be premature to attribute these predictors as possible causes of poor mental health in migrant children. It is equally possible that poor mental health leads to deteriorated academic performance and conduct problems in school, thereby engendering more parent–child conflicts, disciplinary measures from teachers and social rejection by classmates. As of 2005, it has been estimated that 20 million migrant school-aged children have accompanied their parents to resettle in cities (Xinhua News Agency, 2005). It is paramount that more rigorous studies be conducted to clarify the relations between these predictors and the mental health of the children of migrant families. The mental health of migrant children is an important public health problem, with a long-lasting impact on society, as evidenced by longitudinal findings that children with poor mental health predict subsequent poor psychosocial functioning and mental health in adulthood (see Ingram *et al.*, 2002 for reviews).

Migration under the direction of the central government: where should the dislocated ones be resettled?

Resettlement of residents to different areas is not a new policy in China. During the period of the Great Leap Forward Movement in the 1950s, many intellectuals were encouraged to resettle in rural areas to contribute their skills and knowledge to improve the education and living standards of rural residents. However, there is no systematic study that explores the psychological adjustment of these intellectuals migrating to rural areas, except for novels written by some intellectuals reporting their personal accounts. Such resettlement of intellectuals was halted completely by the end of the Cultural Revolution in 1976.

A more recent effort of large scale migration under government direction occurred with the construction of the Three Gorges' Dam on the Jangtze River ('Changjiang'). Because of the construction project of the dams, the inhabitants close to the banks of the upper stream of the river were resettled in two ways. Some inhabitants were resettled in nearby villages located higher up in altitude ('houkao yimin'), while other inhabitants were resettled in other provinces ('weiqian yimin'). There are several well conducted case–control studies that confirm that the immigrants had poorer mental health then the local inhabitants (Jiang *et al.*, 2009; Liu *et al.*, 2009; Wang *et al.*, 2009b). Predictors of poor mental health included disrupted social network, poor coping strategies and adverse life events among the migrants (Jiang *et al.*, 2009; Wang *et al.*, 2009b). Furthermore, related study also found that immigrants resettled in other provinces ('weiqian yimin') had more psychological problems compared with those resettled in nearby villages ('houkao yimin') (Wang *et al.*, 2009a). The reasons cited for better mental health for those resettled nearby include similar regional culture in the resettled region, preserved social network of the migrants with en bloc resettlement of whole villages in nearby areas, and re-provision of farmland and preservation of original jobs as farmers after resettlement (Wang *et al.*, 2009a). Although some studies

Steel, Z., Silove, D., Phan, T., Bauman, A. (2002). Long term effect of psychological trauma on the mental health of Vietnamese refugees resettled in Australia: a population-based study. *Lancet*, **360**, 1056–62.

Sun C. (2007). Investigation and analysis of mental health status of Northeast peasant workers. *Chinese Journal of Health Psychology*, **15**, 460–2 (in Chinese).

Tam, V. C., Lam, R. S. (2005). Stress and coping among migrant and local-born adolescents in Hong Kong. *Youth & Society*, **36**, 312–32.

Tan, S. (2000). The relationship between foreign enterprises, local governments, and women migrant workers in the Pearl River Delta. In L. A West, Y. H. Zhao (eds) *Rural Labour Flows in China*. University of California, Berkeley: Institute of East Asian Studies.

Wang, L., Cong, J., Wang, Y. *et al.* (2009a). Influences of different resettlements on mental health of immigrants. *Chinese Journal of Public Health*, **25**, 259–61 (in Chinese).

Wang, Q., Wang Y., Li, Q., Huang, B. (2009b). Study for the correlation between psychological well-being and psychological stress of external resettlement in migrants from Three Gorges Reservoir Area. *Journal of Chongqing Medical University*, **34**, 221–3 (in Chinese).

Wong, D. F. K., He, X., Leung, G., Lau, Y., Chang, Y. (2007). Mental health of migrant workers in China: prevalence and correlates. *Social Psychiatry & Psychiatric Epidemiology*, **43**, 483–9.

Wong, D. F. K., Chang, Y. L., He, X. S. (2009). Correlates of psychological well-being of children of migrant workers in Shanghai, China. *Social Psychiatry & Psychiatric Epidemiology*, **44**, 815–24.

Xie, Z. Q., Pan, J. (2007). Children of migrant workers on the move between city and countryside. *People's Tribune*, **16**, 34–7.

Xinhua News Agency (2005). Foundation to fund education of migrant workers, 14 January 2005.

Zahid, M. A., Fido, A. A., Razik, M. A., Mohsen, M. A., El-Sayed, A. A. (2004). Psychiatric morbidity among housemaids in Kuwait. *Medical Principles and Practice*, **13**, 249–54.

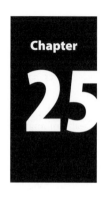

Chapter

25

Immigrant and refugee mental health in Canada: lessons and prospects

Laura Simich and Morton Beiser

Editors' introduction

Different countries face different levels of migration and varying numbers. Each country deals with the issues related to migration in its own way, and the focus varies from multiculturalism in the UK to the melting pot in the USA and the rainbow nation in Canada. The reception granted to migrants varies according to social policy and political ideologies. Psychiatrists must be aware both of social policy and political views in the new culture so that adequate, appropriate and accessible services can be provided to migrants as well as other ethnic and cultural groups. These services will depend upon resources made available in the healthcare system. In this chapter, Simich and Beiser highlight the Canadian experience of migrants and refugees to illustrate rates of mental health problems, subpopulations at risk and social determinants of risk and resilience. Using migrant and refugee settlement programmes, multiculturalism and social policy appear to be welcoming; inevitably, however, increasing the local labour market will place newcomers at a disadvantage. The authors describe and review the data which demonstrates resettlement-related mental health risk factors, especially unemployment. Rates of disorders will vary as social and health inequalities grow. Simich and Beiser conclude that specific interventions are helpful and needed.

Introduction

When immigrants arrive in Canada, they are, on average in better mental health than native-born Canadians (Ng *et al.*, 2008). This chapter focuses on two decades of Canadian migrant mental health research, some of it devoted to exploring personal and social factors that jeopardise this initial mental health advantage, some of it to explicating the factors that contribute to maintaining it. As is the case for the population at large, some immigrants develop frank psychiatric disorders. The availability and effectiveness of mental health services for this subpopulation is another major research trend reviewed in this chapter. A description of immigration, demographic, and social trends in Canada opens the chapter and provides a backdrop for considerations about mental health. The review of *After the Door Has Been Opened* (Canadian Task Force on Mental Health Issues Affecting Immigrants and Refugees, 1988), a landmark Canadian document on immigrant and refugee mental health that follows, provides a context for evaluating developments over the subsequent two decades. The chapter then reviews selected migrant mental health research findings to highlight the extent of mental health problems, subpopulations of immigrants and refugees at particular risk, and the social

Migration and Mental Health, ed. Dinesh Bhugra & Susham Gupta. Published by Cambridge University Press. © Cambridge University Press 2011.

determinants of risk and resilience. A brief discussion of emerging issues, suggestions for future research, and service and policy recommendations concludes the chapter.

Immigration, demographic and social trends in Canada

Canada's first immigrants were English, French and other European colonisers who began trading and settling on native lands in the sixteenth century. Immigrant intake peaked in the first decade of the twentieth century, retreated during the Great Depression and post World War 2 years, and then rebounded in the latter half of the century. By the opening decade of the twenty-first century, Canada had become one of the most culturally diverse places on Earth. The country's multiculturalism policies (Kymlicka, 1995) and refugee resettlement programmes have been favourably contrasted with more problematic integration scenarios in Europe or with the USA's 'sink or swim approach' (Van Selm, 2003). Although a comparative analysis of the history of immigration in North America is beyond the scope of this chapter, some trends provide a backdrop to understanding immigrant integration, social determinants of mental health and migrant mental health research in Canada.

Comparisons between immigrant integration in Canada and in the USA suggest the advantages of certain Canadian policies, while others are grounds for concern. Immigrants in Canada are, on average, much more likely eventually to become citizens than their US counterparts and to acquire citizenship much faster (Bloemraad, 2002). Although there is no research addressing a possible relationship between mental health and becoming a citizen, this action on the part of new settlers may be an indicator of a sense of belonging and inclusion. As described later, however, this is only one indicator of settlement and integration success; demographic changes and economic outcomes also have the potential to affect immigrant mental wellbeing.

The last half of the twentieth century was a time of profound changes in Canadian immigration. Prior to 1960, a frankly discriminatory admissions policy helped ensure that immigrants would be predominantly Northern European and white. The Immigration Act of 1976, which introduced a colour-blind points system based on human capital characteristics such as education, linguistic fluency and occupational skills geared to government-defined labour force needs, changed everything. Of the 250 000 immigrants admitted to fill Canada's annual immigration target (Citizenship and Immigration Canada, 2009), many now come from areas other than the so-called 'traditional' source countries. Over half (52%) of immigrant admissions in 2007 came from 10 source countries: People's Republic of China, India, Philippines, USA, Pakistan, UK, Iran, Republic of Korea, France and Colombia.

Approximately one of five persons living in Canada is foreign-born. However, since the vast majority (70%) of recent immigrants to Canada settle in the country's major cities, the immigrant presence is felt even more profoundly in places such as Toronto, Montreal and Vancouver than in the country's rural areas (Statistics Canada, 2008). Over half Toronto's population is foreign-born, with a mother tongue other than English or French, Canada's two official languages.

Unlike its immigrant intake, which is overtly driven by self-interest, Canada's admission of refugees is based on humanitarianism, and by the country's voluntary participation in the UN Convention on Refugees. Between 1980 and 2001 Canada received a total of 535 131 refugees from a wide variety of source countries. The annual numbers ranged from a high of 40 000 in 1980 (at the height of the 'boat people' crisis in South-east Asia, an event that stimulated the largest admission of refugees in Canada's history) to a low of 15 000 in 1983 (DeVoretz *et al.*, 2005). Between 1999 and 2009, the number of refugee arrivals stabilised at roughly 25 000 per year, approximately 10% of all immigrant admissions (CIC *Facts and Figures*, 2009). About half of Canada's refugee admissions come from refugee camps abroad, the other half as a result of successful claims for refugee status by persons who manage to come to Canada on their own and establish a refugee claim under international agreement. Canada's widely admired reputation for refugee resettlement practices derives from the South-east Asian refugee experience, for which the UN awarded Canada the Nansen medal for humanitarianism. On a per capita basis, Canada continues to accept more refugees for permanent resettlement than any other country.

After immigrants are admitted to Canada, responsibility for their healthcare falls under the jurisdiction of the provinces. Although Canada boasts universal healthcare, services for immigrants are uneven and dependent upon provincial policies. Some provinces, for example, impose a 90-day waiting period before immigrants become eligible for insured services. Under the Interim Federal Health Program, Citizenship and Immigration Canada provides limited direct healthcare for refugees and refugee claimants covering emergency and essential medical services – including short-term mental health consultations – but there are many gaps in entitlements and coverage.

With its well established immigrant and refugee settlement programmes, multicultural-ism policies and good record of citizenship acquisition, Canada presents the surface appearance of a nearly ideal resettlement country. Beneath the surface, however, is an increasingly competitive domestic labour market which is placing recent newcomers at an increasing disadvantage (Badets and Howatson-Leo, 2000; Kunz et al., 2002; Li, 2000; Reitz, 1998; Smith and Jackson, 2002). As a result of labour market difficulties, poverty, with its attendant risk for mental health, has reached unprecedented levels among new Canadians (Kazemipur and Halli, 2001). In 2004, more than one in five recent immigrants of working age was living in poverty compared to fewer than one in ten other Canadians (Fleury, 2007: 25).

Immigrants to Canada also tend to be under-paid and under-employed. Regardless of national origin, recent immigrants aged 25–54 experience more difficulties in the labour market than the Canadian-born (Gilmore, 2009). In 2006, the unemployment rate for the Canadian-born was 4.4%, while the rate for recent immigrants was 11%. In 2008, the average hourly wage of an immigrant worker was 90% that of a working age (25–54-year-old) Canadian-born employee. For immigrants present in Canada for less than 5 years, the corresponding figure was 80%. Canada's selection policies ensure that most immigrants are well educated. Educational advantage does not, however, translate into labour force benefit. In 2008, 42% of immigrants were under-employed; that is, working at jobs at a lower level than would be expected based on level of education (Gilmore, 2009). Lack of recognition of immigrants' educational credentials and discrimination in the labour market are two major contributors to this problem. Visible minorities are more likely to be in low-wage jobs than are white Canadians and to receive lower pay when occupying jobs comparable to non-minorities (Pendakur and Pendakur, 2007). Thwarted ambitions and unmet expectations take an emotional toll on migrants (Beiser et al., 1981; Simich et al., 2006a).

Multiculturalism, a policy of supporting cultural retention while at the same time encouraging successful integration (Berry, 1984), has likely had salutary effects on migrant mental health in Canada. Implementing less discriminatory admissions criteria for immigrants in the 1970s did not, however, guarantee fair treatment after admission. Resettlement stress is an ongoing problem, as is the disconnect between immigration and health policy and practice. In 2002, the Immigration and Refugee Protection Act opened Canada's doors to refugees with serious health problems. Although this laudable humanitarian gesture obviously required additional healthcare resources, none were provided.

The Canadian Task Force on Immigrant and Refugee Mental Health

Immigrant and refugee mental health rocketed to national prominence in 1986 with the formation of a national Task Force on Mental Issues Affecting Immigrants and Refugees in Canada, followed by the release of the task force report, *After the Door has been Opened*, in 1988. The task force was created by two federal government departments: the Multiculturalism Sector of the Department of the Secretary of State, and Health and Welfare Canada. The government action was a response to concerns raised by a great number of community, service and advocacy groups across the country. The 12 members of the task force included psychiatrists, psychologists, nurses, social workers and academics, as well as front line workers, drawn from across the entire country.

Based on an extensive review of the literature as well as written and oral submissions from more than 300 organisations, the task force reached consensus on a central point. *It is not the experience of migration per se that jeopardises mental health: instead, it is the contingencies surrounding migration and resettlement that determine whether relocation creates mental health risk, or new opportunities for personal and economic fulfilment.*

After the Door has been Opened identified resettlement-related mental health risk factors, emphasising among these the deleterious effects of unemployment and under-employment, separation from family, inability to speak English or French and negative public attitudes towards immigrants in general and ethnocultural minorities in particular. The report also called attention to the supportive contribution of the like-ethnic community. Groups requiring special attention, either because of special needs, or because they had been neglected by researchers, policy-makers and service providers, included children and youth, women, seniors and victims of torture and other catastrophic stressors. The report included 27 recommendations. These included broad policy issues such as accelerating the process of family reunification to prevent loneliness, parent–child separations, and family breakdown, ensuring access to language training, and creating at least three centres dedicated to immigration research and to professional training. The recommendations also included specific preventive and intervention strategies, such as professionalising the training of interpreters and creating materials for newcomers that addressed the process of resettlement, its frustrations and disappointments, and that made recommendations about coping with them.

Two decades of immigrant mental health research in Canada

Since the 1980s, the migrant mental health field in Canada has continued to grow in depth and breadth, and has benefited from interdisciplinary and policy-orientated research approaches. Going beyond a narrow biomedical perspective, and using both quantitative and qualitative methods, Canadian researchers have investigated social and cultural determinants of immigrant mental health. In a reprise of the earlier task force initiative, the new Mental Health Commission of Canada's Task Group on Diversity undertook a review of Canadian research literature about migrant and ethnoracial mental health as of 2009, and including an examination of which, if any, of the recommendations in *After the Door Has Been Opened* had been implemented. The task group reported that only six recommendations had been implemented in full. However, more than 50 studies in the two decades since *After the Door Has Been Opened* have investigated mental health or mental health problems among ethnoracial groups in Canada (Mental Health Commission Task Group on Diversity, 2009). Most of these studies focus on rates of mental illness, healthcare for immigrants and refugees, and risk and protective factors for mental health.

The studies make clear that neither the migration process nor migrants themselves are inherently unhealthy; rather, migrant mental health depends to a large extent on post-migration conditions in the resettlement society. Because they are young, self-selected for migration, and have passed an entrance health examination, newcomers to Canada are generally healthy on arrival. Although it is important to recognise this initial immigrant health advantage, it does not justify complacency.

Rates of mental illness and changes over time

According to research carried out under the so-called 'healthy immigrant effect', immigrants tend to lose their health advantage over time. Immigrants from non-European source countries seem to be at greater risk than immigrants of European origin for developing chronic health problems (Ng *et al.* 2005); Figure 25.1.

The data for mental health are not as clear. Results from the Canadian Community Health Survey suggest that immigrants have significantly lower rates of anxiety, depression and alcohol dependence than Canadian-born residents, and that this effect is stronger among more recent than among longer stay immigrants, an observation that has led some researchers to conclude that the 'healthy immigrant effect' applies to mental health (Ali, 2002). However, the cross-sectional survey methods used in the Canadian Community Health Survey are not sensitive to the heterogeneity of immigrant populations, to regional variations, or to complex interactions and changes in social and cultural factors over time (Beiser, 2005). Specific subpopulations such as women and refugees may be more vulnerable and experience particular stresses (Ahmad *et al.*, 2004; Rousseau *et al.*, 2001).

Canadian national surveys also include some data relevant to migrant mental health, but aggregate population data do not always allow fine-grained or in-depth exploration of issues. Local studies with specific immigrant and refugee or ethnic groups may provide more meaningful, specific information for the development of mental health services (Mental Health Commission Task Group on Diversity, 2009). National surveys tend to

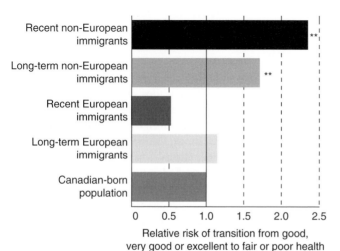

Figure 25.1 Non-European immigrants are more likely than the Canadian-born to report a deterioration in health (Ng *et al.*, 2005).

compare immigrants in general with non-immigrants, and to lump diverse immigrant groups together. The data do not reveal important variations by immigration classes, source areas, ages or gender. For example, as part of Canada's commitment to developing a national children's agenda, the government-initiated the National Longitudinal Survey of Children and Youth (NLSCY), a longitudinal investigation of the development and wellbeing of more than 35 000 Canadian children from birth to early adulthood. This still-ongoing study is producing valuable information about factors influencing children's social, emotional and behavioural development. However, because immigrant and refugee children are severely under-represented in the sample, insights gleaned from the NLSCY tell only part of their story.

An article based on NLSCY data with a surprising finding illustrates the importance of data based on adequate samples of immigrants and refugees (Beiser *et al.*, 2002). Since poverty is one of the most potent of all factors that place children's mental health at risk, and since recently arrived immigrant families are more than twice as likely as non-immigrants to be living in poverty, the guiding hypothesis was that immigrant children would have higher rates of distress and disturbance. The findings were the exact opposite: foreign-born children had fewer emotional and behavioural problems than their native-born counterparts. Further probing of this epidemiological paradox highlighted the role of the immigrant family as a source of resilience. Poor immigrant families were much less likely than poor native-Canadian families to be broken families, and poor immigrant parents were less likely to be ineffective or dysfunctional parents.

Service utilisation

Immigrants are less likely than Canadian-born residents to use mental health services (Kirmayer *et al.*, 2007). Social conditions that affect migrant mental health include perceptions of the formal mental health system and existing professional practices in Canada, where reasons for immigrants' reluctance to use mental health services include negative perceptions of current practices, such as doctors' lack of time for patients and over-reliance on medications in treatment (Simich *et al.*, 2009a; Whitley *et al.*, 2006). Other studies have focused on unmet mental health service needs and barriers, including new settlers' lack of knowledge about where to get help and concerns about stigma (Hsu and Alden, 2008; Li and Browne, 2000).

Risk, resilience and mental health

An interactive paradigm that includes both risk and resilience factors for immigrant mental health is essential for research, policy and practice. The resettlement stress and resilience model in Figure 25.2 has guided epidemiological studies among South-east Asian refugees in Vancouver, British Columbia, Tamil refugees in Toronto, immigrant and refugee children across Canada, and cross-national studies involving Canada, Ethiopia and Israel.

Intuition and theory would predict considerable mental health salience for pre-migration stressors, particularly among refugees. However, research demonstrates that the mental effects of pre-migration tend to disappear shortly after permanent resettlement has been attained, perhaps to reappear many years later (Beiser, 2009). Suppression of memory probably helps refugees deal with the mental health risk of past trauma, at least during the early and mid term years of resettlement (Beiser and Hyman, 1997). Thus, suppression can be a coping strategy that helps preserve mental health rather than the pathological defence

RESETTLEMENT AND
MENTAL HEALTH

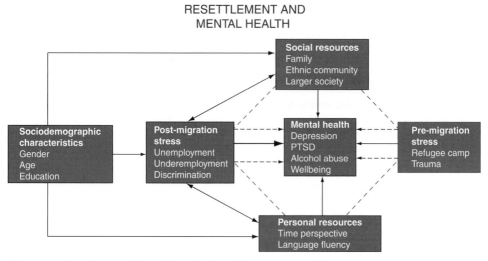

Figure 25.2 Resettlement and mental health. Adapted from Beiser, M. (1999). *Strangers at the Gate: The Boat People's First Ten Years in Canada.* Toronto; University of Toronto Press.

mechanism it is often considered. As people age, however, the recall of memory, both painful and pleasant, is probably ineluctable. Research (Beiser and Wickrama, 2004) demonstrates that, although such recall constitutes a risk for depression, a stable work history and a stable relationship each act as protective mental health factors.

To promote migrant mental health, it is as important to identify protective factors as it is to ascertain vulnerabilities. Sometimes, a particular factor can be both. For example, unemployment is a risk factor for depression among immigrants just as it is among the population at large (Beiser *et al.*, 1993; Wickrama *et al.*, 2002). Stable employment, on the other hand, mitigates the mental health risk invoked by refugees' recall of painful memory (Beiser and Wickrama, 2004). Social support and social networks have been shown to decrease the isolation of African refugee and Asian immigrant groups (Beiser, 1999; Stewart *et al.*, 2008). For some mental health problems, such as suicide, rates among immigrants are generally half that of the non-immigrant population in Canada, and closer to the rates reported in the countries of origin. Although the rates increase among immigrant seniors, they decrease among immigrants living in such major cities as Montreal, Toronto and Vancouver, probably because of the protective effect of cultural and community ties (Malenfant, 2004).

On the other hand, immigrants can become cocooned by the like-ethnic community, with such long-term deleterious effects as decreased probability of learning the language of the receiving society, decreased social contact outside the ethnic community, and heightened risk of entering employment tracks with little prospect for upward mobility (Beiser, 1999, 2009). The possible mental health effects of non-ethnic support, for example through sponsorship and hosting programmes, has received less research attention. Canadian immigration law permits private sponsorship of refugees. As part of its strategy of responding to the South-east Asian Boat People crisis of 1979–1981, the Canadian government encouraged private citizens to become private sponsors, thereby assuming financial as well as other responsibilities during the first year of resettlement in return for which the government brought in refugees under government sponsorship. Studies (Beiser, 1999, 2009) suggest that sponsorships that involved misunderstandings between sponsors and refugees jeopardised mental health. On the positive side, sponsorships appeared to enhance long-term language acquisition, employment and contact with the larger community (Beiser and Johnson, 2003). Theory suggests that a strongly held sense of ethnic identity promotes self-esteem and social belonging. However, research suggests a complex interaction: a strong sense of ethnic identity can be protective for immigrants and refugees who experience difficulty in acquiring tools such as language that permits them to participate in the larger society, but it can, on the other hand, amplify the deleterious effects of perceived discrimination (Beiser and Hou, 2006).

Aside from contributing indirectly to mental health problems by creating barriers to employment, discrimination affects migrant mental health directly (Beiser *et al.*, 2002; Dion, 2001; Noh *et al.*, 1999). According to Canada's Ethnic Diversity Survey (Badets *et al.*, 2003; Statistics Canada, 2003), 20% of people reported experiencing discrimination 'sometimes or often' in the 5 years prior to being interviewed. Almost one-third (32%) of blacks reported experiencing discrimination, compared to 21% of South Asians and 18% of Chinese in Canada. The survey also found that perceived discrimination does not lessen with the passage of time or among the ranks of second generation immigrants.

The study of mental health among the small cohort of immigrant children included in Canada's National Longitudinal Survey of Children and Youth raised a number of intriguing and important questions; for example, Did the good news about mental health apply to all children, refugee and immigrant alike? To visible minority as well as non-visible minority children? and, did factors such as the circumstances of migration or region of resettlement in Canada affect mental health? The NLSCY immigrant child sample was too small to permit the required analyses. To help answer such questions, researchers from 10 universities across Canada, most of them affiliated with the national metropolis centres of excellence for research on immigration, together with ethnocultural community and service groups, created the New Canadian Children and Youth Study (NCCYS), a longitudinal investigation of health and development involving more than 4000 immigrant and refugee children and their families living in six cities across Canada.

A publication from the NCCYS (Beiser *et al.*, 2009) demonstrates that, in many ways, immigrant children's mental health is affected by the same factors that affect the mental health of children in general. Immigrant boys are more likely than immigrant girls, and younger children more likely than older, to display physical aggression. As is the case for children in general, maternal depression increases the probability that an immigrant child will have emotional problems. However, factors more or less specific to the immigrant experience affect children's mental health, net of universal risk and protective factors. Immigrant children whose parents speak little or no English or French are more distressed than children whose parents have better degrees of linguistic fluency, and immigrant children whose parents suffer a good deal of resettlement stress and who experience discrimination have an elevated risk of emotional problems and of physically aggressive behaviour. In addition, the region of resettlement in Canada has apparent mental health salience. Children living in Toronto and Montreal had more mental health and behavioural problems than children living in Winnipeg, Calgary, Edmonton or Vancouver. There were different reasons for these regional differences. Immigrant parents living in Montreal were less fluent in the dominant society language than those living elsewhere, and this accounted for Montreal's relatively poor showing. Toronto, on the other hand, apparently offered poorer institutional responses, for example through its service agencies and its schools, as well as a less welcoming environment for newcomers (Beiser, unpublished data).

Among other contributions, *After the Door Has Been Opened* foreshadowed the need to include immigrants in consultation and research. Three decades later, participatory action research has become an effective and empowering method for engaging immigrant groups in Canada in the design, execution and dissemination of immigrant mental health research. For example, the recently completed Community–University Research Alliance Study, *Taking Culture Seriously in Community Mental Health*, brought together over 40 community, university, service agency and umbrella organisation partners (Maiter *et al.*, 2008; Simich *et al.*, 2009a, b; Westhues *et al.*, 2008) to explore, develop and pilot community mental health initiatives in five ethnocultural communities in Ontario, Canada's most populous province. Such qualitative research studies have helped to 'flesh out' an understanding of migrant mental health by describing subjective experiences of mental health during settlement that are meaningful for understanding unmet needs, cultural values and community-based solutions. Innovative participatory research projects have also come out of non-university settings, such as community health centres and other community agencies serving immigrants and refugees. Employing community-based research methods has also been beneficial in creating partnerships among researchers and service providers. *A Community in Distress*, a mental health survey in Toronto's Tamil diaspora, the largest in the world, was conducted from 2001 to 2004 (Beiser *et al.*, 2003). The research partnership of community professionals and academics, an essential component of the project, outlasted the study itself. The partnership catalysed a community-wide response to combat mental distress and feelings of helplessness among Tamils in the diaspora, who were confronted with daily news about the devastating impact of the December 2004 Asian tsunami on family and friends in Sri Lanka (Simich *et al.*, 2008). In sum, university–community research partnerships can help make migrant mental healthcare initiatives more informed and effective.

Emerging issues in immigrant mental health in Canada

As already noted, the 1988 landmark National Task Force on Mental Health of Immigrants concluded that migration may be stressful, but it does not necessarily threaten mental health unless post-migration stresses overcome the personal and social resources available to cope with them. Data about the incidence and prevalence of mental disorders is still limited for most specific immigrant or refugee populations in Canada, but what evidence there is points consistently to the association of mental distress with post-migration contingencies. For example, the 28% rate of depression among Ethiopians in Toronto is much higher than depression rates for Ethiopians in their homeland, a finding strongly suggesting a combination of high risk and depleted resources for Ethiopian immigrants (Fenta *et al.*, 2004). One might not expect the 'healthy immigrant' effect to apply to refugees as it does to their carefully selected immigrant counterparts. However, the South-east Asian refugees who came to Canada during the 'boat people' crisis (1979–1981) had lower rates of depression than native-born Canadians (Beiser, 1999). Such apparent discrepancies highlight the need for future studies to employ standardised, culturally appropriate methods, and for more investigations comparing mental health among immigrants and their counterparts in home countries, as well as among immigrants and native-born residents of receiving countries.

The match between mental health need and availability of services is another important area for further research. Mental healthcare systems commonly lack the cultural and linguistic competence and will to respond to mental healthcare challenges resulting from immigration (Bhui *et al.*, 2007; de Jong and Van Ommeren, 2005; Ingleby and Watters, 2005). In both Canada and the United States, minority and ethnolinguistic communities are underserved (James and Prilleltensky, 2003; Kirmayer *et al.*, 2007; United States Department of Health and Human Services, 2002). Despite Canada's universal healthcare system, equitable access to good quality mental healthcare for immigrants and refugees is far from guaranteed (Canadian Task Force on Mental Health Issues Affecting Immigrants and Refugees, 1988; Gagnon, 2002; Standing Senate Committee on Social Affairs, Science and Technology, 2006). For example, Toronto is home to the largest Tamil diaspora in the world, and a mental health survey has shown that Toronto Tamil refugees experience PTSD at a rate of 12% (which is comparable to other refugee populations), yet only one in 10 persons qualifying for a diagnosis of PTSD has received treatment of any sort (Beiser *et al.*, 2003). Studies have revealed language barriers and incompatibility between the values, help-seeking strategies and expectations of migrants and the Canadian mental health system (Sadavoy *et al.*, 2004; Wang *et al.*, 2008). More critical analyses of how the medical system and migrants interact are required. Finally, research on the mental health of irregular or undocumented migrants and lack of access to health services in Canada is still in its infancy (Simich, 2006b; Simich *et al.*, 2007), but has the potential to precipitate humanitarian responses despite the difficult social and economic context.

Summary of lessons and prospects

Canada has an enviable reputation as a destination country for immigrants and refugees. To maintain its reputation, more attention needs to be paid to migrant mental health. In the 1980s and 1990s, Canadian migrant mental health research demonstrated that even the most disadvantaged migrants can achieve good health and social integration over the long term under favourable settlement conditions. Multiculturalism, though sometimes criticised, has probably had a salutary effect on migrant mental health. Like-ethnic community support is especially important in the early years of settlement, and well designed and well executed welcoming and sponsorship programmes can probably aid long-term integration and play a significant role in protecting mental health.

Social and health inequities in Canada are, unfortunately, growing. Recent research has shown that discrimination and slower economic integration are having a deleterious impact on migrants, but disillusionment and mental distress are not inevitable. Given the lessons learned from the Refugee Resettlement Project and other studies in the past two decades, it is time to acknowledge that migrant mental health is an important aspect of human capital (Beiser, 2009), and to invest accordingly in culturally appropriate services, illness prevention and community mental health promotion (Mental Health Commission Task Group on Diversity, 2009).

Several specific initiatives would be helpful. For example, language interpretation services are not currently mandatory in Canada's health system, although they are in the courts. Given the relevance of language in delivering good quality mental health services, this should change. National immigration policy is seldom congruent with provincial health service delivery, so migrant mental healthcare tends to be neglected. This problem is slowly being addressed by current research, such as the Refugee Mental Health Practices study, and pilot settlement sector programmes. Mental health literacy and anti-stigma campaigns under consideration by federal and provincial agencies, if funded and implemented well, would also help to bridge the medical and social divide in migrant mental health.

The depth and breadth of migrant mental health research in Canada has expanded, not only in academic settings, but also with greater participation from immigrant communities and agencies, as well as increasing interest from policy-makers. Past research suggests the importance of pursuing longitudinal and mixed methods studies in migrant mental health, and of doing research that takes into account important distinctions such as gender and legal status. Studies that investigate social determinants of mental health in addition to the complexities of trauma and recovery are increasingly the norm. Most migrants in Canada do not become mental health casualties, a fact that provides the opportunity to investigate what keeps migrants mentally healthy and to translate this knowledge into improved policy and practice.

References

Ahmad, F., Shik, A., Vanza, R., Cheung, A. M. U. G., Stewart, D. (2004). Voices of South Asian women: immigration and mental health. *Women's Health*, **40**, 113–30.

Ali, J. (2002). Mental health of Canada's immigrants. In *Supplement to Health Reports Statistics Canada*, vol. **13**, 1–11.

Badets, J., Howatson-Leo, L. (2000). Recent immigrants in the workforce. *Canadian Social Trends*, **3**, 15–21.

Badets, J., Chard, J., Levett, A. (2003). Ethnic Diversity Survey: Portrait of a Multicultural Society Catalogue no: 89–593–XIE.

Beiser, M. (1999). *Strangers At The Gate: The 'Boat People's' First Ten Years in Canada.* Toronto: University of Toronto Press.

Beiser, M. (2005). The health of immigrants and refugees in Canada. *Canadian Journal of Public Health*, **96**, 30–45.

Beiser, M. (2009). Resettling refugees and safeguarding their mental health: lessons learned from the refugee resettlement project. *Transcultural Psychiatry*, **46**, 539–83.

Beiser, M., Hou, F. (2006). Ethnic identity, resettlement stress and depressive affect among Southeast Asian refugees in Canada. *Social Science and Medicine*, **63**, 137–50.

Beiser, M., Hyman, I. (1997). Refugees' time perspective and mental health. *The American Journal of Psychiatry*, **154**(7), 996–1002.

Beiser, M., Johnson, P. (2003). Sponsorship and resettlement success. *Journal of International Migration and Integration*, **4**(2), 203–16.

Beiser M., Wickrama K. A. S. (2004). Trauma, time and mental health: a study of temporal reintegration and depressive disorder among Southeast Asian refugees. *Psychological Medicine*, **34**(5), 899–910.

Beiser, M., Collomb, H., Reval, J. L. (1981). Mastering change: epidemiological and case studies. *American Journal of Psychiatry*, **138**(4), 455–9.

Beiser, M., Johnson, P. J., Turner, R. J. (1993). Unemployment, underemployment and depressive affect among Southeast Asian refugees. *Psychological Medicine*, **23**, 731–43.

Beiser, M., Hou, F., Hyman, I., Tousignant, M. (2002). Poverty and mental health among immigrant and non-immigrant children. *American Journal of Public Health*, **92**(2), 220–7.

Beiser, M., Simich, L., Pandalangat, N. (2003). Community in distress: mental heath needs and help-seeking in the Tamil community in Toronto. *International Migration*, **41**(5), 233–45.

Beiser, M., Hamilton, H., Rummens, J. A. *et al.* (2009). Predictors of emotional problems and physical aggression among children of Hong Kong Chinese, mainland Chinese and Filipino immigrants to Canada. *Social*

Psychiatry and Psychiatric Epidemiology (in press).

Berry, J. W. (1984). Multicultural policy in Canada: a social psychological analysis. *Canadian Journal of Behavioural Science*, **16**, 353–70.

Bhui, K., Warfa, N., Edonya, P., McKenzie, K., Bhugra, D. (2007). Cultural competence in mental health care: a review of model evaluations. *BMC Health Services Research*, 7: 15 doi: 10.1186/1472-6963-7-15.

Bloemraad, I. (2002). The North American naturalizationgap: an institutional approach to citizenship acquisition in the United States and Canada. *International Migration Review*, **36**(1), 193–228.

Canadian Task Force on Mental Health Issues Affecting Immigrants and Refugees (1988). *After the Door Has Been Opened: Mental Health Issues Affecting Immigrants and Refugees in Canada*. Ottawa: Ministry of Supply and Services Canada.

CIC (Citizenship and Immigration Canada) (2009). *Facts and Figures 2008 – Immigration overview: Permanent and Temporary Residents*. http://www.cic.gc.ca/english/resources/statistics/facts2008/permanent/01.asp (accessed 27 April 2009).

de Jong, J., Van Ommeren, M. (2005). Mental health services in a multicultural society: interculturalization and its quality surveillance. *Transcultural Psychiatry*, **42**(3), 437–56.

DeVoretz, D., Beiser, M., Pivenako, S. (2005). The economic experiences of refugees in Canada. In P. Waxman and V. Colic-Peiskes, eds. *Homeland Wanted: Interdisciplinary Perspectives on Refugee Resettlement*. New York: Nova Science Publishers, 1–21.

Dion, K. L. (2001). The social psychology of perceived prejudice and discrimination. *Canadian Psychology*, **43**, 1–10.

Fleury, D. (2007). *A Study of Poverty and Working Poverty Among Recent Immigrants to Canada: Final Report*. Ottawa: Human Resources and Skills Development Canada.

Fenta, H., Hyman, I., Noh, S. (2004). Determinants of depression among Ethiopian immigrants and refugees in Toronto. *Journal of Nervous and Mental Disease*, **192**, 363–72.

Gagnon, A. (2002). *Responsiveness of the Canadian Health Care System Towards Newcomers: Discussion Paper No. 40*. http://www.hc-sc.gc.ca/english/pdf/romanow/pdfs/40_Gagnon_E.pdf (accessed 8 October 2009).

Gilmore, J. (2009). The 2008 Canadian immigrant labour market: analysis of quality of employment. *The Immigrant Labour Force Analysis Series*. Ottawa: Statistics Canada.

Hsu, L., Alden, L. E. (2008). Cultural influences on willingness to seek treatment for social anxiety in Chinese and European-heritage students. *Cultural Diversity and Ethnic Minority Psychology*, **14**, 215–23.

Ingleby, D., Watters, C. (2005). Mental health and social care for asylum seekers and refugees: a comparative study. In I. David (ed.) *Forced Migration and Mental Health: Rethinking the Care of Refugees and Displaced Persons*. New York: Springer Publishing Co, 193–212.

James, S., Prilleltensky, I. (2003). Cultural diversity and mental health: towards integrative practice. *Clinical Psychology Review*, **22**, 1133–54.

Kazemipur, A., Halli, S. (2001). Immigrants and 'New Poverty:' The case of Canada. *International Migration Review*, **35**(4), 1128–56.

Kirmayer, L. J., Weinfeld, M., Burgos, G. *et al.* (2007). Use of health care services for psychological distress by immigrant in an urban multicultural milieu. *Canadian Journal of Psychiatry*, **52**, 295–304.

Kunz, J. L., Milan, A., Schetagne, S. (2002). *Unequal Access: A Canadian Profile of Racial Differences in Education, Employment and Income*. Toronto: Canadian Race Relations Foundation.

Kymlicka, W. (1995). *Multicultural Citizenship: A Liberal Theory of Minority Rights*. Oxford: Clarendon Press.

Li, H. Z., Browne, A. J. (2000). Defining mental illness and accessing mental health services: perspectives of Asian Canadians. *Canadian*

Journal of Community Mental Health, **19**, 143–59.

Li, P. (2000). Earning disparities between immigrants and native-born Canadians. *Canadian Review of Sociology and Anthropology*, **37**(3), 289–311.

Maiter, S., Simich, L., Jacobson, N., Wise, J. (2008). Reciprocity: an ethic for community-based participatory action research. *Action Research*, **6**(3), 305–25.

Malenfant, É. C. (2004). Suicide in Canada's immigrant population. *Health Reports*, **15**(2), 9–17.

Mental Health Commission Task Group on Diversity (2009). Understanding the issues, best practice and options for service development to meet the needs of ethno-cultural groups, immigrants, refugees, and racialized groups. Calgary, AB: Mental Health Commission of Canada.

Ng, E., Wilkins, R., Gendron, F., Bethelot, J-M. (2005). Healthy today, health tomorrow? Findings from the National Population Health Survey. *Dynamics of Immigrants' Health in Canada: Evidence from the National Population Health Survey, Statistics Canada*. Ottawa: Ministry of Industry. http://www.statcan.gc.ca/pub/82-618-m/82-618-m2005002-eng.htm.

Noh, S., Beiser, M., Kaspar, V. H. F., Rummens, J. (1999). Perceived racial discrimination, depression, and coping: a study of Southeast Asian refugees in Canada. *Journal of Health and Social Behavior*, **40**, 193–207.

Pendakur K., Pendakur, R. (2007). Minority earnings disparity across the distribution. *Canadian Public Policy/Analyse de Politiques*, **33**(1), 41–61.

Reitz, J. G. (1998). *Warmth of the Welcome: The Social Causes of Economic Success for Immigrants in Different Nations and Cities*. Boulder, CO: Westover Press.

Rousseau, C., Medkki-Berrada, A., Moreau, S. (2001). Trauma and extended separation from family among Latin American and African refugees in Montreal. *Psychiatry*, **64**(1), 40–59.

Sadavoy, J., Meier, R., Ong, A. (2004). Barriers to access to mental health services for ethnic

seniors: the Toronto study. *Canadian Journal of Psychiatry*, **49**, 192–9.

Simich, L. (2006). Hidden meanings of health security: migration experiences and systemic barriers to mental wellbeing among non-status migrants. *International Journal of Migration, Health and Social Care*, **2**(3/4), 16–27.

Simich, L., Hamilton, H., Baya, B. K. (2006). Mental distress, economic hardship and expectations of life in Canada among Sudanese newcomers. *Transcultural Psychiatry*, **43**(3), 418–44.

Simich, L., Wu, F., Nerad, S. (2007). Status and health security: an exploratory study among irregular immigrants in Toronto. *Canadian Journal of Public Health*, **98**(5), 369–73.

Simich, L., Andermann, L., Rummens, J. A., Lo, T. (2008). Post-disaster mental distress relief: health promotion and knowledge exchange in partnership with a refugee diaspora community. *Refuge*, **25**(1), 44–54.

Simich, L., Maiter, S., Moorlag, E., Ochocka, J. (2009a). Ethnocultural community perspectives on mental health. *Psychiatric Rehabilitation Journal*, **32**(3), 208–14.

Simich, L. Maiter, S., Ochocka, J. (2009b). From social liminality to cultural negotiation: transformative processes in immigrant mental wellbeing. *Anthropology & Medicine*, **16**(3), 253–66.

Smith, E., Jackson, A. (2002). *Does a Rising Tide Lift all Boats? The Labour Market Experiences and Incomes of Recent Immigrants, 1995–1998*. Ottawa: Canadian Council on Social Development.

Standing Senate Committee on Social Affairs, Science and Technology (2006). *Out of the Shadows at Last: Transforming Mental Health*. Ottawa: Mental Illness and Addiction Services in Canada.

Statistics Canada (2003). *Canada's Ethnocultural Mosaic, 2006 Census: Findings*. http://www12.statcan.ca/census-recensement/2006/as-sa/97-562/index-eng.cfm?CFID=3632529&CFTOKEN=11121264 (accessed 13 July 2010).

Statistics Canada (2008). *Canada's Ethnocultural Mosaic, 2006 Census*. Ottawa: Minister of Industry. http://www.statcan.gc.ca/cgi-bin/

af-fdr.cgi?l=eng&t=Canada's%
20Ethnocultural%20Mosaic,%202006%
20Census&loc.=http://www12.statcan.ca/
english/census06/analysis/ethnicorigin/pdf/
97-562-XIE2006001.pdf. (accessed 2 April
2008).

Stewart, M., Anderson, J., Beiser, M. *et al.* (2008).
Multicultural meanings of social support
among immigrants and refugees.
International Migration, **46**(3), 123–59.

United States Department of Health and Human
Services (2002). Mental health: culture, race,
and ethnicity – a supplement to mental
health: a report of the Surgeon General.
Rockville, MD: US Department of Health
and Human Services, Substance Abuse and
Mental Health Services Administration,
Center for Mental Health Services.

Van Selm, J. (2003). Public–private partnerships
in refugee settlement: Europe and the US.
*Journal of International Migration and
Integration*, **4**(2), 157–76.

Wang, L., Rosenberg, M., Lo, L. (2008).
Ethnicity, accessibility, and utilization of
family physicians – a case study of mainland
Chinese immigrants in Toronto. *Canada
Social Science and Medicine*, **67**(9), 1410–22.

Westhues, A., Ochocka, J., Jacobson, N. *et al.*
(2008). Developing theory from complexity:
reflections on a collaborative mixed method
participatory action research study.
Qualitative Health Research, **18**(5), 701.

Whitley, R., Kirmayer, L. J., Groleau, D. (2006).
Understanding immigrants' reluctance to
use mental health services: a qualitative
study from Montreal. *Canadian Journal of
Psychiatry*, **51**, 205–9.

Wickrama, K. A. S., Beiser, B., Kaspar, V. (2002).
Trajectories of economic integration and
depression of Southeast Asian refugees: an
application of growth curve strategy in
psychiatric research. *International Journal
of Methods in Psychiatric Research*,
11(4), 161–75.

Chapter 26

Conclusions

Dinesh Bhugra and Susham Gupta

The ability of migrants to settle down and adjust in the new society will influence their physical and mental health. Some vulnerability factors will pre-exist and may even encourage the individual to migrate, but other factors, such as political or economic, may act as extruding or 'push' factors, and economic and educational factors may also act as 'pull' factors. The experience of migration is not homogeneous, and depends upon a number of factors. It is inevitable that stress related to migration will be managed in different ways, using a number of strategies. Different groups – whether related to religion, age, gender or sexual identity – will experience the process of migration in different ways. Cultural, social and sexual identities may overlap. It is imperative that policy-makers and politicians be aware of issues that migrants face, and there is a need to be conscious of the fact that a vast majority of migrants contribute to the economy of the new country and carry out jobs which may not be generally popular. The policies related to multicultural values, the rainbow nation or melting pot identities of the new countries will also influence individuals and how they are welcome, perceived and received.

Migrants, whether they migrate singly or in groups, with or without families, will experience a degree of stress which will depend upon a number of factors.

In this volume we have looked at rates of different illnesses in different migrant groups in different countries. A few common strands begin to emerge which indicate that some mental disorders are more prevalent in some migrant groups and not others. Coping strategies and resilience among some migrant groups are worth noting and exploring further. The interaction between the individual migrant and the society they leave behind, and with the society to which they move, may produce ambivalent feelings which will influence post-migration adjustment and acculturation.

Migration is a process of social change where individuals face a degree of change and, depending upon the purpose underlying such a process, the subsequent adjustment may occur related to aspirations and achievements. Migration is multifaceted and may occur within the same country, from rural to urban areas or urban to rural. Across national and cultural boundaries the process of migration will bring with it elements of stress. Not all migrants go through stress and develop psychiatric illness. Any such process of movement will produce social change, in that the individual will leave culture, home, family (extended or joint), social networks, kinships, peers and friends behind, and in a very small proportion this may lead to cultural bereavement. An interpretation that sees the new culture as an exciting adventure and endeavour will enable the migrant to adjust quicker and better. A series of factors in the new society, combined with personality style and factors, will influence adjustment and acculturation. These social factors include policy, society's welcoming attitude, racialism, racism in the new

Migration and Mental Health, ed. Dinesh Bhugra & Susham Gupta. Published by Cambridge University Press. © Cambridge University Press 2011.

society and availability of social support and social networks. The individual's responses to these adjustments and perceptions will affect how migrants manage. Cross-national migration is more likely to be for social, political, economic or educational reasons; intra-national migration may also be affected by these factors, but is more likely to be owing to educational or economic factors. Cultural identity and learning or coping with a new language, prior preparation and expectations will all play a role in enabling the migrant to settle down. Heterogeneity of the process and the stress experienced, along with the ability to adjust as a result of age, gender, purpose and preparation, are key factors of which clinicians need to be aware.

Policy-makers must lead on clear policies which take into account the human rights of migrants, refugees and asylum seekers. They must be aware of the healthcare needs of the groups of migrants and the countries from which they originate. The services for migrants need not be separate, though occasionally this may be indicated, but they must be culturally sensitive and emotionally and geographically accessible, which will require adequate funding and resources for training and support. Different departments in the government, such as home, justice, education and health, need to work closely and to coordinate efforts. Access to services should be clearly delineated and widely disseminated. For any kind of service provision, public mental health components must be clearly articulated. Targeting migrants using appropriate languages and modes of communication using accessible pathways, messages can be delivered more effectively. Awareness of local agencies and primary and secondary services should be disseminated widely.

Service providers should be able to inform stakeholders about local services and potential barriers. These barriers will include political and policy factors, structural barriers to help-seeking and emotional barriers which relate to different models of illness. Service planners and providers, along with clinicians, must be aware of what the needs of migrants are and how these can be met by overcoming these barriers. Service providers must provide cultural competence training, and models such as culture brokership. Epidemiological assessment of local needs must be supplemented by qualitative research to understand cultural context and monitor psychopathology. For both service providers and clinicians, regular audits are a must, and these should explore all kinds of treatment interventions.

Clinicians must have access to adequate resources for training and cultural competence. They need to be aware of the resources they can access to inform themselves. Cultural awareness training (although a part of good clinical practice) must be mandated, and regularly updated. Interpreters should be used appropriately, and services based on appropriate linguistic and cultural needs should be available. The service delivery model may be culture-based, gender-based or diagnosis-based, but the communication across borders must be made easy so that team members are aware of what is going on. Managing physical and mental illnesses and distress among refugees, asylum seekers and migrants must be part of the curriculum, and all trainees must be made aware of the components of cultural awareness. Multidisciplinary training should be encouraged. Good practice means involving the family and the community leaders, and must take into account the patient's religious and cultural preferences, and encourage patients to fulfil their social/cultural obligations. Migration provides a useful opportunity to study not only the role of cultural factors in the aetiology of mental illness and whether these factors are causative or protective, but also whether these factors can be understood for the non-migrant groups as well. By understanding these factors it should be possible to understand the role of resilience and coping, which can then be used in managing patients irrespective of their cultures. Cultural congruity and the role of cultural conflict will allow us to look at ecological models of mental and emotional distress.

Index

Note: page numbers in *italics* refer to figures and tables